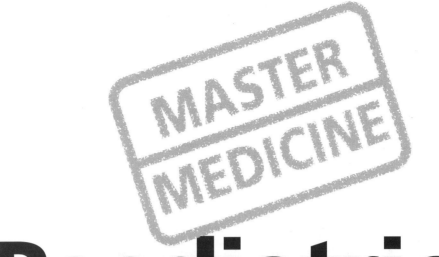

# Paediatrics

## A core text with self-assessment

### SIMON ATTARD-MONTALTO

MBChB MD(Liverpool) FRCP FRCPCH DCH
Chairman, Clinical Department of Paediatrics and Head,
Academic Department of Paediatrics, The Medical School,
The University of Malta, Malta

### VASKAR SAHA

MBBS DCH MD FRCPCH PhD
Head, Cancer Research UK, Children's Cancer Group,
and Professor of Paediatric Oncology, Institute of Cancer,
Barts and The London School of Medicine and Dentistry,
Queen Mary University of London, London

SECOND EDITION

ELSEVIER
CHURCHILL
LIVINGSTONE

Edinburgh  London  New York  Oxford  Philadelphia
St Louis  Sydney  Toronto  2006

## ELSEVIER
### CHURCHILL
### LIVINGSTONE

First edition      1999
Second edition   2006

ISBN 0443 07495X

**British Library Cataloguing in Publication Data**
A catalogue record for this book is available from the British Library

**Library of Congress Cataloging in Publication Data**
A catalog record for this book is available from the Library of Congress

**Notice**
Neither the Publisher nor the Authors assume any responsibility for any loss or injury and/or damage to persons or property arising out of or related to any use of the material contained in this book. It is the responsibility of the treating practitioner, relying on independent expertise and knowledge of the patient, to determine the best treatment and method of application for the patient.
The Publisher

Printed in the UK

# Paediatrics

*For Jane and Usha*

*Commissioning Editor:* Ellen Green
*Project Development Manager:* Barbara Simmons
*Project Manager:* Emma Riley
*Designer:* George Ajayi

# Acknowledgements

We would sincerely like to thank Dr Denis Azzopardi, Dr Mehul Dattani and Dr Andrew Winrow, who provided chapters for the first edition of this book. Furthermore, we are very grateful to numerous colleagues who kindly reviewed chapters, offered constructive criticism and suggested changes to the second edition, including Ms Audrey Camilleri, Dr Paul Cuschieri, Mr Chris Fearne, Dr Victor Grech, Dr Roger Harris, Dr Charles Mallia Azzopardi, Professor John Portelli, Dr Anu Shankar, Dr Delaine Shingadia, Dr Sara Stoneham, Dr John Torpiano, Dr Paul Vassallo Agius and Dr Cecil Vella. Finally, we are indebted to all those undergraduate students who read the first edition and provided helpful feedback that, we hope, has contributed to significant improvements in the second edition.

# Contents

Using this book      *1*

1. Nutrition, normal growth and development      *7*
2. Diseases of the fetus and newborn      *23*
3. The respiratory system      *49*
4. The cardiovascular system      *73*
5. The digestive system      *105*
6. Neuromuscular disease      *123*
7. The urinary system      *145*
8. The endocrine system      *163*
9. Hereditary and metabolic diseases      *189*
10. Infectious diseases      *207*
11. Blood disorders and neoplasia      *233*
12. General surgery, orthopaedics, ENT and dental problems      *261*
13. Behavioural disorders, social paediatrics, injuries and ethics      *291*

Index      *309*

# Using this book

## Philosophy of this book

Undergraduate medical teaching is changing from a lecture-based, didactic theoretical curriculum relying heavily on memorising facts to an applied, problem-orientated approach. This translates into a far more interesting curriculum that mirrors what actually happens in 'real-life' clinical practice. Ultimately this approach is designed to produce new graduates who have a true understanding of clinical medicine and who are not left floundering with a chasm that spans medical theory and reality.

Whatever approach is adopted, a sound background knowledge of the subject is necessary. Inevitably, this will entail some basic reading and fact finding. This core knowledge should then form the basis upon which applied clinical medicine can be developed. This book has been designed to provide the essential core knowledge of paediatrics and to present this in a problem-orientated fashion. It is by no means a comprehensive or all-inclusive tome of paediatrics, which is only necessary for further reading, research or sheer curiosity. At undergraduate level the student is expected to grasp basic principles, have clear ideas of common conditions and have a sensible approach to their management. One needs to appreciate what constitutes a normal child and what symptoms and signs may be indicative of serious illness requiring urgent intervention. Hence, in this book, paediatric emergencies and common problems are covered in detail whereas less common diseases are mentioned only briefly, and esoteric rarities are omitted altogether. The information is presented in a format conducive to revision, and approximately a quarter of each chapter is devoted to self-assessment. The questions in this section are designed to reflect standards in current undergraduate examinations and cover the most important topics in each chapter. In some instances, additional topics that are not discussed in the text feature in the self-assessment, and this section should not be considered an 'optional extra'. Likewise, self-assessment should not be approached with trepidation but should be used to confirm and consolidate one's understanding of the subject while uncovering the inevitable weak points and gaps in knowledge, which can then be addressed by further reading.

## Book design and layout

The book is divided into chapters each covering the major systems in paediatrics. Individual chapters are organised with an introductory 'key' that briefly highlights the goals of each chapter and the essential information the student is expected to gain after reading the chapter. In general, the common symptoms and signs pertaining to the individual system are discussed and their clinical relevance outlined. This is then followed by a discussion of various disease states and conditions that affect the system in question. Where relevant, important facts regarding anatomy, physiology and basic science are included. Individual topics are presented in a standardised format, with attention given to maintain the sequence: aetiology, history, examination, differential diagnosis, investigation, management and outcome. Discussion of treatment is limited to the most important measures: excessive detail (e.g. drug dosages) and anecdotal or pure research-based therapeutic approaches are excluded, or alluded to only very briefly.

Tables and boxes are designed not only to consolidate essential lists but also to insert information. Figures are used to clarify topics that may be easier to comprehend when presented in graphic or pictorial form.

The sections on self-assessment include multiple choice questions, data interpretation, short notes, case histories, viva voce examinations, picture, objective structured clinical examination (OSCE) and construct questions. Each of these examination formats tests knowledge from a different angle. They are representative of similar questions posed in undergraduate examinations. Factual answers as well as detailed explanations are provided for each question. For those topics previously covered in the text, the questions generally address the problem from a different angle and the answers serve as revision. However, many questions are not covered in the text, and for those the detailed answers provide an important extension to the basic information supplied in the book.

## Approaching the examinations

Sadly, one is repeatedly asked by undergraduates whether a topic or item of information is 'necessary for the exam?' Presumably, if the answer is no, then the implication is that the topic will simply be omitted altogether during revision. In many ways this attitude is not surprising, given the way undergraduates are constantly inundated with examinations. However, it is important that students are not reduced to automata who simply live to get past the next examination hurdle (and having done so, rapidly forget all!). Medical education should be an enjoyable process with the aim of – ultimately – producing safe clinicians. Indeed, the latter entails more than simply passing exams.

Despite all their faults, examinations remain an integral part of assessing students. There are several options open to examiners, all of which test knowledge and understanding of the subject in different ways, and all require different skills in order to optimise performance. Some general measures are useful prior to any medical examination:

- Discover the format of the exam: length, question format, i.e. multiple choice, essays etc.
- Plan revision to dovetail with the exam format.
- Read instructions *carefully* before attempting questions.
- Be absolutely clear about the instructions, e.g. choice offered, timing etc.
- Allocate *equal* time to each question (or according to weighting of marking if known).

## Multiple choice questions

Multiple choice questions (MCQs) test factual recall. They cover a broad spectrum of topics, allowing a wide-ranging assessment of the student's knowledge. Given the right approach, even those with a fairly threadbare knowledge can obtain a pass in MCQ examinations as they generally include a sufficient number of straightforward questions. The 'trick' is to maximise one's score on the easier questions while avoiding unnecessary risks on those that are more difficult. MCQs are made up of a stem statement followed by a series of secondary statements. In the usual format, the second statement is true or false in the context of the stem and (as in almost all examinations) *negative* marks are awarded for incorrect answers. Despite the common stem, each subsidiary statement must be assessed in isolation. Guidelines to the MCQ examination would include the following 'dos and don'ts':

**DO**
- read and understand the stem extremely carefully, two or three times.
- leave out questions where reasonable uncertainty exists.
- beware of sweeping statements such as 'never', 'always' etc.

- beware of results given in abnormal units.
- plan your timing: calculate the average time to allocate to each stem at the outset and stick to this.
- practise mock MCQs several times over – you can never do enough MCQs.

**DO NOT**
- guess or take risks at any time: this is usually fatal.
- answer too many or too few questions.
- forget the negative marking format.

## Essay questions

Essay questions are now infrequently used in medical examinations because of their reliance on skills relating to 'written prose' rather than subject matter. Nevertheless, essay questions require a comprehensive grasp of the topic. The answer needs to be laid out in a logical, flowing pattern with an introduction, sequential discussion and conclusion. Time spent on outlining one's train of thought beforehand in a simple list or flow diagram is well spent. It is advisable to annotate these notes alongside your script as insurance in case you run out of time. Essay questions generally cover common broad topics and can be revised by listing the more likely topics within each system and producing a schematic essay outline for each. The use of headings and subtitles will help to divide the essay into ordered, manageable sections and focus the examiner's thoughts. Guidelines to the essay examination would include the following 'dos and don'ts':

**DO**
- read and understand the question carefully.
- be absolutely sure about any choice of questions offered.
- time yourself carefully.
- construct the essay logically.
- outline the essay plan before starting to write.

**DO NOT**
- allocate time disproportionately.
- indulge in verbose prose or repetition.
- digress and answer out of context.

## Short notes

Short notes provide an ideal method for covering several topics in reasonable depth and are more objective than essay questions. Marks are awarded for relevant facts; none are given for extra or superfluous detail. One should aim to produce a structured, ordered list in a logical sequence. However, as there is no negative marking in 'short notes', it is not unreasonable to include details even if there is some doubt to their relevance to the question in hand. Guidelines to the short notes would include the following 'dos and don'ts':

**DO**
- read and understand the question extremely carefully.
- be absolutely sure about any choice.
- answer succinctly, while avoiding irrelevant facts.
- ensure a logical sequence of related facts.

**DO NOT**
- include irrelevant detail.
- digress from the issue at hand.
- allocate time disproportionately.

## Data interpretation

Questions of data interpretation generally test the understanding of basic principles, normal values and pattern recognition. The student would do well to look at all the clues provided. Unless a single diagnosis comes to mind, then draw up a list of possible options and, depending on the clues available, decide on the best-fit scenario. This type of question does not usually include negative marking, so it is important to provide an answer even if you are terribly unsure of its validity. Guidelines to the data questions would include the following 'dos and don'ts':

**DO**
- read and understand the question extremely carefully.
- look at all the clues provided.
- choose the best-fit diagnosis.

**DO NOT**
- rush an answer before all the clues fit.
- leave out any question.
- allocate time disproportionately.

## Viva voce

Many candidates expect an oral to be the most harrowing experience of the examination. The idea that the examiners 'are out to get you' is, frankly, a misconception. It is important to listen carefully to the questions asked, take time to construct your thoughts, and speak clearly. Examiners are trying to ascertain your depth of knowledge and not to trap you. They are human, and you will gain sympathy by being courteous and maintaining eye contact. They will be irritated by a *sotto voce* mumble aimed at the general direction of the floor. Avoid illogical statements, anecdotes, and naming rare syndromes about which you know precious little. The last is invariably going to whet the examiners' interest, and they will promptly ask about the syndrome! Above all, never bluff. The certainty of being caught out making things up is 100%. You will be much better off admitting that you do not know the answer to a certain question and moving on to some other, safer ground. Guidelines to the viva voce would include the following 'dos and don'ts':

**DO**
- concentrate on the question.
- structure your thoughts.
- admit to not knowing.

**DO NOT**
- mumble, or talk incoherently.
- mention issues about which you have little knowledge.
- bluff, or invent answers that you think the examiners want to hear.

## Slide or picture examination

Slide and picture questions rely on recall and pattern recognition. A systematic approach is required and the whole picture, X-ray etc. should be scrutinised very carefully for all the clues. This applies to any accompanying text, notes, captions etc. Consider common problems first, and query the possibility of a rare diagnosis only when you are in a distinction situation. Guidelines to slides or pictures would include the following 'dos and don'ts':

**DO**
- look at and understand all the clues extremely carefully.
- focus on any obvious abnormality.
- focus on the centre of the slide/picture, then work outwards.
- consider common conditions first.
- base your answer on what you see and not what you think you should see.

**DO NOT**
- rush an answer before you have looked at all the clues.
- guess or make up signs.

## Problem-oriented questions

Problem-orientated questions present a mock real-life situation via a brief history. The pattern of questioning may vary. In one method a series of questions is provided and a story unfolds. These questions epitomise the problem-orientated approach to examinations and test the candidate's ability to comprehend the salient clues provided and deal with the clinical situation. In another approach, you will be asked to manage a common medical problem. This may range from prescribing therapy or obtaining consent to advising a patient about their condition. This question asks for a constructed answer. In some cases, the various categories will be obvious from the question and should be dealt with accordingly. In others, you will be left to plan out a logical sequence of events. The guidelines for these types of question are:

**DO**

- make a stepwise plan before you start answering.
- focus on the main problem in question.
- identify investigations and procedures relevant to the case.
- formulate a plan of management.
- evaluate the short- and long-term implications of the case.
- consider the main issues for communication and discussion with parents.

**DO NOT**

- get bogged down by detail.
- repeat your observations disguised under different headings.

In this book we have attempted to provide different examples of these questions in different chapters. Remember, the answers to these questions are only examples of how they can be answered. You are free to make your own strategy, and as long as it is logical and practical you will be rewarded.

## *Objective Structured Clinical Examination (OSCE)*

OSCEs provide a platform for covering a large number of diverse clinical topics in a totally structured format so that students can be assessed objectively. These examinations are very time-consuming and laborious to design and set up but, ultimately, are more objective and, therefore, more fair to the students. The OSCE generally utilises a range of examination formats, including picture cards, slides, data, X-rays, ECGs etc., as well as practical sessions which may test history taking, practical demonstrations and clinical skills. Marks are weighted such that the clinical hands-on and practical stations are given priority. Virtually anything can be written into an OSCE format! However, all questions are organised into set stations with a finite time interval, generally lasting from 4 to 6 minutes. Hence, the number of questions asked on a particular topic must be focused but limited. The majority of OSCE questions will generally cover the core issues and, unless one's knowledge is threadbare across a wide range of topics, it is very difficult to fail an OSCE. Very few questions would be particularly difficult, and these would be

included to identify the distinction candidates! The guidelines for these types of question are:

**DO**

- read the questions carefully.
- answer all questions (there is no negative marking).
- focus on the main problem being questioned.
- be concise – 4 minutes pass quickly.
- concentrate on the clinical stations and stick to the task at hand.
- consider the main issues for communication and discussion with parents.

**DO NOT**

- get bogged down by detail.
- get 'stuck' on a particular question.
- allow yourself to be distracted by colleagues completing their OSCE nearby.
- reminisce on a previously difficult question – focus on each question in the time allocated.

## Self-appraisal and examination technique

Passing examinations does not depend solely on having sufficient core knowledge of the subject and being able to use this knowledge in applied clinical situations. It also relies on an understanding of the examination format and presentation, both on paper and verbally. This improves with confidence, which comes after sufficient reading around the subject and repeated practice of mock examinations. It is important to plan the revision for any examination and adjust the emphasis of the revision after gauging one's own depth of knowledge. An honest self-scoring exercise alone or with like-minded friends who are not hell bent on one-upmanship can be very useful. It is far better to have a working knowledge of most issues rather than an in-depth understanding of a few esoteric facts. Hence, revision should be planned with a broad list in mind and time allocated equally to all the major topics. A readable, medium-sized text is preferable to a comprehensive paediatric 'bible' or a text comprising endless lists with little reference to clinical settings. Often personalised notes taken from lectures and texts leave a lasting impression and provide an efficient method for revision. At all times we would encourage participation during teaching sessions. Tutors welcome and respond to active dialogue, the two-way process generally enhancing the quality of the teaching as well as the impression left on the students.

Finally, theory needs to be backed up with clinical skills and, in this regard, the dictum 'practice makes perfect' is so true! We cannot stress enough the need for students to repeatedly practise their hands-on skills on 'real' patients. Indeed, most children (and their parents) generally welcome the 'distraction' offered by inquisitive and interested medical students and, in the vast majority of cases, do not bite!

## Conclusion

The vast majority of undergraduates pass all the examinations set throughout the curriculum and eventually graduate successfully. Indeed, the system is designed to pass rather than to fail at this level. Those who do not succeed generally do so because they have not made a sufficient effort with background reading or have planned their revision badly. We hope that this book will help to address both these issues, while still allowing the student to appreciate the fascination of clinical paediatrics outside the examination setting.

# Nutrition, normal growth and development

**1.1** Introduction     7

**1.2** Nutritional requirements     7

**1.3** Normal physical growth     10

**1.4** Normal development     13

**1.5** Nutritional disorders     15

Self-assessment: questions     18

Self-assessment: answers     21

## Overview

In order to grow and develop normally, infants and children depend on an adequate nutritional intake. This chapter will review nutritional requirements as they vary with the various stages of development, from the neonatal period, throughout infancy, and later on in childhood. Although the more common deficiency states will be highlighted, it is important to remember that obesity is the commonest nutritional disorder in 'developed' countries. You will need to know what the normal nutritional requirements are for the different age groups, and how to assess the nutritional status of a child. Before you can begin to understand the diseases of childhood, you need a basic understanding of the normal child. This chapter also describes the normal patterns of physical and developmental growth, and will provide you with an understanding of the normal developmental milestones of childhood and how they are assessed.

## 1.1 Introduction

Childhood is a time of active growth in terms of physical size, mental, emotional and sexual maturation, and psychological development. Normal growth is dependent on adequate nutrition and encompasses major transformations from birth to adulthood, progressing in an ordered, stepwise fashion. Although specific stages in physical and psychosocial maturation are attained at relatively fixed times in development, wide variations are observed from one individual to another. Despite these variations, there are acceptable limits for the acquisition of developmental milestones, outside of which progress is considered to be delayed. The recognition of such delay is based on the identification of several absent or abnormal milestones following a comprehensive assessment of the whole child, taking into account several modalities of function and performance.

Major congenital anomalies, chromosomal defects and damage to the growing central nervous system (CNS) are likely to result in significant neurodevelopmental delay. The latter is associated with major disruptions in the normal processes of growth and development, especially those affecting the central nervous system. Hence, severe hypoxic and hypotensive episodes, infections and metabolic derangement, especially if associated with intercurrent curtailment of adequate nutrition, can result in neuropsychomotor delay.

## 1.2 Nutritional requirements

### Learning objectives

You should understand:

- the normal nutritional requirements of the newborn and infant
- the principles of intravenous feeding

### Normal requirements

After birth, the fastest growth velocity (length increase per year) is observed in the newborn period. As shown in Figure 1, this rate falls steadily throughout childhood until a second growth surge at puberty, just before linear growth ceases. Consequently, newborns require more energy (measured in calories or joules) per kilogram weight than at any other stage in childhood (Table 1).

Preterm babies who have 'lost out' on the benefits of 9 months of in-utero feeding have increased calorific needs. As a result of their increased metabolic rate, large surface area and excessive heat loss, preterm babies have increased energy requirements and obtain the

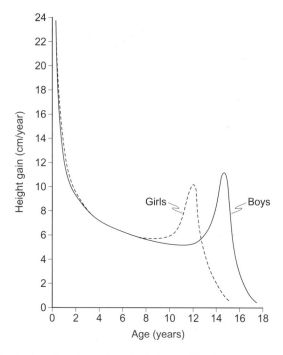

**Fig. 1** Growth velocity from birth to adulthood.

**Table 1** Changes in energy and protein requirements with age

| Age (years) | Energy requirement | | Protein requirement (g/kg) |
|---|---|---|---|
| | (kcal/kg) | (kJ/kg) | |
| 0–1 | 120–90 | 500–380 | 3.5 |
| 1–7 | 90–75 | 380–300 | 2.5 |
| 7–12 | 75–60 | 300–250 | 2.0 |
| 12–18 | 60–30 | 250–125 | 1.5 |

**Table 2** Daily intake of milk with weight and age

| Weight (kg) | Daily intake of milk on days 1–14 after birth (ml/kg)* | | | |
|---|---|---|---|---|
| | 1 | 3 | 10 | 14 |
| <1.5 | 90 | 120 | 180 | 200 |
| 1.5–2.5 | 60 | 110 | 130 | 150 |
| 2.5–4.0 | 60 | 90 | 110 | 120 |
| 4.0–10.0 | 100 daily | | | |
| 10.0–20.0 | 1000 mL + 50 mL/kg per kg over 10 kg | | | |
| >20.0 | 1500 mL + 25 mL/kg per kg over 10 kg | | | |

\* Breast milk contains up to 74 kcal/100 mL (300 kJ/ 100 mL), whereas average formula milk contains 67 kcal/100 mL (280 kJ/100 mL).

additional calories via an increased milk volume intake relative to their size (Table 2).

## Milk feeds

The dictum *breast is best* remains true for almost all cases. Mature breast milk provides about 70–74 kcal/ 100 mL, presented in the ideal proportion of carbohydrate, fat and protein to ensure normal growth. Vitamins and minerals are provided in sufficient quantities and in absorbable forms to ensure deficiencies do not arise. Bonding is easier in breastfed babies. 'Modern' *formula milks* emulate breast milk to a high degree (Table 3). Preterm infants require more calories, protein, vitamins and minerals (including sodium, calcium, phosphorus, magnesium, trace elements) in proportion to their weight, and this is indeed reflected in the composition of expressed breast milk. Preterm formulae are designed to take these needs into account.

Breastfeeding is only contraindicated in mothers who are HIV positive (in so-called developed countries only), have active hepatitis B or C, or are taking lithium, immunosuppressants, cytotoxics or radiopharmaceuticals.

## Timing and route of feeds

Feeding should be commenced within the first 2 hours and continued 2-hourly in preterm and small-for-dates babies (especially if less than 1.5 kg) because of the risk of hypoglycaemia. Term infants can be fed within 4 hours. *Enteral* feeding, preferably via the oral route, is ideal. Nasogastric tube feeding by gravity over 20 minutes is useful, especially in sick infants and those born at less than 33–34 weeks' gestation, when the sucking reflex is poorly developed. *Parenteral feeding* is reserved for infants who, as a result of illness or prematurity, are unable to tolerate enteral feeding (Table 4). In newborn infants, if enteral feeding is still not possible, intravenous dextrose/saline solutions should only be used for about 48 hours before total parenteral nutrition (TPN) is commenced.

Remember that many feeding problems have their origin in rigid feeding regimens instituted at an early age. For the healthy term baby, demand feeding is the best, i.e. the baby should be fed when hungry. Normally a term baby will feed at the breast shortly after birth and then sleep for a few hours.

## Weaning

Semisolid food, usually a cereal with added iron and vitamin D, is introduced at around 6 months. By 6 months, infants can chew and drink from a beaker, and semisolid food, fruit juices etc., can be given. At 1 year, chopped

**Table 3** Breastfeeding

**Advantages**

| | |
|---|---|
| Cost | Free |
| | Does not need warming |
| | Readily available |
| Anti-infective | Secretory IgA comprises 90% of immunoglobulin in human milk |
| | Contains cellular macrophages and lymphocytes |
| | Lactoferrin inhibits growth of *E. coli* in the infant intestine |
| | Bifidus factor promotes the growth of lactobacillus and prevents colonisation with other bacteria |
| | Interferon and lysozymes present |
| Nutritional | More easily digested curd, higher lactalbumin content than cow's milk |
| | Hypoallergenic |
| | Rich in essential and polyunsaturated fatty acids and contains lipase to aid digestion |
| | Calcium:phosphate ratio (2:1) aids absorption of calcium |
| | Bioavailable iron and decreased solute load to kidney |
| Social | Promotes bonding |
| | Contraceptive effect |
| | Reduction in disease later on in life such as diabetes |

**Disadvantages**

| | |
|---|---|
| Infections | Transmission of HIV, CMV and hepatitis |
| Transmission of drugs and other agents | Antithyroid, antimetabolites, alcohol, caffeine |
| Nutritional deficiency | Vitamin K; delayed weaning may lead to nutritional deficiencies |
| Breast milk jaundice | Mild, self-limiting in the early neonatal period |
| Others | Breastfeeding may be difficult to establish, especially where mother is unwell or stressed |

**Table 4** Contraindications to enteral feeding

| Contraindication | Examples |
|---|---|
| Prematurity | In severe prematurity delay for 24–48 hours* |
| Birthweight | Less than 1 kg, delay for 24–48 hours* |
| Gastrointestinal problems | The 3-hourly gastric aspirate is greater than the volume of milk given |
| | Ileus |
| | Mechanical obstruction |
| | Necrotising enterocolitis |
| | Severe malabsorption syndromes |
| | Severe short gut syndrome |
| Neurological problems | Feeding-associated apnoeas |
| | Uncontrolled convulsions |
| General illness | Acute phase of any major illness |
| | Septicaemia |
| | During major procedures (e.g. exchange transfusion) |

* The delay varies from one unit to the next; many will commence enteral feeds within a few hours of birth (as there are no data to suggest which is better).

or liquidised adult food, including doorstep milk, provides an adequate diet.

## Special feeds

**Antireflux (AR)** feeds are standard feeds that contain a thickener and are useful to reduce excessive posset-ting or vomiting in those with troublesome gastric reflux.

**Soy-based feeds** may be useful in proven cases of cow's milk allergy, although 30% of children with cow's milk allergy are also allergic to soya milk. Soy protein provides less energy than breast milk, and a corresponding 10% increase in volume is needed to make up the equivalent calorie content. Hydrolysed casein milk (e.g. Nutramigen) may be a better alternative.

**Elemental feeds** contain partly predigested, absorbable nutrients and are therefore useful in children with short bowel syndrome and problems of absorption.

**Specialised feeds** are custom-made for patients with food intolerance (e.g. lactose-free milks for lactose intolerance), specific malabsorption (e.g. milk containing medium-chain triglycerides in certain postoperative situations) or metabolic disorders (e.g. low-phenylalanine milk for phenylketonuria).

## Intravenous feeding

Intravenous feeding is given to children who are unable to tolerate enteral feeds: 10% dextrose can be given to preterm babies for 1–3 days and term infants for 4–6 days, after which body energy stores are exhausted. Older children can be given combinations of 5–10% dextrose and 0.45–0.9% saline, with appropriate electrolyte supplementation (e.g. daily potassium, 2 mmol/kg/day). If intravenous feeding is prolonged, a compre-

---

**Box 1** Total parenteral nutrition

**Relative contraindications to TPN**
Uraemia
Jaundice
Acidaemia
Sepsis
Hypoxia
Thrombocytopenia.

**Complications of TPN**
Catheter-related sepsis
Thromboses
Extravasation and scarring
Cholestatic jaundice
Hyperlipidaemia
Hyperglycaemia
Acidosis
Metabolic derangement

---

**Box 2** Causes of failure to thrive

**Neonatal period**
Inadequate calorie intake: insufficient volume, incorrect formula, poor feeding technique
Infection (e.g. urinary tract)
Acidaemia
Anaemia

**Childhood**
Poor feeding: brain damage, endocrinopathy
Excess vomiting
Malabsorption: milk intolerance, coeliac disease, inflammatory bowel disease, cystic fibrosis
Systemic illness: heart failure, respiratory failure, renal disease, liver failure
Chronic infection
Social deprivation

---

hensive feed that includes a nitrogen and a fat source should be used.

## Total parenteral nutrition

Total parenteral nutrition is tailor-made for the age, weight and needs of the individual patient. It provides calories in the form of carbohydrate, protein and fats, together with mineral requirements, vitamins and trace element supplements. It should be administered through an indwelling central venous (or umbilical) catheter, preferably used solely for TPN. Regular assessment of the serum glucose, pH, electrolyte and trace elements, urinary glucose and liver and renal function is necessary while TPN is being delivered (Box 1).

## 1.3 Normal physical growth

### Learning objectives

You should:

- know how to differentiate between normal and abnormal growth patterns
- Appreciate the changes that occur at puberty

### Weight gain

Neonates lose up to 5–10% of their birthweight, though this is regained by 10 days (up to 3 weeks in preterms). Weight gain generally progresses at about 15 g/kg/day.

In full-term infants the birthweight is doubled around 5 months of age and tripled by 12 months. Steady weight gain is a reliable guide to the wellbeing of the child, and should always be documented on an appropriate centile chart (Fig. 2a). Excess weight for age is the most common nutritional disorder in developed countries. The major causes for *failure to thrive* (also known as faltering growth), as manifest by insufficient weight gain resulting in a 'falling off' downwards across centile lines, are social deprivation and feeding problems. Other causes are listed in Box 2.

### Obesity

Obesity is clinically defined as a weight of >98th centile for age. There has been a rapid increase in the incidence of childhood obesity, with a prevalence of approximately 15% in the UK and 20% in the USA. Up to 30% or more of these children become obese adults. The risk is greater with a family history of obesity, affluence, higher socioeconomic group, urban existence, and an increase in the time spent on sedentary activities (e.g. watching television). This disorder is generally caused by excessive food intake coupled with insufficient energy expenditure during exercise. Pathological causes contribute less than 1% of cases. Obese children are often teased and may have psychological problems. Advice on dietary curtailment, exercise and lifestyle modification should be given. The help of a dedicated, experienced dietitian is essential, but treatment is rarely successful unless there is a firm commitment of both the child and the family to adhere to the recommended diet.

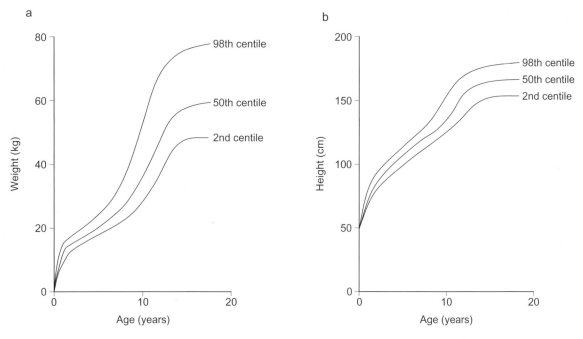

**Fig. 2** Increase in (a) weight and (b) height from birth to adulthood.

## Linear growth

Linear growth progresses in a steady fashion throughout childhood, with a surge at puberty followed by a total cessation in the late teenage years. This is depicted graphically on centile charts, compiled from a large cohort of normal children and showing the growth 'lines' for the mean of the population (50th centile), as well as for normal short and tall individuals (Fig. 2b). A normal growth curve is one that runs approximately parallel to a centile line. Children whose height plots outside these lines, or rapidly crosses the percentile lines, warrant investigation for the causes of tall or short stature.

## Sexual maturation

Gonadotrophins and growth hormone released from the anterior pituitary initiate puberty, which is accompanied by an acceleration in linear growth in both sexes. The latter starts earlier in girls and begins in the peripheries, giving adolescents a gawky appearance. Gonadotrophins stimulate the release of oestrogens and androgens from the respective gonads, which, in turn, orchestrate pubertal development.

### Girls

The appearance of breast buds heralds puberty and usually occurs at the age of 8–9 years (Fig. 3). This constitutes Tanner stage I breast development and is followed by an increase in breast tissue (stage II), an increase in areolar size (stage III), an increase in breast size and areolar pigmentation (stage IV), and the adoption of the adult breast (V). Pubic hair follows the appearance of breast buds. Hair is usually fair and downy (stage I), then darkens (II), becoming curly (III) and more abundant (IV) until the adult triangular pubic pattern is assumed (V). Labial, clitoral, uterine and ovarian development is under the influence of oestrogen and follicle-stimulating hormone. Menstruation is usually a late feature, when linear growth is decelerating, and early periods are often anovulatory and irregular. On average, girls have approximately 12 months of linear growth after the appearance of menses.

### Boys

An increase in testicular size is the first sign of male puberty, usually occurring by the age of 10 years (Fig. 3). These organs increase in volume from 1–3 mL in infants to 12–20 mL in adults. Penile enlargement follows: initially an increase in length (stage I), then thickness (II), pigmentation (III) and skin rugosity (IV), before the adult form is attained (V). Pubic hair develops in tandem, as it does in females. The seminiferous tubules, epididymis, seminal vesicles and prostate gland develop under the influence of luteinising hormone and testosterone. Changes in body build, hirsutism, acne, vocal cords and dentition complete the process.

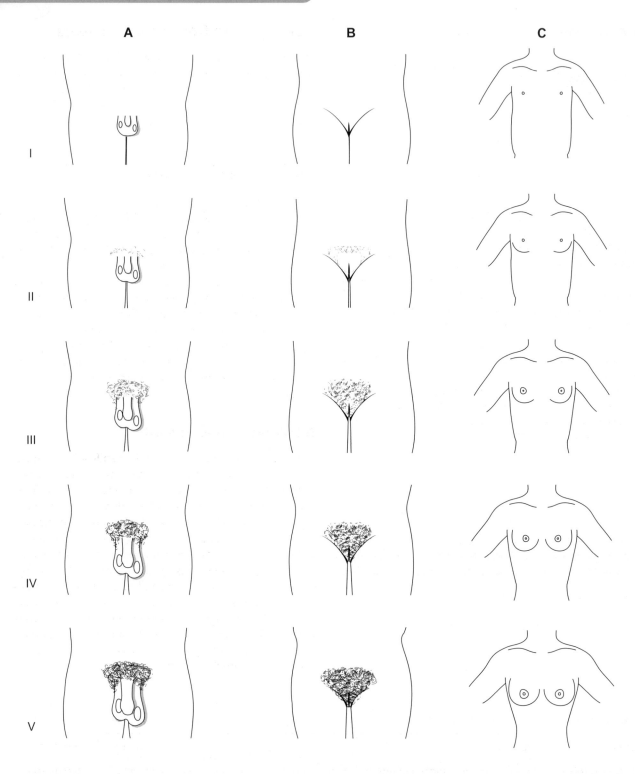

**Fig. 3** Sexual maturation in boys and girls. I–V A show the changes in sexual maturation in boys. An increase in testicular volume is followed by increase in penile length and girth. Pubic hair increases from a few pale straight hairs to assume the adult appearance with dark, curly hair in both boys and girls (A and B). I–V C show the progression in breast buds and areolae to the adult shape and size.

## 1.4 Normal development

Human development progresses through a sequence of events, during which specific functional skills are acquired. Despite individual variation, these landmarks ('milestones') should occur at approximately the same age for normal children, and are therefore essential in the assessment of neurodevelopmental progress (Box 3).

It is easier to grasp development by using these major categories while focusing on specific key age groups, rather than trying to remember a progressive continuum of developmental parameters throughout childhood.

Primitive reflexes appear and disappear in sequence during specific periods of development. Their absence or presence beyond a specific timeframe signifies dysfunction of the CNS (Table 5).

---

**Box 3** Categories for assessing developmental milestones

Gross motor
Fine motor
Special senses (vision, hearing, language)
Psychosocial
Educational

---

## Development: from birth to 4 years

Motor skills are acquired primarily during the first few months of life, whereas psychosocial and educational milestones assume greater importance after the first 2 years. Table 6 shows important milestones that, on average, are attained at birth, 6 weeks, 6, 10, 13, 18 months, and 2, 3 and 4 years.

## Development: 4–6 years

Children generally commence school at the age of 4 years, by which time they should be independent with regard to feeding, dressing, washing and toilet care. They are now more gregarious, mischievous and sociable, appreciating the need to share and play together. They consolidate their understanding of colours, numbers and drawing skills. Their depiction of 'a man' and 'a house' improves steadily (Fig. 4). The vocabulary escalates and speech becomes more complex, so that by 7 years 'baby talk' has disappeared. They become ever more inquisitive and questioning and, as their understanding and imagination increases, so does the complexity of play.

## Abnormal development

Developmental delay in infancy is manifest by a failure to acquire motor milestones, such as adequate head control, the ability to sit and bear weight, as well as social non-responsiveness, lack of interest in surroundings, and an inability to respond to audiovisual stimuli. Persistence of premature reflexes, such as the Moro reflex, beyond 2–3 months is also abnormal. These and a delay in milestones require review and follow-up by a specialist neurodevelopmental team. This team normally comprises paediatrician, child psychologist, orthoptist, audiologist, physiotherapist, speech, occupational and educational therapists, and social workers, who perform a comprehensive assessment of motor, functional, audiovisual and cognitive ability.

---

**Table 5**

| Reflex | Characteristic | Appears | Duration |
|---|---|---|---|
| Stepping reflex | Lifting infant to rub dorsum of foot over edge | At birth | 1–2 months |
| Rooting reflex | Stroking of cheek will result in head turning to same side | At birth | 2 months |
| Palmar grasp | Infant will grasp object in open palm | At birth | 2–3 months |
| Tonic neck | Manual turning of head to one side produces ipsilateral flexion and contralateral extension of the extremities | At birth | 3–4 months |
| Moro | Place infant semiupright. Allow head to fall backwards momentarily. There is symmetrical abduction and extension of the arms, with flexion of the thumbs, followed by flexion and adduction of the upper limbs | At birth | 3–6 months |
| Parachute | Sudden 'fall' in the prone position produces spontaneous extension of extremities | 7–8 months | Lifelong |

**Table 6** Developmental milestones from birth to 4 years

| Age | Category | Acquired skill |
| --- | --- | --- |
| Birth | Gross motor | Complete head lag, lies prone, hips flexed |
| | Fine motor | Sucking reflex, fisting |
| | Vision | Blinks to light |
| | Hearing | Startles to noise |
| 6 weeks | Gross motor | Improving head control, prone, hips extended |
| | Fine motor | Hands often open |
| | Vision | Focuses object in 90° arc |
| | Hearing | Settles to mother's voice |
| | Psychosocial | Smiles |
| 6 months | Gross motor | Good head control, press-up if prone, sits using hands |
| | Fine motor | Transfers between hands, palmar grasp |
| | Vision | Focuses object in 180° arc |
| | Hearing | Whisper at short distance |
| | Language | Chuckles, babbles |
| | Psychosocial | Indicates likes, dislikes |
| 10 months | Gross motor | Creeps, cruises around furniture, sits and pivots |
| | Fine motor | Index finger approach |
| | Vision | Small objects other side of room |
| | Hearing | Whisper at a distance |
| | Language | Vocalising, da-da, ma-ma |
| | Psychosocial | Waves, plays pat-a-cake |
| 13 months | Gross motor | Walks unaided, casting of objects |
| | Fine motor | Offers objects in play, places cube |
| | Vision | Small objects end of room |
| | Hearing | Distraction test |
| | Language | 1–2 words; jargon commences |
| | Psychosocial | Stops mouthing, slobbering |
| 18 months | Gross motor | Walks upstairs, jumps |
| | Fine motor | Uses spoon, tower three cubes, scribbles with pencil |
| | Language | Two to three word sentences |
| | Psychosocial | Dry by day, partly dresses self |
| | Education | Identifies one picture, points to some objects/parts of body |

**Table 6** *(cont'd)*

| Age | Category | Acquired skill |
|---|---|---|
| 2 years | Gross motor | Runs, kicks ball |
| | Fine motor | Screws top, tower six cubes, copies vertical line |
| | Language | Four to six word sentences |
| | Psychosocial | Dry by day and night, dresses self well |
| | Education | Points four parts of body, identifies five pictures; names three |
| 3 years | Fine motor | Tower nine cubes, copies cross, circle |
| | Language | Vocabulary accelerates |
| | Psychosocial | Dresses self fully except laces |
| | Education | Points ten parts of body, identifies 12 pictures and names eight, names three colours |
| 4 years | Fine motor | Cubes: imitates gate, copies square, places shapes into slots |
| | Psychosocial | Dresses self fully |
| | Education | Identifies, names several pictures, names several colours |

## 1.5 Nutritional disorders

### Learning objectives

You should:

- understand the physical changes that occur in malnutrition
- know the signs, symptoms and management of the common mineral and vitamin deficiencies

### Protein–energy malnutrition

Protein–energy malnutrition (PEM) follows a prolonged period of nutritional deprivation. Total body protein and muscle mass decrease as a result of catabolism outstripping anabolic processes. Total body fat is decreased, though its deposition in the liver may be increased. Minerals, especially potassium, are reduced. Total body water is increased, especially in the extracellular space. PEM often arises after weaning, and presents with marasmus or kwashiorkor, or both. Patients with marasmus are alert and hungry but severely wasted and stunted, with a lack of subcutaneous fat. Children with kwashiorkor are lethargic, miserable, apathetic, and have severe hair and skin changes. There is a lack of muscle bulk, generalised oedema, ascites and hepatomegaly. Both are associated with secondary anaemia, endocrinopathies, immunosuppression and vitamin deficiencies. Electrolyte disturbances, hypoglycaemia, hypothermia, dehydration, anaemia, infection and vitamin deficiencies (especially A, D, E) must be corrected, together with nutritional supplementation. Intravenous fluids should be replaced by oral replacement as soon as possible. A high-calorie diet (150–200 kcal/kg/day) with a minimum of 2–3 g/kg milk or animal protein and vitamin and mineral supplements is required. Recovery is characterised by the 'nutritional recovery syndrome', with a progressive gain in weight (10 g/kg daily) and an increased interest in the surroundings.

### Iron deficiency

Iron deficiency is the most common deficiency in developed countries. In the inner cities of the UK around 20% of children are iron deficient – in cities with large Asian

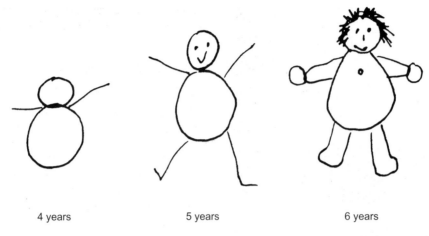

| 4 years | 5 years | 6 years |

**Fig. 4** Depiction of a man by a child of 4, 5 and 6 years, respectively.

communities this proportion is greater. Iron deficiency is usually a consequence of an inadequate dietary intake of foodstuffs rich in iron, including meat and green vegetables, and delayed weaning. Iron stores are primarily built up toward the end of uterine life, so that preterm babies often lack this important element. Iron-deficiency anaemia is common after prolonged feeding with breast or cow's milk, as neither contains sufficient iron. Chronic blood loss, especially in those with oesophageal reflux and gastrointestinal ulceration, ultimately leads to depletion of iron stores and symptoms of anaemia, including pallor, lethargy and, occasionally, cardiac failure and pica. Investigation shows a microcytic, hypochromic anaemia associated with low ferritin levels. In patients from the Mediterranean basin and Indian subcontinent thalassaemia should be excluded. Treatment involves a daily replacement of 6 mg elemental iron, given orally as a ferrous salt.

## Vitamin D deficiency (rickets)

Vitamin D is essential for the normal mineralisation of bone. Its deficiency results from a diet inadequate in dairy products, a lack of sunlight, malabsorptive states, and liver and renal disease. The skin contains 7-dehydrocholesterol, which is converted to vitamin $D_3$ by ultraviolet light. Dietary vitamin can be obtained from plant sources (ergocalciferol or $D_2$) or animal sources (cholecalciferol or $D_3$). The provitamin is first metabolised in the liver to the monohydroxy derivative, and in the kidney to the active metabolite 1,25-dihydroxy cholecalciferol ($1,25(OH)_2D_3$) or the inactive metabolite $24,25(OH)_2D_3$.

Deficiency results in the decreased absorption of calcium and phosphate, with decreased mineralisation of the bones, especially at the growth plate. Affected patients develop softened bones (e.g. craniotabes in infants, bowing of tibiae), distension of the growing ends of the bones (wrists, knees and ribs, producing a rickety rosary), short stature and generalised hypotonia. Investigation shows a decrease in phosphorus, low or normal calcium and increased alkaline phosphatase. As a result the metaphyses of the long bones are demineralised and the epiphyseal plates widen and become cupped (Fig. 5). An intake of 10 µg vitamin D daily prevents rickets; treatment requires 250 µg daily.

## Other vitamin deficiencies

### Vitamin A deficiency

Vitamin A is fat soluble. It is plentiful in liver, milk, coloured vegetables and wheat. Vitamin A deficiency is common in rice-eating populations who rarely consume animal fat. Retinol is the active derivative of vitamin A and contributes the photosensitive pigment to the rods (light) and cones (colour) of the retina.

Vitamin A deficiency results in night blindness, later conjunctival xerosis and corneal scarring. Dry silver plaques may appear on the bulbar conjunctiva (Bitot spots). In parts of the world where vitamin A deficiency is a major problem, 30 mg should be given orally at least twice a year. In children with corneal involvement (keratomalacia), initially 3 mg/kg is given intramuscularly, then 1.5 mg a day by mouth until healing is complete. Vitamin A also plays a role in keratinisation, spermatogenesis, and the epithelialisation of the respiratory and gastrointestinal systems. Subclinical deficiencies in malnourished children with diarrhoea and respiratory tract infections have been associated with increased morbidity in developing countries.

### Vitamin $B_1$ deficiency

Thiamine is absent in boiled rice. Thiamine deficiency results in beri-beri in infants, presenting with cardiac

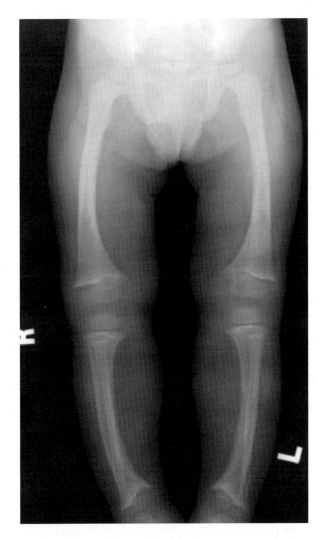

**Fig. 5** Radiological changes in rickets.

failure, laryngeal oedema and distal nerve degeneration. With Vitamin $B_1$ deficiency, up to 100 mg thiamine is given first, followed by 5–10 mg daily.

## Vitamin $B_2$ deficiency

Riboflavin deficiency is usually associated with other coenzyme deficiencies. It causes an angular stomatitis, cheilosis and keratitis. Treatment of deficiency is with 3–10 mg daily.

## Niacin deficiency

Niacin is present in small quantities in cereals. Hence, maize-eating communities may lack this coenzyme and develop pellagra, which consists of a symmetrical dermatitis on exposed surfaces, glossitis, fissuring of muco-cutaneous junctions, and neurological sequelae. Treatment of deficiency requires 50 mg daily.

## Vitamin $B_6$ deficiency

Adequate functioning of the nervous system depends on pyridoxine, and its deficiency results in seizures and peripheral neuropathies and, occasionally, cheilosis and seborrhoea. Vitamin $B_6$ deficiency may occur in newborn infants and later, following malabsorption and the destruction of pyridoxine by overheating milk and cereals. Treatment is with 100 mg intramuscularly for neonatal seizures, whereas a daily intake of 10–100 mg by mouth generally suffices for pyridoxine-dependent children.

## Vitamin $B_{12}$ deficiency

Vitamin $B_{12}$ deficiency is seen in patients taking a strictly vegan diet and in those with terminal ileal disease (e.g. Crohn's disease). It results in a macrocytic anaemia.

## Vitamin C deficiency (scurvy)

Breast and formula milk, but not cow's milk, provide the daily requirement of 10 mg vitamin C. Deficiency results in symptoms initially observed at 6–12 months, with fretfulness, easy bruising, pseudoparalysis owing to subperiosteal haematomas, and bleeding gums. Investigation shows a hypochromic anaemia, bony atrophy, decalcification and subperiosteal calcification. Scurvy is effectively treated with 200 mg vitamin C daily.

## Vitamin E deficiency

Vitamin E deficiency follows malabsorption and presents with haemolytic anaemia in preterm infants, and weakness, sometimes ataxia and neuropathy in children. Preterm babies are given 20 IU vitamin E supplements per day.

## Vitamin K deficiency

Vitamin K deficiency occurs in newborns, and in children with liver disease and malabsorption. Breast milk does not contain vitamin K and, as a result, breastfed babies are more prone to develop haemorrhagic disease of the newborn (HDN). In order to prevent HDN all babies are given an intramuscular injection of 1 mg of vitamin K. This is repeated at 7 days in those at particular risk, and then again at 28 days, either orally or by intramuscular injection.

# Self-assessment: questions

## Multiple choice questions

1. The following statements describe developmental milestones:
   a. Infants do not smile socially before the age of 3 months
   b. Infants do not sit unaided till the age of 12 months
   c. Children walk without help at around 12–14 months of age
   d. Slobbering generally stops at 2 years of age
   e. An index finger approach is typical in a 10-month-old child.

2. The following statements describe child development:
   a. Children voice words into simple sentences at around 18 months of age
   b. Children cannot build a tower of six bricks till they are about 6 years old
   c. Children can copy a circle at 18 months
   d. Picture cards provide a poor assessment of the power of comprehension
   e. Toilet training should begin at 12 months of age.

3. With regard to normal growth in childhood:
   a. Growth velocity decreases in the first decade of life
   b. The pubertal growth spurt starts earlier in boys than in girls
   c. Birthweight is doubled at 12 months
   d. Weight loss is the most common nutritional disorder in developed countries
   e. Puberty is commenced by the appearance of menstrual periods in girls.

4. With regard to milk feeding in infancy:
   a. Preterm formulae contain additional calories compared to breast milk
   b. Breast milk is extremely rich in iron
   c. Expressed breast milk is usually sufficient to cater for the infant's needs
   d. Preterm infants require feeding at longer intervals to allow for slower gastric emptying
   e. Cow's milk is adequate for term but not for preterm babies.

5. With regard to nutritional requirements and deficiencies in childhood:
   a. Iron deficiency may be associated with pica
   b. Rickets of prematurity presents with osteopenic bones, sometimes fractures
   c. Vitamin A deficiency is the commonest form of blindness worldwide
   d. Infants require 4 mmol/kg body weight of potassium daily
   e. Protein and fat provide 4 kcal/g compared to 9 kcal/g from carbohydrate.

## Short notes

List the benefits and problems associated with breastfeeding.

## Viva voce question

Describe how you would perform a distraction test for hearing assessment in an 18-month-old boy.

## Case history

You are the senior house officer in paediatrics and have seen a 4-year-old girl in the outpatient department, referred by her general practitioner for poor weight gain. She is brought to clinic by her mother, who is 8 months pregnant, her 2-year-old brother, and her mother's friend. From the dietary history you note that she has always been a 'difficult feeder'. She dislikes (and will throw up) almost all vegetables and most meat-containing foodstuffs, but likes potatoes, eggs, milk and fruit juice. She was breastfed for 1 week and then started on a standard formula milk and weaned on to semisolids at 2 months. She is fully immunised. Her mother kept an accurate record of her weight measurements and you note that she plotted on the 40th centile for weight at birth, and on the 10th centile at 3 months, when she was changed to a soy-based preparation. Nevertheless, she plotted on the 3rd centile at 6 and 12 months. Her weight is now below the 3rd centile and her height on the 25th centile. A system review was unhelpful and examination confirms an unkempt, pale, boisterous, scrawny but otherwise normal girl.

Her mother is seriously concerned that her daughter has worms and would like X-rays, including a contrast study, of her bowels.

The child is not returned for follow-up on two occasions, but returns unexpectedly to outpatients with both parents after another 7 weeks. In the interim her mother has been delivered of a baby boy, and her father claims he had misplaced the appointment card.

You arrange to review the child in 1 month's time, at which time you discover that the haemoglobin is 8.5 g/dL, white cell count $16 \times 10^9$/L, MCV (mean cell volume) 72 fL and MCHC (mean corpuscular haemoglobin concentration) 25 g/dL. Urinalysis by dipstick showed 1+ protein and there were $10^4$ cells per high-power field, with a mixed growth on culture.

1. What is the initial diagnosis?
2. What further details would you request about the child?
3. What further details would you request from the family and social history?
4. How would you counsel the mother at this point?
5. What investigations are indicated?
6. What is the most likely diagnosis at this stage?
7. What therapeutic and follow-up arrangements are appropriate?
8. What important indices would you measure on this occasion?
9. What additional measures should you take for this child?
10. What additional measures should you take for this family?

## OSCE questions

### OSCE 1

Examine the prints taken from this 2-year-old child, who had walked at the age of 14 months but who, over the past 2 months, had refused to bear weight on the lower limbs:

a. What abnormality is shown in Figure 6?
b. What abnormalities are shown in Figure 7?
c. What is the most likely diagnosis?
d. What tests would confirm this?

### OSCE 2

Indicate the appropriate age of the following children (in months or years):

a. sits unsupported and holds bottle with two hands
   age:_____
b. approaches small objects with palmar grasp and walks, two hands held
   age:_____
c. talks incessantly using simple sentences
   age:_____
d. copies an X and a large O
   age:_____

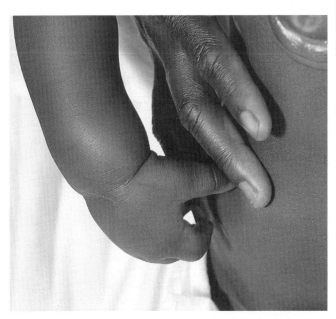

**Fig. 6**

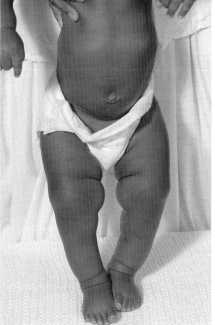

**Fig. 7**

## Data question

A 15-month-old girl was seen by her general practitioner, who was concerned about her pallor and ordered a full blood count. He phones you with the following result:

| | | |
|---|---|---|
| Hb | 7.2 g/dL | |
| MCV | 64 fL | (N = 70–85 fL) |
| MCH | 20 pg | (N = 24–30 pg) |
| MCHC | 27 g/dL | (N = 30–36 g/dL) |
| White count | $9.1 \times 10^9$/L | (normal differential) |
| Platelet count | $178 \times 10^9$/L | (N 150–250 $\times 10^9$/L) |

a. What does the full blood count show?
b. Comment on the white cell and platelet counts.
c. What is the most likely diagnosis?
d. What treatment would you commence?
e. What other test would you order in a child of North African descent?

# Self-assessment: answers

## Multiple choice answers

1. a. **False**. Smiling usually occurs at 6 weeks.
   b. **False**. Infants can usually sit unaided at 6 months.
   c. **True**. The average age for unassisted walking is 13 months.
   d. **True**. Slobbering starts at 3–4 months and stops by 2 years.
   e. **True**. The primitive grasp reflex at birth disappears at 12 weeks; desire to go for objects is fulfilled by an inaccurate palmar grasp at 4 months. Deliberate, accurate grasp develops at 5 months. This improves steadily to enable picking up of ever-smaller objects from 5–10 months, when the index finger approach is established.

2. a. **True**. 'Da da' and 'ma ma' are voiced at around 8 months, followed by single words from 10 months, culminating in simple, two-word sentences at 18 months.
   b. **False**. This occurs at around 2 years.
   c. **False**. A child can copy a circle at about 3 years.
   d. **False**. Picture cards test vision, recognition, association and speech and provide an excellent means of assessing comprehension.
   e. **False**. Toilet-training should not start before 18 months.

3. a. **True**. There is a second spurt at puberty.
   b. **False**. On average, the pubertal growth spurt starts 1–2 years earlier in girls.
   c. **False**. Birthweight is doubled at 5 months.
   d. **False**. Overweight and obesity are far more common in developed countries.
   e. **False**. Breast bud development is the first sign of puberty; periods appear toward the end of puberty.

4. a. **True**. Preterm formulae have 80 kcal/100 mL compared to 70 kcal/100 mL in breast milk.
   b. **False**. Breast milk is low in iron supply, but its iron is readily absorbed.
   c. **True**. Although milk fortifiers may be added for preterm infants.
   d. **False**. Short intervals are used to prevent hypoglycaemia caused by increased requirements and low glucose stores in preterms.
   e. **False**. Cow's milk is not introduced before 12 months.

5. a. **True**. Inappropriate ingestion of inert material or faeces (pica) may be a presenting feature in children with iron deficiency.
   b. **True**. Generalised osteopenia, sometimes rendering bones virtually invisible on X-ray, and widespread fractures, especially of the ribs, are classic features of neonatal rickets.
   c. **False**. This is the most common cause of blindness in rice-dependent populations.
   d. **False**. They have a daily requirement of 2 mmol/kg potassium, 4 mmol/kg sodium and 1 mmol/kg calcium.
   e. **False**. Protein and carbohydrate provide 4 kcal/g; fat provides 9 kcal/g.

## Short notes answer

The advantages of breastfeeding include:

- Correct amounts of protein, fat and carbohydrate for daily requirements
- Appropriate ratio of casein to lactalbumin
- Correct amounts of electrolytes
- Iron presented in absorbable form
- Contains vitamins, folic acid
- Contains lipase, which helps digestion
- Improved maternal bonding
- Immune properties (e.g. IgA, lactoferrin, white cells, lysozyme)
- Low pH encourages beneficial probiotic bacteria such as bifidobacteria and *Lactobacillus acidophilus* rather than *Escherichia coli* in stool
- Economical, cheap.

Problems associated with breastfeeding include:

- Inability to assess exact amounts of feed taken
- Increased unconjugated jaundice in the neonatal period, though never to kernicteric levels
- Transfer of maternal medications and infections to infant.

## Viva voce answer

The child should be seated on his parent's lap in a quiet room, preferably without too many visible distractions. The distractor positions himself (seated comfortably) a metre or so in front of the child, and the controller of the test stands behind the parent, out of sight of the child. The distractor is then told to gain the child's attention using a bright coloured object. Once the child's concentration is focused on this toy, the controller signs to the distractor to hide the toy. At the moment when the child has lost the focus of his attention and is not yet distracted by some other object, the controller mouths a high-pitched (e.g. SSSHHH) or low-pitched (e.g. GGGOOO) noise at the level of the child's ear (while still out of sight). A positive distraction test is indicated by a clear appreciation of the sound by the child, who then turns his head to seek out its origin. The test can be repeated for both ears using different sounds. The test is not applicable to children whose head and truncal control is underdeveloped such that they are unable to sit up (i.e. before 6 months), and it usually fails beyond 18 months or so when the child cannot be 'fooled' so easily.

## Case history answer

1. Failure to thrive owing to an inadequate diet and probably a deficiency syndrome (especially iron). She was weaned too early and is now on an inadequate diet, mostly sustained with milk and fruit juice.
2. In addition to her medical history, it is important to enquire about her general behaviour, the presence of pica, global development, especially speech, language and learning, and social skills such as toilet training.
3. It is important to know the family set-up, i.e. number of children and their ages, the father's employment and family income, housing situation and social benefits, if any. The medical history of other family members and their heights and weights should be recorded.
4. Advise the mother that the child's problem is likely to be related to her poorly balanced diet, and that she is probably low in iron stores. Explain that this is not serious and is easily reversed with appropriate therapy and a good diet. Gently point out that X-ray imaging is unlikely to be helpful and would expose the child to unnecessary irradiation. Go on to explain what investigations are necessary, what they entail and why.
5. The following investigations are appropriate:

   - Full blood count, differential and indices
   - Electrolytes, calcium, phosphate, alkaline phosphatase, magnesium
   - Ferritin, folate
   - Albumin, total protein
   - Renal and liver function
   - Urinalysis
   - Bone age (X-ray left wrist and hand).

6. Iron-deficiency anaemia.
7. Commence iron supplements, repeat urinalysis and culture from a clean-catch specimen (initial sample was contaminated). Arrange follow-up to monitor weight and response to treatment.
8. Check weight, (height), full blood count, ferritin and urinalysis.
9. Refer the child to a professional dietitian and, if appropriate, to a child guidance clinic.
10. Refer the family to social services to maximise state support and to supervise progress of the patient and siblings. The problem appears to be one of a chaotic family held together by a caring but overworked mother with several young children. Her concern, fastidious recording of weight measurements, and maintenance of an up-to-date vaccination schedule argue against child abuse by neglect.

## OSCE answers

### OSCE 1
A. Figure 6 shows swelling of the wrist.
B. Figure 7 shows swelling of the knees and bowing of the legs.
C. Rickets.
D. Biochemical tests to confirm low/normal calcium level, low phosphate level and elevated alkaline phosphatase.

### OSCE 2

| Q: | Ideal answer | others | score (max 15) |
|---|---|---|---|
| A: | 6–8 months | | 4 |
| | | 9–10 months | 2 |
| | | less 6; more 10 months | 0 |
| B: | 10–12 months | | 4 |
| | | 9–10 months | 2 |
| | | 12–13 months | 1 |
| | | less 8; more 13 months | 0 |
| C: | 18–24 months | | 4 |
| | | 24–30 months | 2 |
| | | less 18 months | 0 |
| D: | 3.0–3.5 years | | 3 |
| | | 2.5–3.0 years | 1 |
| | | 3.5–4.0 years | 1 |
| | | less 2.5; more 4 years | 0 |

## Data question

| | | |
|---|---|---|
| A. | Microcytic, hypochromic anaemia | 3 points |
| B. | These are both normal | 1 point |
| C. | Iron deficiency anaemia | 2 points |
| D. | Iron replacement and an iron-rich diet | 2 points |
| E. | Haemoglobin electrophoresis for thalassaemia | 2 points |

# 2 Diseases of the fetus and newborn

**2.1** Introduction     23

**2.2** The fetus     24

**2.3** Assessment of the newborn     26

**2.4** Congenital anomalies     27

**2.5** Birth asphyxia     29

**2.6** Respiratory disease     31

**2.7** Infections     32

**2.8** Jaundice in the newborn     35

**2.9** Neonatal convulsions     37

**2.10** Low birthweight     37

Self-assessment: questions     40

Self-assessment: answers     43

## Overview

There is now an increasing ability to monitor the health of the fetus. This has been largely due to the refinement of ultrasound technology and the dramatic increase in our knowledge of fetal physiology and the changes that occur at birth. A team approach permits the optimal management of fetal health and the subsequent problems faced during the neonatal period. Neonatal care has developed into a major subspecialty and contributes significantly to the workload in any paediatric unit. You will need to understand the normal growth of the fetus, the factors that can influence this, and the techniques used for assessment. Prematurity and its complications, and especially surfactant deficiency, inherited and congenital diseases, all contribute to a significant morbidity and mortality in this age group. Similarly, ante- and postpartum infection can have devastating effects on the outcome of premature and newborn infants, and students would be expected to be confident in the management of this problem. Birth asphyxia remains a common problem despite great strides in neonatal care and, like

jaundice of the newborn, should be managed by a systematic approach if late complications are to be avoided. Remember that over 90% of pregnancies are uneventful and that mostly the parents are only seeking reassurance that their baby is well. Therefore, the key learning objective of this chapter is to understand the resuscitation of and perform a physical examination of the newborn.

## 2.1 Introduction

### Learning objective

You should:

- be familiar with the normal definitions relating to growth and outcome of the newborn

Of the 600 000 babies born each year in the UK, 1600 die during the first week of life. The causes of death are listed in Box 4. Although prematurity is the leading cause of morbidity, the outcome of premature birth has improved dramatically: 90% of those born after 28 weeks of gestation can be expected to survive without serious complications.

### Definitions

#### Definitions related to growth

**Term infant:** infant born between 38 and 42 weeks of gestation (i.e. after 37 completed weeks)

**Preterm infant:** infant born before 37 completed weeks of gestation

**Post-term infant:** infant born after 42 weeks of gestation

**Low birthweight (LBW):** infant weighing 2500 g or less at birth

**Very low birthweight (VLBW):** infant weighing 1500 g or less at birth

**Small for gestational age (SGA):** infant weighing less than the 10th percentile

**Large for gestational age (LGA):** infant weighing more than the 90th percentile

**Box 4** Causes of neonatal death

| Fetal | Preterm infants | Term infants |
|---|---|---|
| Congenital anomalies | Congenital anomalies | Congenital anomalies |
| Chromosomal problems | Chromosomal problems | Perinatal asphyxia |
| Placental insufficiency | Severe prematurity | Perinatal trauma |
| Placental abruption | Surfactant deficiency | Meconium aspiration |
| Umbilical cord accident | Bronchopulmonary dysplasia | Persistent fetal circulation |
| Hydrops fetalis | Intraventricular haemorrhage | Infection |
| Intrauterine infection | Infection | Metabolic diseases |
| | Necrotising enterocolitis | |

**Appropriate for gestational age (AGA):** infant weighing >10th and <90th percentile for weight.

Causes of reduced intrauterine growth include maternal disease, placental dysfunction, fetal abnormalities and congenital infections. The most important cause of excessive growth is poorly controlled maternal diabetes.

### Definitions related to outcome

**Stillbirth:** infant born dead after 24 weeks of gestation (UK figures: 5.6/1000 births)

**Abortion:** fetal death before 24 weeks of gestation

**Perinatal mortality:** the number of stillbirths and deaths during the first 1–6 complete days per 1000 total births (UK figures: 8.3/1000 births)

**Neonatal mortality:** deaths in the first 28 days of life (UK figures 3.5/1000 live births)

**Infant mortality:** deaths occurring from birth to 12 months (UK figures 5.2/1000 live births).

The perinatal period is the first 7 days after birth; the neonatal period is the first 28 days after birth; and the postneonatal period spans 28 days to 12 months of life. The perinatal mortality rate for the UK has reduced greatly during the 1980s and 1990s, and was approximately 8/1000 in 1993. The postneonatal mortality rate has also fallen, because of a great reduction in the number of cot deaths, probably as a result of the introduction of the supine sleeping posture.

The perinatal mortality rate is a measure of the quality of the antenatal care, management of labour, and immediate resuscitation and care of the newborn. It also reflects the socioeconomic conditions affecting the general health of the mothers and the surroundings into which the babies are born. The infant mortality rate provides a more comprehensive overview, and is low in the developed countries (fewer than 10 per 1000 live births) and high in some developing countries (30–200/1000 live births).

## 2.2 The fetus

### Learning objective

You should:

* know the investigations performed antenatally to assess fetal wellbeing

### Maternal factors

A successful outcome to pregnancy is linked to the mother's state of health and nutrition, living standards and quality of healthcare. A full medical and obstetric history is essential. Maternal factors that may affect fetal health are given in Table 7. This is by no means a comprehensive list.

### Antenatal screening

At the first booking visit (10–13 weeks) the blood pressure will be checked and the urine analysed for infection, protein and glucose. A blood sample is taken to check for blood group and type; haemoglobin; screening for infections such as hepatitis B and C; syphilis or HIV (with consent); and for immunity to rubella. Other blood tests may be done, as required. The triple test is optional and is carried out at 16 weeks' gestation. It measures maternal serum α-fetoprotein, human chorionic gonadotrophin and unconjugated oestriol. Adjusted to maternal age, the results can be predictive of Down syndrome or neural tube defects, but will need confirmation with other tests.

### Ultrasound

This is a non-invasive test that has no known effect on the fetus. Apart from the high-resolution 2D scans now available, 3D and 4D scanning is faster and provides a clearer image of the baby's external anatomy, including the face, hands and feet, as well as activity in the womb. Normally a dating scan is offered at 8–12 weeks and a detailed scan at 20 weeks. At the dating scan the thickness of the skin of the back of the neck, or 'nuchal translucency' is estimated. If this is increased it suggests Down syndrome. The detailed scan establishes the biophysical profile (fetal heart variability, movements of respiration and body, tone and amniotic fluid volume).

Where these scans suggest an abnormality, detailed anomaly scans and/or invasive tests are performed. Doppler studies are helpful in assessing intrauterine growth rate (IUGR) and in predicting the development of eclampsia. Examples of abnormalities detected on ultrasound are given in Table 8.

Once anomalies are suspected on ultrasonography, a sample of fetal tissue may be required to confirm the diagnosis. Other methods of prenatal diagnosis are used to obtain fetal cells for DNA or biochemical analysis, allowing a large (and constantly increasing) number of metabolic, chromosomal and genetic disorders to be identified before birth. All invasive methods are now performed under ultrasound guidance, and are listed in Table 9.

## Disorders associated with maternal abnormalities

Maternal disease (e.g. diabetes, thyroid disease, phenylketonuria and systemic lupus erythematosus), teratogens (e.g. alcohol, warfarin, phenytoin) and

**Table 7** Maternal factors that affect fetal health

| | |
|---|---|
| Age | IUGR and premature labour more common in teenage pregnancies. Increased risk of IUGR, pregnancy-induced hypertension, chromosomal anomalies and multiple pregnancy in those older than 35 years |
| Parity | Higher perinatal mortality rate in those who have had five or more previous pregnancies |
| Socioeconomic | Poor socioeconomic conditions associated with low birthweight and prematurity
Single parenthood |
| Employment | In general this is not a risk to fetal development |
| Illnesses | Diseases such as diabetes, hypertension, sickle cell disease, autoimmune disorders may all affect fetal wellbeing |
| Drugs | There is a long list of drugs that may affect the fetus. For example, phenytoin is associated with cleft lip and palate, valproate with spina bifida. Drugs of abuse such as cocaine readily cross the placenta, resulting in congenital abnormalities and features of neonatal addiction and withdrawal |
| Maternal infection | Congenital and perinatal infections |

**Table 8** Examples of abnormalities detected on ultrasound

| | |
|---|---|
| CNS | Hydrocephalus, spina bifida, anencephaly |
| Cardiovascular | 60% of cardiac chamber anomalies; congestive cardiac failure |
| Gastrointestinal | Exomphalos, gastroschisis, diaphragmatic hernia, meconium peritonitis, bowel obstruction |
| Urogenital | Hydronephrosis, dysplastic/polycystic kidneys, bladder outflow obstruction |
| Skeletal | Skeletal dysplasias, talipes, cleft lip and palate |
| Others | Chromosomal anomalies (Down syndrome), hydrops |

**Table 9** Invasive procedures for antenatal diagnosis

| Procedure | Timing | Risk of fetal loss | Indication |
|---|---|---|---|
| Amniocentesis | Usually at 15–16 weeks | 1 : 100 | Chromosome analysis |
| | Early at 11–12 weeks | Higher | α-Fetoprotein, acetylcholinesterase, bilirubin, enzyme analysis[a] |
| Chorionic villus sampling | 9 weeks onwards | 2 : 100 | Chromosome analysis, enzyme analysis, DNA analysis[b], congenital infections |
| Fetal blood sampling | 20 weeks onwards | 1 : 100; higher if fetus is unwell | Congenital infections, rapid chromosome analysis, severe Rhesus and isoimmune analysis |
| Fetal tissue sampling | Skin biopsy | | Enzyme analysis |

[a] For inborn errors of metabolism.
[b] For genetic disorders such as thalassaemia, haemophilia, cystic fibrosis.

infection (e.g. cytomegalovirus, toxoplasmosis, rubella) may all result in a congenital abnormality in the fetus.

**Infants of insulin-dependent diabetic** mothers have an increased risk of hypoglycaemia in the neonatal period, are generally large for dates, and may have associated malformations such as cardiovascular (cardiomyopathy), genitourinary and neural tube defects. Sacral agenesis results in a patulous anus and urinary incontinence.

**Fetal alcohol syndrome** results from maternal chronic alcoholism and is indicated by characteristic facies (long philtrum and thin smooth upper lip), growth retardation and microcephaly.

**Congenital infections** may cause hydrocephalus or microcephaly, cataracts, chorioretinitis, deafness, generalised neurodevelopmental delay, pneumonitis, congenital heart disease, hepatosplenomegaly, osteitis and myelosuppression, depending on the type of infection (see Section 2.6).

## 2.3 Assessment of the newborn

### Learning objectives

You should:

- be able to carry out the examination of a normal newborn
- be able to appreciate the signs of prematurity

All newborn infants should be carefully examined after birth to exclude abnormalities and to reassure the parents. This first examination is also a good opportunity to encourage the mother to breastfeed the infant. The assessment should begin with a careful review of the maternal history and of the infant's behaviour. The examination is best done from 'top to toe', with the aim of excluding congenital abnormalities and searching for signs of ill health.

### The history and examination

#### Maternal history

The following areas should be covered:

- Social, e.g. smoking, alcohol, drug abuse
- Genetic or familial disease, e.g. Down syndrome, cystic fibrosis
- Obstetric history, e.g. previous pregnancy loss
- Current pregnancy, e.g. blood loss, hypertension
- Results of investigations, e.g. ultrasound, serology, α-fetoprotein.

### Neonatal examination

The examination should be carried out with the infant undressed in the presence of the mother. Observe the infant's posture, movements and colour, and exclude any characteristic disorder, e.g. Down syndrome. The infant's weight and head circumference should be plotted on appropriate centile charts.

**Head and neck**
**Swellings** may be caused by caput, a boggy swelling present from birth, subperiosteal cephalhaematoma, which is limited by sutures, or a subaponeurotic haematoma, an extensive boggy swelling that may cause hypovolaemia.

**Abnormal shape** may be caused by premature fusion of cranial sutures (craniosynostosis).

The **head circumference** may be abnormally small (microcephaly) or large (macrocephaly), for example as caused by hydrocephalus.

**Clefts of lip and/or palate** should be assessed with the mouth fully open.

**Preauricular sinuses** may be associated with branchial arch and renal malformations.

**Swellings, cysts or sinuses** in the neck may be related to the thyroid gland if midline, or to branchial cleft malformations if situated in the anterior triangle.

**The eyes** should be carefully examined to exclude cataracts or other abnormalities.

**Chest**
A **respiratory rate** greater than 60 breaths/minute, or central cyanosis, nasal flaring and costal recession should be investigated urgently.

**Cardiovascular examination** includes palpation of the peripheral pulses, including the femoral pulses (which may be reduced or absent in coarctation of the aorta) and auscultation for heart murmurs. However, a heart murmur may not be present even in major congenital heart abnormalities (see Chapter 4).

**Abdomen**
An **exomphalos** caused by failure of the midgut to return into the abdomen during fetal life, or a gastroschisis resulting from herniation of abdominal contents through an anterior abdominal wall defect, will be evident at birth. A simple umbilical hernia does not require treatment.

**Abdominal distension** may result from an enlarged organ or be caused by intestinal obstruction, e.g. from intestinal atresia or secondary to Hirschsprung's disease.

The **genitalia** should be examined, the testicular position noted in males, and the anus checked for patency.

## Hips

These should be examined for *congenital dislocation of the hips* (see Section 2.3).

## Back

A *myelomeningocoele* (*spina bifida*) is usually diagnosed before birth, but less severe spinal abnormalities may be suspected because of a hairy patch or a lipoma on the lower back. A sacral dimple is not significant. A large swelling over the sacrum may be caused by a *sacrococcygeal teratoma*, which will require surgical excision shortly after birth.

## Skin and mucous membranes

In dark-skinned babies, and occasionally in Caucasians as well, blue-black pigmented areas or Mongolian spots are seen on the base of the back and buttocks. These usually fade after the first year. Urticaria, heat rash and white pimples (milia) are common transient phenomena. Often babies have small cysts in their mouths: Epstein pearls on the palate and epulis on the gums. Occasionally natal teeth may be present.

## Neurological assessment

A simplified neurological assessment is shown in Table 10. Spontaneous movements, posture, tone, the response to light, bright objects and to sounds should be noted and recorded. Tendon reflexes should be elicited. Clonus is often present in newborn infants. The Moro reflex, an 'embrace' elicited by removing support from under the infant's head, should be symmetrical and complete. Neurological disturbance may cause apathy or irritability and may result from cerebral malformations or is secondary to systemic illness such as infection or metabolic disease. Reduced tone and movements may be caused by neuromuscular diseases.

**Table 10** Simplified neurological assessment

| Examination | Observation |
| --- | --- |
| Spontaneous movements | Frequent |
| Posture | Flexed arms, extended legs |
| Upper limb tone | Resists lifting of arms |
| Lower limb tone | Resists hip abduction, popliteal extension |
| Truncal tone | Attempts to straighten back when lifted prone |
| Tendon reflexes | Brisk; some clonus common |
| Moro response | Abduction and extension then adduction and flexion |
| Response to objects | Fixes on bright objects |
| Response to sounds | Quietens or startles |

## Assessment of maturity

Maturity may be assessed by physical and neurological examination during the first 7 days of life. The method described by Dubowitz and colleagues in 1970 is commonly used, and a simplified score is shown in Figure 8 and Table 11. Normal findings in the newborn are listed in Table 12.

## 2.4 Congenital anomalies

### Learning objective

You should:

- understand the basis for congenital structural defects

Congenital anomalies result from genetic, environmental or multifactorial causes. Structural defects of prenatal onset can be separated into those arising from a single primary defect in development and those representing multiple malformations, often associated together into characteristic *syndromes*.

## Introduction

The most common *single primary defects* include congenital dislocation of the hip (p. 273) talipes equinovarus (p. 274), cleft lip with or without cleft palate (p. 280), cardiac septal defects (pp. 77–82) and neural tube defects (p. 125). Most single defects are acquired through multifactorial inheritance (p. 192). Although the aetiology is often unknown, many can be categorised according to the error in morphogenesis. A specific, localised error results in a *malformation* (e.g. cardiac septal defect), whereas an alteration in shape or structure in a part that has already differentiated normally results in a *deformation*. The latter generally occur in the neuromuscular system and are probably caused by intrauterine moulding. For example, reduced amniotic fluid results in a restriction in fetal movements, and in the first instance may precipitate an abnormal presentation (e.g. breech). However, deformations such as talipes, hip dislocation, abnormal moulding of the head (e.g. dolichocephaly, plagiocephaly), underdevelopment or distortion of the chin (micrognathia, mandibular asymmetry) and torticollis may also arise.

Sometimes a single primary defect can result in a cascade or *sequence* of secondary and tertiary errors in morphogenesis. For example, in the Pierre–Robin sequence there is an error in the development of the mandible, with micrognathia. As a result, the tongue is relatively large for the distorted oral cavity and falls

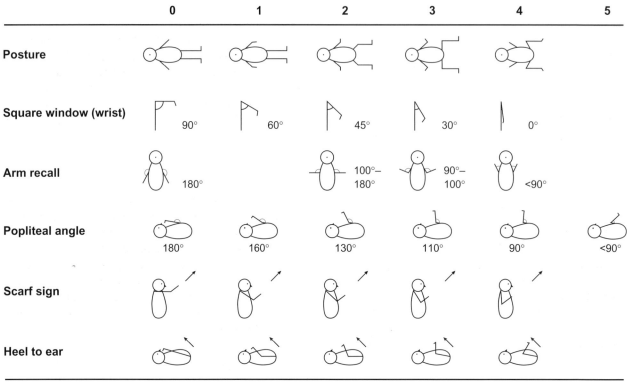

**Fig. 8** Assessment of neuromuscular maturity. Score is used in the scale outlined in Table 11 to indicate maturity.

| Table 11 Assessment of physical maturity | | | | | | |
|---|---|---|---|---|---|---|

**Assessments to produce maturity score**

| | Score | | | | | |
|---|---|---|---|---|---|---|
| | *0* | *1* | *2* | *3* | *4* | *5* |
| Skin | Gelatinous, red, transparent | Smooth, pink, visible veins | Superficial peeling and/ or rash, few veins | Cracking, pale area, rare veins | Parchment, deep cracking, no vessels | Leathery, cracked, wrinkled |
| Lanugo | None | Abundant | Thinning | Bald areas | Mostly bald | |
| Plantar creases | No crease | Faint red marks | Anterior transverse crease only | Creases anterior two-thirds | Creases cover entire sole | |
| Breast | Barely perceptible | Flat areola, no bud | Stippled areola, 1–2 mm bud | Raised areola, 3–4 mm bud | Full areola, 5–10 mm bud | |
| Ear | Pinna flat, stays folded | Slightly curved pinna, soft, slow recoil | Well-curved pinna, soft but ready recoil | Formed and firm with instant recoil | Thick cartilage, ear stiff | |
| Genitals | | | | | | |
| Male | Scrotum empty, no rugae | Testes descending, few rugae | Testes down, good rugae | Testes pendulous, deep rugae | | |
| Female | Prominent clitoris and labia minora | Majora and minora equally prominent | Majora large, minora small | Clitoris and minora completely covered | | |

**Use of score to indicate maturity rating**

| | Score | | | | | | | | | |
|---|---|---|---|---|---|---|---|---|---|---|
| | **5** | **10** | **15** | **20** | **25** | **30** | **35** | **40** | **45** | **50** |
| Maturity rating (weeks) | 26 | 28 | 30 | 32 | 34 | 36 | 38 | 40 | 42 | 44 |

**Table 12** Normal findings in the newborn

Peripheral cyanosis of the hands and feet and circumoral cyanosis
Swollen face and eyes post delivery
Subconjunctival haemorrhages
Epstein pearls – small milky white cysts along the midline of the palate
Cysts of the gums
Breast enlargement – occasionally may discharge milk ('witch's milk')
White vaginal discharge
Capillary haemangioma or 'stork bites' – usually fade with age
Neonatal urticaria
Milia – white small vesicles on nose, cheek and sometimes on the trunk
Mongolian blue spot – blue/black macular discoloration of the skin, usually over buttock, spine and legs; can be mistaken for bruising. Mainly seen in Mediterranean, Asian or Afro-Caribbean babies and disappears with age
Umbilical hernia – resolves within 2–3 years
Positional talipes – foot can be fully dorsiflexed, unlike in talipes equinovarus
Harlequin colour change – difference in colour between the two sides of the trunk and limbs
Caput (succedaneum)

backwards (glossoptosis), blocking the closure of the posterior palatal shelves and giving rise to a large, U-shaped cleft palate. In Potter syndrome, renal agenesis/hypoplasia leads to oligohydramnios, which results in breech and other abnormal presentations, together with pulmonary hypoplasia.

Destruction of a normally formed part results in a *disruption*. This arises through amputation of a normal structure (e.g. a digit by an amniotic band) or infarction caused by interruption of the blood supply in utero (e.g. ileal atresia).

Malformations involving two or more systems usually have a common aetiological cause and are caused by related chromosomal and genetic defects, or are the result of a common teratogen. Specific chromosomal disorders are discussed in Section 9.4.

## 2.5 Birth asphyxia

## Learning objectives

You should:

- know how to assess and the steps taken to resuscitate an asphyxiated baby

- know the common complications of severe asphyxia

Birth asphyxia is defined as a reduction of oxygen delivery and an accumulation of carbon dioxide owing to cessation of blood supply to the fetus around the time of birth. The incidence is about 1:600 births, but the most serious consequence, brain injury, occurs in about 1:1000 births. Birth asphyxia may occur in a previously well infant, or follow neuromuscular, metabolic or infectious disease.

## Diagnosis

Birth asphyxia is often first suspected when the infant unexpectedly fails to establish respiration after birth. In *primary apnoea*, the circulation is maintained and the heart rate is >100 beats per minute (bpm). Cessation of asphyxia at this stage is followed by spontaneous recovery of respiration. However, if asphyxia continues, *secondary apnoea* and circulatory failure develop. The heart rate is now <100 bpm and immediate resuscitation is needed (Box 5).

### Apgar score

The Apgar score is commonly used to describe the condition at birth (Table 13), but a detailed clinical description is preferable. Details of any resuscitation required, particularly the time taken to establish respiration, should be recorded. The cord arterial and venous blood gases should be measured to determine the occurrence of metabolic acidaemia. The Apgar score is usually recorded at 1, 5 and 10 minutes. A low Apgar score at 1–2 minutes indicates the need to initiate resuscitation, whereas a low score at 10 minutes is an indicator of a poor neurological outcome.

## Management at birth

Most newborn infants will breathe vigorously by 1–2 minutes after birth and will not require resuscitation. The infant should be wiped dry, quickly inspected to

**Box 5** Diagnosis of birth asphyxia

The diagnosis of birth asphyxia is based on the presence of:
1. Evidence of fetal distress, such as an abnormal cardiotocograph
2. Fetal metabolic acidosis, i.e. a pH <7.0 and a base deficit >15
3. Abnormal neurological state, e.g. seizures, abnormal tone at and after birth
4. Multiorgan involvement, e.g. transient renal failure.

**Table 13** The Apgar score

| Score | 0 | 1 | 2 |
|---|---|---|---|
| Heart rate | 0 | <100 | >100 |
| Respiration | Absent | Irregular | Regular |
| Muscle tone | Limp | Reduced | Normal |
| Response to stimulation | None | Grimace | Cough |
| Colour of trunk | White | Blue | Pink |

**Table 14** Resuscitation of the newborn

Keep the baby warm, give gentle oral suction and stimulate

| | |
|---|---|
| **A**irway | open by placing the head in the neutral position |
| **B**reathing | keep head slightly extended and ensure face mask covers nose and mouth connect to bag and oxygen and establish a respiratory rate of 30–40/min with chest wall movement (15–25 cmH₂O) (note that first few breaths may require more pressure – >30 cmH₂O) reassess every 30 s; |
| | if no response, intubate – if intubation does not improve oxygenation and respiratory movement, consider: displaced or blocked endotracheal tube, equipment failure, problems such as pneumothorax, diaphragmatic hernia, shock, pulmonary hypoplasia etc. |
| **C**irculation | start external cardiac compression if heart rate <60 bpm (often best appreciated by the umbilical cord pulsations). Ratio 3:1 (90 compressions to 30 bpm) |
| **D**rugs | if there is profound bradycardia give adrenaline (epinephrine) via the endotracheal tube |
| | if no response, cannulate the umbilical vein and give adrenaline intravenously intravenous fluids (saline, gelofusin, blood), dextrose |
| | if profound bradycardia, consider intravenous bicarbonate |
| | naloxone may be given if mother has received opiate |

exclude a major malformation, and placed in the mother's arms. A breastfeed may be offered after a few minutes. Approximately 1% of infants do not establish regular breathing, and are still cyanosed after 1–2 minutes or develop secondary apnoea. These infants will require resuscitation, which should be initiated by those at the delivery, who, in turn, should also request assistance (Table 14).

## Complications of birth asphyxia

Birth asphyxia can lead to complications affecting different organ systems.

**Central nervous system**. Asphyxia may cause hypoxic–ischaemic encephalopathy (HIE) and impaired brainstem function, with or without seizures.

**Cardiovascular system**. Ischaemic injury results in cardiac dysfunction and failure.

**Pulmonary system**. Pulmonary congestion and haemorrhage can occur.

**Renal system**. Transient renal failure is common.

## Outcome following birth asphyxia

Clinical assessment and further investigations are needed to determine the neurological outcome following asphyxia.

### Hypoxic–ischaemic encephalopathy

This is the neurological syndrome that may develop following asphyxia. The severity of the neurological abnormality is variable and is related to the subsequent neurological outcome. Three grades are identified:

I. Mild: infant is alert, irritable, but has normal tone and no seizures
II. Moderate: infant is lethargic, hypotonic, often has seizures
III. Severe: infant is stuporous, flaccid, often apnoeic, with persistent seizures.

Infants who only develop mild HIE recover completely, whereas about 20% of infants with moderate HIE have neurological complications. Most infants with severe HIE die or develop severe brain injury.

### Brain activity

A normal electroencephalogram (EEG) during the first few days after asphyxia indicates a probable normal outcome, whereas a suppressed EEG or frequent seizure activity indicates a poor prognosis.

### Brain damage: imaging assessment

Cranial ultrasound examination may demonstrate haemorrhage, infarction, or suggest cerebral oedema. Cerebral artery blood flow velocity may be abnormally reduced following asphyxia. More detailed information can be obtained by nuclear magnetic resonance imaging (MRI) and spectroscopy.

## 2.6 Respiratory disease

### Learning objectives

You should:

- know the common causes for respiratory distress in the neonatal period
- know the principles of diagnosis and management of respiratory illnesses in the newborn

Apnoea (cessation of breathing for >20 seconds, usually accompanied by bradycardia) and tachypnoea (respiratory rate >60 breaths per minute) indicate respiratory difficulty and require investigation. Central cyanosis may be difficult to recognise unless it is severe, and oxygen saturation should always be measured by pulse oximetry in infants with respiratory difficulties. A 'grunting' sound and/or whining cry are commonly heard in an infant with respiratory distress. The sound is caused by the infant breathing against a partially closed glottis, probably in an attempt to produce positive end-expiratory pressure and prevent atelectasis (pulmonary collapse).

## Causes of respiratory problems in the neonate

Respiratory distress is manifest by central cyanosis, tachypnoea, grunting, nasal flaring, and intercostal and subcostal recession. Auscultation is often unhelpful in the premature and term infant. Respiratory distress is a sign of pulmonary disease, but may also be a prominent feature of non-pulmonary pathology (Box 6).

---

**Box 6** Pathology of respiratory distress

| Pulmonary | Non-pulmonary |
|---|---|
| Surfactant deficiency | Infection |
| Pneumonia | Asphyxia |
| Aspiration: meconium, milk | Neuromuscular disease |
| Pneumothorax | Metabolic diseases with acidosis |
| Congenital abnormalities | Cardiac disease: |
| Lung cysts | Left to right shunts |
| Tracheo-oesophageal fistula | Obstructed circulation |
| Diaphragmatic hernia | Arrhythmia (e.g. SVT) |

---

### Pneumonia

Pneumonia may present within hours of birth as a consequence of antepartum infection, or it may be acquired several days after birth as a complication of other illness. The most important cause of early-onset pneumonia is infection with group B haemolytic streptococci. The infected infant develops increasing respiratory distress, with tachypnoea and grunting. Generalised pulmonary opacification is present on the chest X-ray film, similar to the appearance observed in surfactant deficiency. Septicaemic shock may develop rapidly, and prompt systemic antibiotic treatment and support of the circulation is essential. Intrapartum antibiotic therapy given to the mother may prevent neonatal infection.

### Meconium aspiration

Meconium aspiration commonly occurs following intrapartum asphyxia. Plugging of the airways by meconium causes distal atelectasis and/or hyperinflation via a ball-valve effect. Inflammation and secondary infection of the affected lung tissue may occur. In severe cases, marked respiratory distress develops as a consequence of the ensuing hypoxia and pulmonary hypertension. In the respiratory-depressed meconium-stained newborn, prompt suction of the airways at birth to remove as much meconium as possible may prevent respiratory complications.

### Surfactant deficiency

Surfactant deficiency (hyaline membrane disease, HMD, or respiratory distress syndrome, RDS) is the most common cause of respiratory distress in premature infants. It is less likely to occur in small-for-gestational age infants because in this condition lung maturation is greater. The condition is caused by a deficiency of pulmonary surfactant, a phospholipid produced by type 2 alveolar cells. Surfactant lowers surface tension, and its deficiency results in reduced lung compliance, increased work of breathing, atelectasis, hypoxia and respiratory acidosis. As a result, the infant develops tachypnoea, nasal flaring, grunting respirations and intercostal recession. The chest X-ray shows a characteristic diffuse granular appearance with a prominent air bronchogram (Fig. 9). Steroids given to the mother 24 hours before premature delivery promote lung maturity, encourage surfactant production and reduce the severity of the neonatal respiratory illness. Surfactant preparations given intratracheally have revolutionised the treatment of surfactant deficiency. Exogenous surfactant is effective in the prevention of this disease; it also reduces its severity, and has decreased the mortality of preterm infants with surfactant deficiency disease by about 40%.

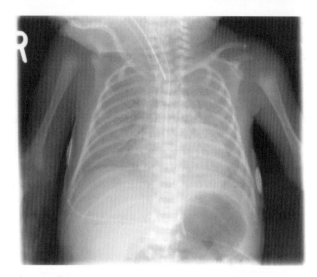

**Fig. 9** Chest X-ray film showing changes occurring in surfactant deficiency disease.

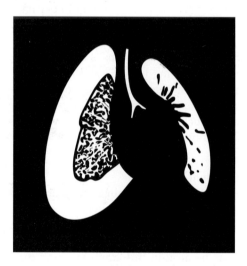

**Fig. 10** Chest X-ray film showing right tension pneumothorax.

**Pneumothorax**

A pneumothorax can occur spontaneously immediately after birth in otherwise healthy infants. The infant may be asymptomatic but may develop tachypnoea and cyanosis. The diagnosis is confirmed by chest X-ray (Fig. 10). The condition often resolves spontaneously, and a pleural drain is necessary only in those infants who develop severe respiratory difficulty.

Tension pneumothorax is an important, serious complication in infants requiring mechanical ventilation, especially preterm infants with surfactant deficiency and those with meconium aspiration. Tension pneumothorax will cause lung compression, mediastinal shift, and impair venous return to the heart. Unless the situation is relieved by the immediate insertion of a

pleural drain, profound hypoxia leading to cardiorespiratory arrest will ensue.

**Chronic lung disease**

This condition, previously called bronchopulmonary dysplasia, is clinically defined by an oxygen requirement at 28 days of life. It generally follows respiratory problems in premature infants, particularly those with surfactant deficiency, but may follow severe pulmonary infections, meconium aspiration, and in those in whom the respiratory condition was exacerbated by a patent ductus arteriosus. The infant is generally managed with oxygen by nasal prongs, which is weaned slowly over a period of weeks or months, as tolerated. Diuretics and, in those where weaning off oxygen remains particularly difficult, a prolonged reducing course of corticosteroids may offer benefit. Severe intractable cases are seriously at risk during any additional respiratory problem, including minor viral infections, and may also go on to develop *cor pulmonale*.

## 2.7 Infections

### Learning objectives

You should:

- know what are the common infections in the neonatal period and why they occur

- appreciate the signs and symptoms that suggest the diagnosis

- understand the process of diagnosis and treatment

Newborn infants commonly develop minor infections such as conjunctivitis and skin pustules and are also more susceptible to serious infections, including septicaemia and meningitis. The early clinical features of serious infections are often non-specific, and an increased awareness is essential if early diagnosis and prompt treatment are to be initiated and complications reduced.

## Common minor infections

### Conjunctivitis

A sticky eye is common after birth and usually results from irritation of the eye during delivery, or is caused by a partially blocked tear duct. No treatment is required. Conversely, a purulent discharge may indicate bacterial or chlamydial conjunctivitis. The discharging eye should be swabbed and treated with appropriate antibiotic eye drops. Chlamydial conjunctivitis infection is an important cause of serious eye disease in developing countries, and may be complicated by chlamydial pneumonitis. It causes a persistent discharge, and a swab obtained by scraping the conjunctiva is required to confirm the diagnosis. Erythromycin given systemically via the oral route is effective treatment for this condition.

## Skin pustules

Skin pustules and paronychia are usually caused by staphylococci. If several lesions are present oral flucloxacillin is indicated to prevent dissemination and septicaemia.

## Candidiasis

*Candida albicans* infection causes white patches on the inside of the cheeks and tongue, whereas candidal dermatitis usually affects the nappy area. Treatment is with oral and topical nystatin.

## Serious infections

Neonates have poor host barriers to infection and an immature immune system. Consequently, infection is a major cause of neonatal morbidity and may arise in utero or in the peri- and postnatal periods (Box 7).

## Congenital infections

Congenital infections occur as a result of maternal infection during pregnancy. Although these infections may go unrecognised in the mother, who is often asymptomatic, they severely affect multiple organs in the fetus and tend to have a similar presentation. The clinical signs include low birthweight owing to prematurity or poor growth, microcephaly, hepatosplenomegaly, prolonged jaundice, petechiae caused by thrombocytope-

nia, choroidoretinitis and cataracts. Imaging may show cerebral atrophy, intracranial calcification, a pneumonitis and osteitis (Fig. 11). The diagnosis is usually confirmed by serological tests.

**Cytomegalovirus infection**
Cytomegalovirus (CMV) is the commonest congenital viral infection. Most infants are asymptomatic, but CMV infection may cause severe pneumonitis and survivors may develop intracranial calcification, microcephaly and severe neurological deficit. The diagnosis is

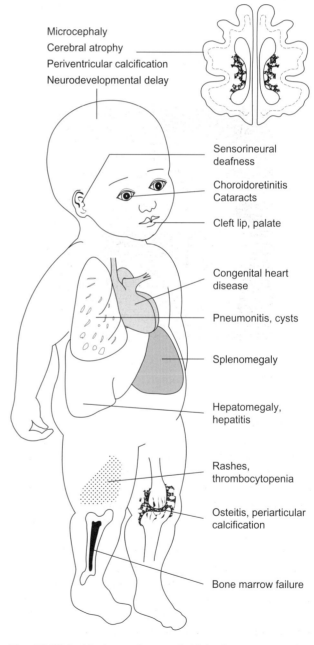

Fig. 11 Clinical features of congenital infection.

**Box 7** Infectious causes of neonatal morbidity

| Congenital | Perinatal | Postnatal |
|---|---|---|
| Toxoplasma (T) | Bacterial | Bacterial |
| Other (O) | septicaemia | septicaemia |
| Rubella (R) | Herpes simplex | Bacterial |
| Cytomegalovirus (C) | HIV | meningitis |
| Herpes, HIV (H) | | |
| Syphilis (S) | | |

The congenital infections are often referred to as TORCHS, reflecting the causes confirmed by the presence of 'owl-eye' inclusion bodies in the urinary sediment, culture of urine for CMV, polymerase chain reaction (PCR) techniques and raised CMV-specific IgM in the serum.

### Toxoplasmosis

Congenital toxoplasmosis is caused by primary maternal infection with the protozoan *Toxoplasma gondii*, following ingestion of meat contaminated by oocysts from cat faeces. The condition is rare in the UK, but is more prevalent in continental Europe. Chorioretinitis may be the only manifestation, but the infection may cause growth retardation, hydrocephalus and intracranial infection; the last two have a poor prognosis despite antibiotic therapy. Repeated serological testing at a reference laboratory may be necessary to establish the diagnosis.

### Rubella

Maternal infection with rubella during pregnancy has become exceptionally rare because of routine vaccination in childhood and routine screening in early pregnancy. Maternal infection in the first trimester poses the greatest risk to the infant. The complications include cataracts, cardiac defects (especially persistent ductus arteriosus), deafness, microcephaly and neurodevelopmental delay.

### Congenital syphilis

Congenital syphilis is a rare illness, as all pregnant women are screened for syphilis at presentation and the treatment of affected mothers is effective in preventing vertical transmission of the spirochaete. However, maternal infection acquired later in pregnancy results in the occasional case of congenital syphilis. The affected newborn develops a rash, periostitis, nasal discharge, hepatomegaly and jaundice (caused by hepatitis). Treatment with penicillin is completely effective.

### Perinatal HIV infection

The majority of HIV infections in children are acquired perinatally from mothers who may be asymptomatic. Infection is usually acquired during the last trimester or during the birth, but there is also a potential risk of transmission by breastfeeding. Without preventive chemotherapy, about 25% of infants born to HIV-positive mothers become infected and may become symptomatic weeks or months after birth. The presenting features are respiratory distress caused by *Pneumocystis carinii* infection or lymphoid interstitial pneumonitis, failure to thrive, enlarged lymph nodes, or recurrent bacterial and fungal infections. Treatment with neverapine or zidovudine (AZT) for the mother who is HIV positive but at low risk, with an adequate CD4 count, during pregnancy and delivery reduces the risk of perinatal infection. In those with low CD4 counts and at high risk of HIV transmission, combination antiretroviral therapy with at least three drugs is indicated. Neonates born to HIV-positive mothers will require neverapine or AZT for at least 6 weeks after birth.

## Acquired infections

Infections acquired during birth are common when there is maternal infection or prolonged rupture of the membranes occurs. They usually present during the first 7 days, often within 48 hours of birth. Later-onset infection occurs particularly in premature infants and hospitalised infants.

Acquired infections may progress rapidly if treatment is delayed, resulting in life-threatening septicaemia. As the initial clinical features indicative of septicaemia are usually non-specific, infection should always be suspected in any infant who becomes unwell or develops symptoms and signs, as listed in Table 15.

Investigations are required to confirm the diagnosis. Thrombocytopenia may be present, and there is increased toxic granulation, with a shift to the left seen on the blood film. Blood and urine should be cultured. A lumbar puncture and culture of the CSF should be considered if there are neurological symptoms or apnoea. Treatment with dual broad-spectrum antibiotics to provide adequate Gram-positive and Gram-negative cover (usually β-lactam plus cephalosporin antibiotics) should be commenced while results of cultures are awaited.

### Group B streptococcal infection

The most common acute neonatal bacterial infection involves group B streptococci. It is usually acquired during delivery from asymptomatic mothers. The infection presents within a few hours of birth, with increasing respiratory distress, which may run a fulminating course unless prompt treatment is commenced. Late-onset disease after 7 days may be acquired in hospital and often presents with meningitis or septicaemia. Confirmed group B streptococcal infection will necessitate

**Table 15** Presenting features suggestive of infection

| Symptoms and signs | Investigations |
|---|---|
| Change in behaviour (irritability, lethargy) | Acidosis |
| Poor feeding | Leukocytosis/-penia |
| Vomiting | Thrombocytopenia |
| Apnoea or respiratory distress | Hypoglycaemia |
| Rash | |
| Unstable temperature | |
| Poor perfusion | |

prophylactic therapy with penicillin for a period of 3 months.

### Herpes simplex infection

Herpes simplex infection may be acquired during birth if the mother has primary genital herpes infection; in this case, delivery by caesarean section is indicated. Early treatment with intravenous aciclovir may prevent the most serious consequences, meningoencephalitis and disseminated disease, which carry a high risk of mortality.

### Hepatitis B infection

Vertical transmission of hepatitis B from mother to infant is likely where the mother is hepatitis B e antigen (HBeAg) positive without having anti-HBe antibodies. Infants born to such mothers should be given both passive and active immunisation, as this offers effective protection in more than 90% of susceptible infants. Hepatitis B immunoglobulin (HBIg) is given intramuscularly into one thigh soon after birth, and hepatitis B vaccine (HBVac) in the contralateral thigh. The latter is repeated 1 and 6 months later.

### Other bacterial infections

Infection with *Listeria monocytogenes* accounts for about 5% of serious neonatal infections. It characteristically causes a severe pneumonia and, occasionally, meningitis. Treatment is with amoxycillin. Gram-negative infections (e.g. with *Escherichia coli*) can cause meningitis and septicaemic shock. Prompt treatment with antibiotics and circulatory support are essential. Repeated coagulase-negative staphylococcal infection is particularly common in preterm infants with an indwelling central venous catheter.

## 2.8 Jaundice in the newborn

### Learning objectives

You should

- be able to differentiate between physiological and pathological jaundice in the newborn
- understand the therapeutic options as well as the potential complications of therapy, as well as the disease itself

Jaundice is very common, occurring in at least 50% of full-term infants and in over 80% of preterm infants during the first week of life. The majority of jaundiced infants have physiological hyperbilirubinaemia and are otherwise healthy. Others are jaundiced as a result of

neonatal illness, such as hepatitis, biliary atresia, infection and haemolytic and metabolic disease. Unconjugated (indirect) bilirubin is fat soluble, may cross the blood–brain barrier and, unlike conjugated (direct) hyperbilirubinaemia, can cause brain injury, especially in the preterm infant with haemolytic disease. Unconjugated bilirubin deposits in parts of the brain, including the basal ganglia, resulting in kernicterus. Initial hypotonia is usually followed by opisthotonus (marked extension of neck and back) and convulsions. Kernicterus has a high mortality rate; survivors may develop sensorineural hearing loss and athetoid cerebral palsy. Conjugated bilirubin is water soluble and excreted in the urine, where it imparts a dark colour (compared to the usual, almost colourless appearance of normal urine in neonates). Hyperbilirubinuria, in conjunction with pale stools, is indicative of a biliary obstruction, with or without an associated hepatitic element.

## Causes of jaundice

### *Physiological*

Neonatal jaundice can be physiological or pathological. Physiological jaundice has multiple causes, including immaturity of liver enzymes, an increased bilirubin load from excessive red cell degradation, and increased absorption of bilirubin from the gut. Physiological jaundice develops after the first day, and although it persists for longer in preterm infants, it generally resolves after 10 days. The bilirubin level rarely exceeds 250 μmol/L. Prolonged physiological jaundice persisting for 3–4 weeks is common in breastfed infants, where the bilirubin level may exceed 250 μmol/L.

### *Pathological*

Pathological jaundice may be unconjugated or conjugated in type (Box 8). Conjugated hyperbilirubinaemia (direct bilirubin >50 μmol/L, or more than 25% of the total bilirubin level) is abnormal and should prompt investigations to exclude biliary atresia.

## Clinical assessment

Slightly jaundiced infants who are otherwise well do not require investigation; however, further investigation is indicated in the following situations:

Jaundice in the first 24 hours after birth (to exclude haemolytic disease and infection)
Moderately severe jaundice (bilirubin >200 μmol/L)
Prolonged jaundice (persisting for more than 1 week).
Important points in the clinical history and examination are listed in Table 16.

**Box 8** Hyperbilirubinaemia

**Unconjugated hyperbilirubinaemia**
Physiological jaundice
Haemolysis
Blood group incompatibility (e.g. Rhesus, ABO, Kell)
Red cell enzyme defects (glucose 6-phosphate
  dehydrogenase (G6PD) or pyruvate kinase deficiency)
Red cell membrane defects (e.g. spherocytosis)
Excess bilirubin
Large bruises/haematomas
Polycythaemia
Inherited disorders of conjugation

**Conjugated hyperbilirubinaemia**
Obstructed biliary tract (e.g. biliary atresia, choledochal
  cyst)
Hepatitis
Hypothyroidism (initially unconjugated)

**Combined hyperbilirubinaemia**
Genetic disorders (e.g. cystic fibrosis, $\alpha_1$-antitrypsin
  deficiency)
Metabolic disorders (e.g. galactosaemia)
Infection (e.g. septicaemia, urinary tract infection)

**Table 16** Important symptoms and signs in the neonate with jaundice

| | Symptoms and signs |
|---|---|
| **History** | |
| Positive family history of jaundice | Breast milk jaundice, congenital spherocytosis, G6PD deficiency (Asian, African and Mediterranean races) |
| Pregnancy and delivery | Maternal diabetes, evidence of congenital infection, operative or traumatic delivery |
| Examination | Apathy or irritability Excessive bruising or cephalhaematoma Hepatosplenomegaly Signs of congenital infection (e.g. cataracts, retinitis, rashes etc.) Colour of urine and stools |

## Investigations

The total, direct and indirect bilirubin levels should be measured. Further investigations will depend on the type of hyperbilirubinaemia.

### Conjugated hyperbilirubinaemia

A conjugated (direct) bilirubin level >50 µmol/L is an indication to investigate for hepatic or biliary tract abnormalities, i.e. ultrasound scan of the liver, tests for biliary excretion, and serological tests for congenital infection. If hepatic or biliary tract disease is suspected, the infant must be referred urgently to a specialist unit for treatment. Metabolic disease should also be considered, and a positive urine test for reducing substances suggests galactosaemia.

### Unconjugated hyperbilirubinaemia

In those with unconjugated (indirect) jaundice, haemolytic disease must be excluded by examining the blood count and film, the maternal and neonate's blood group and the Coombs' test. Glucose 6-phosphate dehydrogenase (G6PD) deficiency should be excluded in infants of Asian, African or Mediterranean origin by measuring G6PD levels in serum.

## Treatment

### Phototherapy

Blue light (wavelength 450 nm) effectively converts unconjugated bilirubin to a non-toxic photoisomer that is excreted in bile. Exposure to blue light is indicated in:

- Haemolytic disease, when it should be started as soon as possible
- Preterm infants with rapidly rising bilirubin levels
- Severe jaundice (bilirubin >250 µmol/L) in well, full-term infants.

Infants receiving phototherapy are often irritable, develop skin rashes and have loose stools. The eyes should be protected with covers and extra volume given to compensate for the increase in fluid losses while receiving phototherapy. Whenever possible the infant should be nursed at the mother's side.

### Exchange transfusion

Exchange transfusion may be required to prevent kernicterus in the at-risk infant with rapidly rising unconjugated bilirubin levels. The procedure consists of repeatedly withdrawing portions of blood from the infant and replacing them with appropriately cross-matched blood. The volume exchanged is usually twice the infant's blood volume (i.e. twice 85 mL/kg). Exchange transfusion may be indicated in the following situations:

- Preterm infants, especially if acidotic or hypoxic
- Severe haemolytic disease, e.g. Rhesus incompatibility, G6PD deficiency.

## 2.9 Neonatal convulsions

### Learning objective

You should

- know the signs of neonatal convulsions

Many normal newborn babies respond to minor stimuli with startle responses. It is often difficult to distinguish these normal jitters from intermittent focal convulsions and generalised tonic spasms. Often neonatal convulsions are subtle, amounting to little more than a transient change in activity associated with minor eye movements, blinking, nystagmus, chewing, salivation, cycling/pedalling movements, blanking episodes, and brief alterations in breathing pattern. Convulsions must be considered in the differential diagnosis of recurrent apnoeas, cyanotic spells and bradycardias. The most common cause for neonatal seizures is hypoxic–ischaemic encephalopathy (HIE). Other causes are given in Box 9. The types of seizures occurring are described in Table 17.

The precise diagnosis of neonatal convulsions requires a detailed neurological examination; metabolic screen, including blood gas, electrolytes, glucose, calcium and magnesium, and bilirubin; septic screen, including blood count, blood, urine and CSF culture; cranial imaging, including ultrasound and possibly CT or MRI scanning; and an EEG.

The management involves supportive care, control of the seizures, and correction or elimination of the underlying defect. Anticonvulsants commonly used include phenobarbitone (phenobarbital), diazepam and phenytoin.

**Box 9** Common cause of neonatal seizures

Hypoxic–ischaemic encephalopathy (HIE): most common
Hypocalcaemia
Hypoglycaemia
Pyridoxine dependency
Infections (including congenital infections and meningitis)
Peri/intraventricular haemorrhage
Kernicterus
Drug withdrawal
Cytoarchitectural abnormalities of the brain
Inborn errors of metabolism

**Table 17** Types and aetiologies of neonatal convulsions

| Seizure type* | Aetiology |
|---|---|
| Focal seizure | Localised structural abnormality, infection, haemorrhage |
| Multifocal clonic | Hypoglycaemia, hypocalcaemia, hypo/hypernatraemia, HIE, drug withdrawal |
| Tonic | HIE, diffuse brain injury, haemorrhage, kernicterus |
| Myoclonic | Multiple causes; usually associated with a poor prognosis |
| Subtle seizures | Drug withdrawal, HIE, haemorrhage, infection |

* Infection, inborn errors of metabolism and kernicterus may manifest any type of seizure.

## 2.10 Low birthweight

### Learning objective

You should:

- know the causes and complications of low birthweight

Low birthweight (i.e. <2.5 kg) may result from prematurity or intrauterine growth retardation (IUGR, i.e. small for gestational age). These two conditions have different causes, clinical features and outcomes.

### Prematurity

Prematurity is more common in poor socioeconomic groups and follows premature rupture of the membranes, infection, multiple pregnancy and maternal disease (e.g. diabetes, pregnancy-induced hypertension). In many cases, no direct cause for the early delivery can be identified. Premature infants develop problems primarily related to the immaturity of their organs (Table 18).

### Infants that are small for gestational age

Intrauterine growth retardation (IUGR) can be symmetrical, when the head circumference and weight are both small and on similar centiles, or asymmetrical, when the head size is appropriate for gestation (i.e. head growth is spared). As shown in Box 10, the symmetrical IUGR is usually caused by congenital abnormalities and infection, whereas asymmetrical retardation is often a consequence of maternal disease.

**Table 18** Complications of prematurity

| System | Effects |
|---|---|
| Respiratory | Surfactant deficiency disease<br>Apnoea<br>Bronchopulmonary dysplasia |
| Cardiovascular | Persistent ductus arteriosus |
| Gastrointestinal | Poor feeding (requiring nasogastric<br>   feeding)<br>Parenteral nutrition |
| Bone marrow | Anaemia of prematurity |
| Neurological | Peri/intraventricular haemorrhage |
| Multisystem<br>  Fluid balance<br>  Biochemical | <br>Salt and water loss<br>Hypoglycaemia<br>Hypocalcaemia |
| Infection | Septicaemia |
| Jaundice | Unconjugated jaundice |

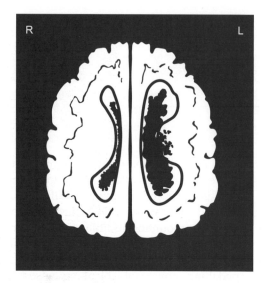

**Fig. 12** Intraventricular haemorrhages: grade II (right) and IV (left).

**Box 10** Intrauterine growth retardation

| Symmetrical | Asymmetrical |
|---|---|
| Congenital malformations | Toxaemia |
| Chromosomal abnormality | Smoking |
| Congenital infection | Maternal disease |

## Clinical problems of low-birthweight infants

Infants with IUGR are often 'stressed' as a result of chronic intrauterine malnutrition or hypoxic–ischaemic injury to vital organs. They may show signs of neurological injury owing to periventricular haemorrhage shortly after birth, and evidence of cerebral injury, with periventricular leukomalacia, during the first few weeks. Passage of meconium ante- or perinatally is common, increasing the risk of meconium aspiration. Hypoglycaemia arises because of reduced glycogen stores in these growth-retarded infants.

### Periventricular haemorrhage

Periventricular haemorrhage is a serious complication of the preterm infant (Fig. 12). The haemorrhage originates in the subependymal germinal matrix, which is present until 32 weeks of gestation. Major periventricular haemorrhage with expansion of the ventricular system and intracerebral extension is often fatal. Less severe cases result in hydrocephalus through obstruction of the ventricular system by blood clot, arachnoidi-

tis, and venous infarction of the periventricular cerebral tissue.

### Periventricular leukomalacia

Periventricular leukomalacia (PVL) describes cystic necrosis of periventricular white matter as a result of hypoxic–ischaemic injury. The injury resulting in PVL may occur before birth, but the risk is greatest for preterm infants with severe respiratory problems requiring prolonged ventilation. Because of the proximity of the corticospinal tracts, spastic diplegia is a common complication of PVL. The cystic changes can be detected and followed up on sequential cranial ultrasound scans.

### Necrotising enterocolitis

Necrotising enterocolitis (NEC) is a condition of uncertain aetiology – possibly infection – that results in intestinal wall necrosis and perforation. NEC occurs mainly in sick preterm infants, but can also arise in healthy full-term infants. It presents with abdominal distension, bile-stained vomiting and loose, blood-stained stools. The diagnosis is confirmed by a plain X-ray of the abdomen, which shows dilated loops of bowel, thickened bowel walls, intramural gas and, if perforation has occurred, pneumoperitoneum (Fig. 13). Treatment is initially conservative, consisting of withholding feeds and giving systemic antibiotics. Surgery is indicated if bowel infarction and perforation are suspected. Severe disease is often fatal; survivors may continue to have problems as a result of intra-abdominal

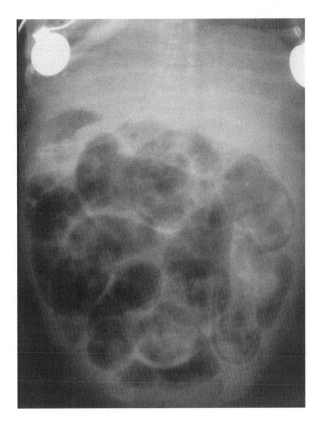

**Fig. 13** X-ray film of necrotising enterocolitis.

adhesions, strictures and, in those who have had extensive resection, malabsorption because of a short bowel syndrome.

## Outcome of the low-birthweight infant

The outcome of preterm infants has improved dramatically in recent years. Outcome is primarily dependent on the severity of prematurity, respiratory complications and periventricular haemorrhage. Infants born before 26 weeks of gestation require ventilation, often for several weeks. Those who develop large periventricular haemorrhages with cerebral involvement have the worst outcome, with a mortality greater than 50%, and neurological complications in about 25% of survivors.

The mortality is increased further in infants who have severe IUGR. Those who survive have an increased risk of poor postnatal growth and further neurological abnormalities. The overall outcome is dependent on the underlying cause for the prematurity and IUGR, and is worst for infants with increasing prematurity and earlier onset of poor head and body growth in utero.

# Self-assessment: questions

## Multiple choice questions

1. The following statements are true:
   a. Perinatal mortality refers to neonatal deaths in the first 28 days of life
   b. Infection is the most important cause of neonatal mortality
   c. The incidence of prematurity has not changed for several decades
   d. Multiple pregnancies have decreased in recent years
   e. Maternal smoking is associated with increased risk of prematurity.

2. During pregnancy:
   a. Low maternal α-fetoprotein indicates an increased risk of neural tube defects
   b. Polyhydramnios may be associated with fetal abnormalities
   c. Uncontrolled diabetes results in small-for-dates infants
   d. Maternal steroid therapy effectively reduces the severity of surfactant deficiency disease
   e. All mothers are screened for syphilis during pregnancy.

3. With regard to the examination of the newborn after birth:
   a. Only newborn infants with a medical problem are routinely examined
   b. The femoral pulses are commonly not palpable in newborn infants
   c. A respiratory rate greater than 60 breaths per minutes is normal
   d. Petechiae on the face and neck suggest a clotting deficiency
   e. Bilateral limb oedema is a feature of Turner syndrome.

4. With regard to congenital abnormalities:
   a. Down syndrome is the most common chromosomal disorder
   b. Sacral agenesis is associated with maternal alcohol ingestion
   c. Maternal infection is associated with congenital anomalies
   d. Trisomy 18 is usually fatal
   e. Infants with Pierre–Robin sequence may suffer respiratory difficulties.

5. The following statements describe congenital dislocation of the hips (CDH):
   a. CDH is more common in boys
   b. Suspicion of dislocated hips is an indication for X-ray examination of the hips
   c. Breech deliveries are associated with an increased risk of dislocated hips
   d. Dislocated hips may be corrected by using double nappies
   e. Routine examination will successfully identify all infants with congenital dislocation of the hips.

6. With regard to congenital abnormalities:
   a. Infants with cleft palate require immediate surgery to facilitate feeding
   b. The risk of recurrence in future pregnancies following the birth of a child with congenital cleft palate is significant
   c. A subaponeurotic haemorrhage is of no significance
   d. Congenital malformations are usually isolated defects
   e. A single palmar (Simian) crease is always indicative of Down syndrome.

7. Birth asphyxia in the newborn:
   a. Is an important cause of cerebral palsy
   b. Is diagnosed on the basis of the Apgar score
   c. Usually results from an underlying fetal abnormality
   d. Indicates a need for immediate intubation and mechanical ventilation
   e. May be associated with several seizure types.

8. In congenital abnormalities of the upper gastrointestinal tract:
   a. Oesophageal atresia is usually diagnosed antenatally
   b. Oesophageal atresia may present with cyanosis soon after birth
   c. Diagnosis of oesophageal atresia may be confirmed by ultrasound examination after birth
   d. Oesophageal atresia is not usually associated with a fistula
   e. Jejunal atresia is characteristic of Down syndrome.

9. In respiratory distress in the newborn:
   a. Pneumonia can be differentiated from surfactant deficiency by the appearance on chest X-ray film
   b. *Pneumococcus pneumoniae* is the most important cause of neonatal pneumonia
   c. Pneumonia can be prevented by maternal antibiotic therapy
   d. Pulmonary hypertension may occur following meconium aspiration
   e. Prompt aspiration of the airway at birth reduces the risk of significant meconium aspiration.

10. In respiratory distress in the newborn:
    a. Meconium aspiration is more common in the small-for-dates infant
    b. Surfactant deficiency disease is particularly severe in small-for-dates infants
    c. The severity of surfactant deficiency disease is reduced by surfactant replacement
    d. Ventilation by face-mask increases the respiratory distress in those with diaphragmatic hernia
    e. Transient tachypnoea of the newborn (TTN) results in respiratory distress that always resolves within 4 hours of birth.

11. The following statements are true:
    a. The correct management of an infant who has bile-stained vomiting but is otherwise well is to withhold feeds and observe
    b. The likeliest diagnosis in an infant who develops bile-stained vomiting and bloody stools is necrotising enterocolitis (NEC)
    c. The risk of NEC is greater with an indwelling umbilical arterial catheter
    d. Gastroschisis is rarely associated with other abnormalities
    e. The most serious problem in infants with renal agenesis after birth is respiratory failure.

12. The following statements describe infections in the perinatal period:
    a. Admission of a newborn infant to the neonatal intensive care unit is not a significant risk factor for infection
    b. Infections in the newborn consistently present with fever
    c. Treatment of infection in newborn infants should await the results of investigations
    d. Congenital infections often have similar clinical features
    e. Most childhood HIV infection occurs after birth.

13. With regard to jaundice in the newborn period:
    a. Jaundice is unusual in premature infants compared with those born at term
    b. Neonatal jaundice should always be investigated
    c. Physiological jaundice appears during the first 24 hours after birth
    d. Jaundice is uncommon in breastfed infants
    e. Conjugated hyperbilirubinaemia is always pathological.

14. With regard to jaundice in the newborn period:
    a. Pale stools in a jaundiced infant suggest haemolytic disease
    b. Phototherapy effectively reduces jaundice by reducing the severity of haemolysis
    c. Exchange transfusion is rarely used for the treatment of neonatal jaundice
    d. Exchange transfusion is indicated for severe conjugated hyperbilirubinaemia
    e. Preterm infants are at increased risk of kernicterus.

## Short notes

Write short notes on the following:

1. Temperature control in the premature infant
2. Hypoglycaemia in the newborn
3. A newborn infant, born by ventouse extraction at term and weighing 3 kg, was noted to have developed respiratory distress at 12 hours of age.
   a. What clinical signs may have been indicative of respiratory distress?
   b. Give a differential diagnosis.
   c. Outline the investigations required at 12 hours.

## Viva voce question

You have been asked to review a newborn infant who is dysmorphic. Outline the key points in your management.

## OSCE questions

### OSCE 1
a. This infant was born with hepatosplenomegaly and respiratory distress. What is also seen in Figure 14? What is the most likely diagnosis? List three other complications.
b. This infant was born to a young prostitute with an illicit drug habit. What is shown in Figure 15? What investigations would you perform on the infant?

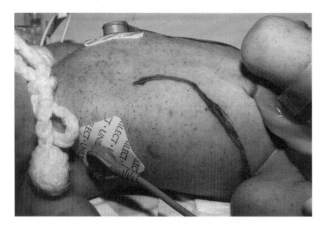

**Fig. 14**

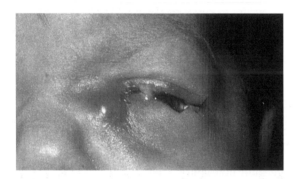

**Fig. 15**

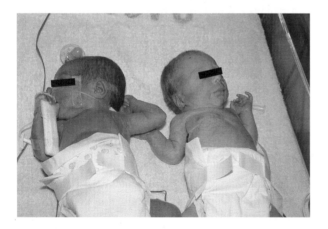

**Fig. 16**

OSCE 2
These twins were both tachypnoeic and distressed at birth (Fig. 16). What is different in the appearance of these two twins? What has occurred perinatally? Why are they tachypnoeic? What are the main issues in their management?

## Case history

A 27-year-old insulin-dependent diabetic woman, whose glycaemic control during pregnancy was erratic, developed premature contractions at 35 weeks' gestation, shortly followed by signs of fetal distress. At this point a female infant weighing 3.7 kg was delivered by uncomplicated emergency caesarian section, and had Apgar scores of 8 and 10 at 1 and 5 minutes, respectively.

A. Comment on the infant's weight relative to the gestation and history during pregnancy.

At 20 minutes of age the infant became tachypnoeic, tachycardic and 'mottled' in air, requiring oxygen by face-mask. An initial blood sugar taken on a heel-prick sample was 1.3 mmol/L and she was transferred to the neonatal unit.

B. Comment on the glucose level and how this can be explained.
C. What other problems could account for the infant's symptoms at 20 minutes?
D. What other investigations would be indicated at this stage?
E. Outline the key issues in management at this stage.

The infant settles and is in 21% oxygen by 3 hours of age. The blood sugar level persists between 1.8 and 2.5 mmol/L, despite a continuous infusion of 10% dextrose.

F. What therapeutic measure may now be administered if the infant's glucose control remains problematic on 10% dextrose?

# Self-assessment: answers

## Multiple choice answers

1. a. **False**. The perinatal mortality rate refers to deaths after 24 weeks' gestation until the first 6 days of life per 1000 total births.
   b. **False**. Congenital malformation and prematurity account for more than 80% of neonatal deaths.
   c. **True**. The incidence of births before 37 completed weeks of gestation has been about 7% since the 1960s.
   d. **False**. The introduction of assisted conception techniques has resulted in a great increase in multiple pregnancies.
   e. **False**. Maternal smoking is associated with fetal growth retardation but not prematurity.

2. a. **False**. Raised maternal α-fetoprotein levels suggest a neural tube defect, whereas low maternal α-fetoprotein may be associated with an increased risk of Down syndrome.
   b. **True**. Polyhydramnios may be associated with fetal intestinal obstruction or neuromuscular disease.
   c. **False**. Infants are usually large, above the 90th centile.
   d. **True**. Maternal steroid therapy during the 24 hours before delivery induces fetal lung maturation, and reduces the severity of surfactant deficiency disease and the incidence and severity of intraventricular haemorrhage (IVH).
   e. **True**. It is routine to screen for rubella, hepatitis and syphilis at booking in the antenatal clinic; in some countries (but not in the UK) the mother is also screened for toxoplasma.

3. a. **False**. It is normal practice for all newborn infants to be examined at least once after birth and before discharge from hospital.
   b. **False**. Femoral pulses should be palpable; absent femoral pulses indicate coarctation of the aorta.
   c. **False**. A newborn infant commonly has a respiratory rate of 30–50 breaths per minute; a rate of greater than 60 per minute suggests respiratory distress.
   d. **False**. Petechiae over the face and neck after birth are usually caused by birth trauma,

particularly if the delivery was difficult, prolonged, or breech.
   e. **True**. A characteristic feature of Turner syndrome (XO).

4. a. **True**. Down syndrome occurs in about 1 in 600–700 children.
   b. **False**. Sacral agenesis characteristically occurs in infants of diabetic mothers, resulting in a patulous anus and urinary incontinence.
   c. **True**. Maternal infection with toxoplasmosis, cytomegalovirus, rubella, syphilis and other infection (TORCHS) can all result in fetal abnormalities.
   d. **True**. Infants with trisomy 18 (Edwards syndrome) characteristically have clenched fingers, low-set ears, and micrognathia, and die soon after birth.
   e. **True**. The Pierre–Robin sequence includes cleft palate, micrognathia and posterior position of the tongue, which causes respiratory obstruction; nursing the infant in the prone position helps, but occasionally a nasopharyngeal airway or fixing of the tongue by suture may be required.

5. a. **False**. It is more common in girls.
   b. **False**. X-ray examination should not be performed during the first few months; ultrasound examination is preferred to exclude dislocated hips.
   c. **True**. A positive family history, breech delivery and postural abnormalities indicate an increased risk of CDH.
   d. **False**. Dislocated hips should be treated by splinting in abduction using a pelvic harness; double nappies are not effective.
   e. **False**. Despite routine examination, congenital dislocation of the hips can still be missed until later owing to poor examination technique and, in some cases, manifests some weeks after birth.

6. a. **False**. Most infants will feed successfully, though occasionally a dental plate may be used to assist with sucking; increasing the size of the opening of the teat or the use of special teats (e.g. Haberman teats) may also facilitate feeding. The lip is repaired at 0–3 months of age and the palate at about 8 months.

b. **True**. The recurrence risk is about 2.5%.

c. **False**. Cephalhaematoma is of no significance but a subaponeurotic haemorrhage, which is not limited by cranial sutures, can cause significant hypovolaemia.

d. **False**. One defect should always prompt the search for others.

e. **False**. Can be an isolated finding of no significance (provided the remainder of the examination is entirely normal).

7. a. **True**. Cerebral palsy (CP) is defined as a non-progressive disorder of motor function caused by antenatal or perinatal cerebral injury; 20% of cases of CP are caused by perinatal asphyxia.

b. **False**. The Apgar score is a convenient, simple way of describing an infant's condition at birth; the diagnosis of birth asphyxia is based on evidence of fetal distress, the presence of a metabolic acidosis, and the condition of the infant at birth.

c. **False**. In most cases of birth asphyxia the fetus is normal; occasionally there is an underlying neuromuscular, metabolic or infectious disease.

d. **False**. Many asphyxiated infants will establish spontaneous respirations after stimulation; intubation is warranted when respiratory depression is associated with bradycardia.

e. **True**. These may take the form of tonic–clonic seizures, limb or facial twitching, subtle seizures (abnormal sucking movements and apnoeic spells).

8. a. **True**. Polyhydramnios and abnormal echogenicity on antenatal ultrasound scan should raise the suspicion of intestinal obstruction, including oesophageal atresia.

b. **True**. If not recognised antenatally, oesophageal atresia causes respiratory difficulty and cyanosis, particularly after feeding.

c. **False**. The diagnosis is confirmed by passing a nasogastric tube and showing that the tube is held up in the oesophagus, as visualised with a chest X-ray.

d. **False**. In 85%, oesophageal atresia is associated with a fistula between the distal oesophagus and the trachea.

e. **False**. It is duodenal atresia.

9. a. **False**. Pneumonia and surfactant deficiency may have an identical appearance on a chest X-ray, i.e. a ground-glass appearance and air bronchogram.

b. **False**. Group B streptococcal infection is the commonest cause of neonatal pneumonia.

c. **True**. Antibiotic treatment of the mother during labour effectively reduces the risk of congenital pneumonia.

d. **True**. Significant pulmonary hypertension often complicates severe meconium aspiration; treatment includes pulmonary vasodilators such as prostacyclin. Nitric oxide may be effective in this condition.

e. **True**. This is the single most important measure to reduce the severity of aspiration in the depressed infant, but is not appropriate for the meconium-covered but lively, vigorous infant.

10. a. **True**. Infants who are small for gestational age are more likely to suffer intrapartum asphyxia and hence meconium aspiration.

b. **False**. Surfactant deficiency disease occurs in immature infants but is less likely to occur in small-for-gestational age infants because lung maturation is enhanced in this condition.

c. **True**. Exogenous intratracheal surfactant reduces the severity of surfactant deficiency disease, reducing the mortality of preterm infants in this condition by about 40%.

d. **True**. This forces air into the bowel lying within the chest and further compresses the underdeveloped lung(s).

e. **False**. TTN is caused by retained lung fluid; in many cases it will resolve within 4 hours, and certainly by 24 hours.

11. a. **False**. Bile-stained vomiting is the cardinal sign of intestinal obstruction and may be intermittent if the cause is malrotation and volvulus of the bowel. Therefore, all cases should be investigated urgently, as a delay in diagnosis may result in vascular impairment and ischaemia of the bowel.

b. **True**. Bile-stained vomiting suggests bowel stasis caused by obstruction or ileus, and bloodstained stools are indicative of mucosal sloughing, both features of NEC.

c. **True**. Especially in neonates with cyanotic congenital heart disease, hypoxia, acidosis and sepsis.

d. **True**. Whereas exomphalos is commonly associated with chromosomal and other malformations, gastroschisis is usually an isolated defect and therefore has a better prognosis.

e. **True**. Renal agenesis results in no fetal urine production; the resulting oligohydramnios interferes with fetal breathing and causes pulmonary hypoplasia, which is usually fatal.

12. a. **False**. Admission to the special care baby unit significantly increases the risk of nosocomial infections.
 b. **False**. Fever is unusual in neonates, even with infections. Hypothermia is more likely, together with non-specific signs, including a change in behaviour, poor feeding, vomiting and apnoea.
 c. **False**. Successful outcome following perinatal infections depends on prompt treatment, which should not be delayed until the results of the investigation are made available.
 d. **True**. Congenital infections have common clinical features, such as a low birthweight, jaundice, hepatosplenomegaly, petechiae owing to thrombocytopenia, and cranial and ophthalmic complications.
 e. **False**. Most children acquire HIV at the time of birth; treatment of the mother with neverapine or zidovudine during the last trimester may prevent neonatal infection.

13. a. **False**. Jaundice occurs in more than half of newborn infants.
 b. **False**. Most neonatal jaundice is mild; investigation or treatment is indicated when jaundice appears during the first 24 hours, increases rapidly, or persists for more than 10 days.
 c. **False**. Jaundice in the first 24 hours is likely to be caused by haemolysis, especially related to blood group incompatibility; physiological jaundice commonly occurs at 48–72 hours of age and resolves by 7–10 days.
 d. **False**. Breastfed infants are more likely to become jaundiced, and this may persist for 2–3 weeks.
 e. **True**. Conjugated hyperbilirubinaemia is always pathological and requires investigation.

14. a. **False**. Pale stools in a jaundiced baby are indicative of conjugated hyperbilirubinaemia resulting from hepatitis or biliary tract obstruction.
 b. **False**. Phototherapy effectively converts unconjugated bilirubin to a non-toxic photoisomer; it does not affect the haemolytic process.
 c. **True**. Most jaundiced infants do not require treatment; phototherapy is effective for moderate jaundice, whereas exchange transfusion is indicated in severe haemolytic disease and in sick preterm infants.
 d. **False**. Conjugated bilirubin is not neurotoxic and is not an indication for exchange transfusion.

 e. **True**. Preterm infants, particularly if acidotic or hypoxic, are especially susceptible to bilirubin encephalopathy, commonly called kernicterus.

## Short notes answers

1. Smaller infants have less subcutaneous fat insulation, a greater relative surface area and a greater problem with heat loss. A cold infant is more likely to develop:

 • Poor peripheral perfusion and a metabolic acidosis
 • Increased respiratory distress and hypoxia
 • Surfactant deficiency disease through insufficient surfactant
 • Hypoglycaemia
 • Excess utilisation of calories and weight loss.

 Hence, rigorous measures must be taken to prevent heat loss. All newborns, and especially premature babies, should be placed in a (pre) warm environment immediately after birth. They should be dried using warm towels and wrapped in a second, warm dry towel to avoid unnecessary exposure. They should not be placed on cold, wet surfaces, nor exposed to a draught. Premature and low-birthweight infants should be transferred to a prewarmed incubator with warmed, humidified air/oxygen. Very low-birthweight infants will require an overhead heater and/or space blankets. Those with exposed mucosae/organs (e.g. gastroschisis, exomphalos, ectopia vesicae) must be wrapped in clean, plastic film. All infusion products should be prewarmed. Finally, the ambient temperature of the neonatal unit must be higher than normal at all times.

2. Hypoglycaemia in the newborn is defined as a blood glucose of <2.6 mmol/L at any age, regardless of body weight or gestation. It is caused by:

 • Exhaustive utilisation of glycogen stores
 • Hyperinsulinism
 • Other diseases.

 Depleted stores of glycogen can occur in:

 • Small-for-dates and premature infants
 • Birth asphyxia, acidosis
 • Hypothermia
 • 'Stress': septicaemia, cardiac failure or arrest, meconium aspiration, necrotising enterocolitis, intraventricular haemorrhage
 • Underfeeding, starvation.

Hyperinsulinism is seen in:

- Infants of diabetic mothers
- Haemolytic disease of the newborn (HDN).

There are also a number of other diseases that cause hypoglycaemia:

- Hypothyroidism
- Beckwith–Wiedemann syndrome
- Glycogen storage disease
- Galactosaemia
- Tyrosinaemia
- Aminoacidopathies.

**Symptoms**. Newborns revert to metabolism of proteins (gluconeogenesis) and, later, fatty acids as a source of energy, and may therefore be asymptomatic but hypoglycaemic for 1–3 hours. Symptoms and signs include increased jitteriness, convulsions and apnoeic spells, pallor, tachy- or bradycardia, hypotension, respiratory distress and increased lethargy.

**Prevention**. Blood glucose 'stix' should be performed routinely at the bedside and at frequent intervals in all at-risk infants before they become symptomatic. If levels are low, the result must be confirmed by estimation of blood glucose in a laboratory. At-risk infants, such as those born to diabetic mothers, small-for-dates and very low-birthweight infants, should be fed every 2–3 hours.

**Treatment**. Asymptomatic infants should be given the next full-strength feed, preferably by the oral or nasogastric route. The glucose 'stix' should be checked 1 hour later and normal feeds continued if the glucose has returned to normal. If glucose is still low, oral feeds have not been established or the baby is symptomatic, then a single dose of 0.5 g/kg 10% dextrose should be given intravenously, followed by a dextrose infusion at 60 mL/kg/day. Rarely, 15–20% dextrose and glucagon is required.

3a. Symptoms and signs of respiratory distress:

- Tachypnoea/breathlessness
- Increased work of breathing
- Head bobbing
- Recession (suprasternal/sternal/intercostal/subcostal)
- Nasal flaring
- Grunting
- Whining cry
- Cyanosis
- Poor feeding
- Vomiting.

3b. Differential diagnosis:

- Infections (chest), septicaemia/other
- Pneumothorax
- Surfactant deficiency
- Congenital anomaly
- Cystic fibrosis
- Hypoglycaemia
- Birth asphyxia
- Drug withdrawal.

3c. Investigations:

- Septic screen
- Full blood count and differential
- Blood gas
- Glucose
- Chest X-ray.

## Viva voce answer

You should introduce yourself to the mother, explaining that you have come to examine her child. Proceed to perform a thorough examination, taking extra care in the assessment of the three 'Hs' – head, hands and heart – where dysmorphic features are most likely to be noted. Note the shape of the head and measure its circumference; note the size of the fontanelles; the hairline; shape, size and position of the eyes, nose, mouth and ears; the presence of a protruding tongue, epicanthic folds and Brushfield spots on the iris; and feel for a cleft palate. Examine the iris and retina with the ophthalmoscope to exclude colobomata. Note the length of the neck and any redundant tissue at the nape. Document the shape, position (and number) of all four limbs and digits. Assess the baby's cry, suck and feeding, general tone and posture, and note any abnormal movements. Look for abnormally shaped or positioned nipples, an abnormal chest and abdomen, and the presence of umbilical/inguinal herniae. Examine the external genitalia for ambiguity, hypospadias and undescended testes. Assess for signs of congenital heart disease, including the absence of femoral pulses. Weigh the infant unclothed and plot on the appropriate centile chart (see Fig. 2 and Table 11).

Reclothe and resettle the baby before sitting down to talk to the parents. Explain your preliminary findings at this point, your concerns (if any), and the reasons why you feel further assessment/investigation is required. You should explain the rationale behind any tests that you may propose. Proceed to investigate as indicated by the signs on examination, but a cranial ultrasound scan, an echocardiogram, renal ultrasound and karyotype are generally essential in those with major dysmorphic features. An appropriate length of time should be spent with the family to discuss the results, and a sympathetic but realistic view of the prognosis/likelihood of future problems given. Repeated discussions with the family, organisation of genetic counselling and support groups are paramount.

## OSCE answers

### OSCE 1

A1: generalised petechiae or petechial rash

A2: Congenital infection, especially cytomegalovirus or toxoplasmosis (or rubella or syphilis)

A3: Encephalitis, meningitis, intracranial calcification, choroidoretinitis, cataracts, pneumonitis, hepatitis, osteitis, nephritis

B1: Purulent conjunctivitis

B2: Chlamydia and gonorrhoea cultures from pus/conjunctival discharge
TORCH screen
Septic screen/blood cultures if systemically unwell.

### OSCE 2

1. One twin is anaemic; the other plethoric.
2. Twin-to-twin transfusion.
3. The paler twin due to severe anaemia; the plethoric twin due to fluid (blood) overload leading to heart failure.

4. Transfuse the anaemic twin with cross-matched blood; treat heart failure and, if necessary, venesect the overtransfused twin.

## Case history answers

| | | | |
|---|---|---|---|
| a. | macrosomia | or | |
| | large for gestational age | or | 2 |
| | *infant of diabetic mother* | | *(1)* |
| b. | low level/hypoglycaemia | | 2 |
| | high glucose levels in mother resulting in | | 1 |
| | hyperinsulinaemia in infant resulting in | | 1 |
| | rebound hypoglycaemia after delivery | | 1 |
| c. | respiratory distress syndrome/surfactant deficiency | | 1 |
| | sepsis/chest infection | | 1 |
| | congenital heart disease | | 0.5 |
| | other metabolic derangement | | 0.5 |
| d. | septic screen/blood cultures | | 1 |
| | formal blood glucose | | 1 |
| | blood gas analysis | | 1 |
| | chest X-ray | | 1 |
| | *echocardiogram* | | *(0.5)* |
| e. | dextrose bolus/infusion | | 2 |
| | oxygen/respiratory support | | 1 |
| | antibiotics | | 1 |
| f. | 20%/concentrated dextrose/glucose infusion | | 2 |
| | *glucagon* | | *(0.5)* |
| Total: | | | 20 |

**3.1** Introduction                                      49

**3.2** Anatomy, physiology and radiology                 49

**3.3** Clinical assessment                               50

**3.4** Infections                                        53

**3.5** Asthma                                            57

**3.6** Cystic fibrosis                                   60

**3.7** Other respiratory disorders                       62

Self-assessment: questions                                65

Self-assessment: answers                                  68

## Overview

Respiratory illnesses account for the majority of clinic visits for young children and contribute to 25–30% of acute admissions to hospital. Asthma has become the most common chronic illness of childhood and cystic fibrosis is the most common inherited disease in Caucasians, leading to chronic disease. The symptoms of respiratory illness are common to many conditions, and a good history and physical examination are vital to making an accurate diagnosis. Roentgenological findings need to be correlated with physical findings. It is vital to recognise the signs of respiratory distress and to know the correct steps in the management of respiratory failure. You need to have a good understanding of the prevention and treatment of chronic bronchial asthma and its acute exacerbations. You will need to be familiar with the use of the pulse oximeter and peak flow meter, and the correct use of metered dose inhalers and nebulisers in all age groups.

## 3.1 Introduction

Acute respiratory tract infections and asthma form a major part of paediatric practice. Because of the frequency of respiratory illnesses in children, problems related to this system are common in medical examina-tions at all levels. An understanding of basic respiratory physiology helps in the correct interpretation of symptoms and physical signs and in the attainment of an age-appropriate differential diagnosis.

## 3.2 Anatomy, physiology and radiology

### Learning objective

You should:

- appreciate the normal anatomy, physiology and radiological appearance of a child's airway

### *Normal anatomy*

The nasal passages, pharynx and ears are examined as part of the respiratory tract. The trachea is supported by a series of incomplete cartilage hoops and divides into two bronchi. The right main bronchus is more vertical than the left, and therefore offers an easier passage for aspirated foreign bodies. The right lung has three lobes (upper, middle and lower), separated respectively by the horizontal and oblique fissures. The left lung has two major lobes (upper and lower) separated by an oblique fissure, though the upper lobe is itself divided into upper and lingular lobes. Both lungs project low down behind the dome of the diaphragm and peak behind the clavicles.

### *Normal physiology*

The extrathoracic components of the respiratory tree tend to collapse inwards during inspiration and open during expiration. Therefore, if the extrathoracic airway is compromised, the obstruction is first evident during inspiration, and as the airway narrows further, obstruction occurs during both phases of breathing (bidirectional).

The intrathoracic airways are actively opened during inspiration by the action of the respiratory muscles. In addition, surfactant reduces the surface tension of the alveoli, thereby reducing the effort necessary to keep the alveoli open during inspiration. During expiration, the airways tend to collapse owing to the natural elasticity or compliance of the lung. Therefore, partial obstruction to the intrathoracic airways causes earlier closure of the airways during expiration and results in 'air trapping', with eventual overinflation of the lung.

## Radiology

In children most chest X-rays are performed in the anteroposterior (AP) position, rather than PA (posteroanterior) views as performed in adults. Figure 17 shows the normal radiological landmarks. It is important to ensure that the film is not rotated (i.e. the ends of the clavicles are equidistant from the midline) and that the course of the trachea is not deviated. The right hemidiaphragm is usually positioned slightly higher than the left. A marked difference in height suggests volume loss on that side, usually caused by lobar collapse. 'Flattened' hemidiaphragms suggest hyperinflation of the lungs. Unilateral hyperinflation associated with increased radiolucency ('blackness of the lung') suggests air trapping, and is most commonly seen with ipsilateral foreign bodies.

Parenchymal lung disease in the lower lobes causes loss of definition of the ipsilateral hemidiaphragm. Right middle lobe or left lingular disease causes loss of definition of the right and left cardiac borders, respectively.

The thymus may drape itself over either side of the cardiac contour, and as there is a sharp cut-off at the lower border, may produce a 'sail sign' on the right side. It may also mimic consolidation of the lung.

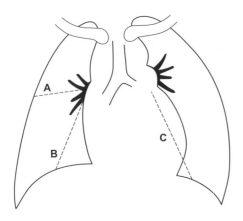

**Fig. 17** Normal radiographic landmarks. The right bronchus is wider and more vertical, the right hilum is lower and the right hemidiaphragm is higher. A, right horizontal fissure; B, right oblique fissure; C, left oblique fissure.

## 3.3 Clinical assessment

### Learning objectives

You should:

- know the common symptoms of upper and lower respiratory tract illnesses of childhood
- be able to examine the respiratory system and assess for signs of respiratory failure

## Symptoms and signs

Unlike adults, children rarely complain about chest pain or dyspnoea. The respiratory symptoms and signs most commonly encountered result from the local effects of the underlying condition, and can be categorised as *cough*, *stridor* or *wheeze*. Generalised effects of respiratory disorders may also be seen, such as growth retardation, poor exercise tolerance and daytime somnolence.

## Cough

The aetiology of a cough may be diagnosed by considering its nature, diurnal variation, chronicity and associated signs (Box 11). The acute onset of a cough can be associated with either an upper or a lower respiratory tract infection, with the inhalation of a foreign body being a possibility. A predominantly nocturnal chronic cough is characteristic of asthma, as is exercise- or laughter-induced coughing. Coughing associated with feeding in babies may indicate recurrent aspiration of milk or gastro-oesophageal reflux. Small children may have a productive cough, but sputum is usually swallowed. Productive coughs are encountered in lower respiratory tract infections or disorders resulting from chronic inflammation. Bloodstained productive coughing is a feature of bronchiectasis. Certain infections may cause characteristic coughing episodes, typified by

| **Box 11** The aetiology of a cough | |
|---|---|
| **Acute** | **Chronic** |
| Upper respiratory tract infection | Asthma |
| | Cystic fibrosis |
| Bronchiolitis | Bronchiectasis |
| Pneumonia | Gastro-oesophageal reflux |
| Foreign body | Aspiration syndromes |
| | Foreign body (long-standing) |

the paroxysms of coughing seen in whooping cough (pertussis).

## Stridor

Stridor is an alteration in the quality of breathing. Many parents describe it as 'noisy breathing', or 'a frightening sound' when their child cannot catch their breath. Stridor implies obstruction to the extrathoracic airway and usually involves the upper airways. It is usually more pronounced on inspiration, when the airways tend to narrow as a part of normal physiology. The intensity of the stridor does not indicate the degree of severity, though severe narrowing will cause stridor during both inspiration and expiration. Indeed, stridor may be soft, as in acute bacterial epiglottitis; in acute viral laryngo-tracheobronchitis (croup) it is coarse and loud. It may be present at birth as a result of a structural anomaly or vocal cord palsy, or may develop soon after, as in congenital laryngeal stridor (congenital laryngomalacia). In this condition, stridor increases with increased activity, crying, and when lying in the supine position. Initially the soft cartilage of the larynx collapses, especially during inspiration, but the stridor resolves as the cartilage calcifies with the infant's growth.

## Wheeze

Wheeze is a breath sound that is usually produced by air passing through partially fluid-filled narrowed intrathoracic airways. It is often audible to parents, who think their child is 'chesty'. It is present when the airways, especially the bronchioles, are narrowed as a result of infection, inflammation or reversible airways constriction. Wheezing in asthma is classically expiratory.

## Other symptoms

Children with a respiratory problem may also present with symptoms related to chronic respiratory insufficiency, including poor growth, short stature, delayed puberty, difficulty in sleeping owing to nocturnal cough, and daytime sleepiness. Chest pain is usually pleuritic in nature, and is therefore worse on deep inspiration. Not infrequently, pleuritic pain may radiate to the upper abdomen.

## Respiratory examination

The examination should begin with an assessment of the child's general health and growth, and should always include plotting their growth parameters on an appropriate centile chart. Many chronic respiratory disorders will slow growth and physical development. As with all paediatric examinations, the maximum amount of information is derived from observing the child. This will identify whether the child is distressed at rest, propped forward to aid the use of accessory muscles, craning the neck to straighten it as a reflex effort to overcome obstruction, or dribbling because of dysphagia associated with serious upper airways obstruction (e.g. epiglottitis).

## Cyanosis

Inspect the lips and the tongue for central cyanosis. This arises when the percentage of desaturated haemoglobin increases, and may be caused by acute or chronic respiratory failure and intrapulmonary shunting of desaturated blood through under-aerated parts of the lung (ventilation–perfusion mismatch). In chronic respiratory failure the child may become polycythaemic, manifest as a plethoric appearance because of the increased circulating erythrocyte mass and haemoglobin concentration.

## Clubbing

Nail clubbing results from cardiac, gastrointestinal and respiratory causes. The latter include *cystic fibrosis*, *bronchiectasis* and other suppurative lung disorders such as an *empyema*. *Fibrosing alveolitis* is a rare paediatric cause.

## Chest wall

The chest wall must be inspected from both front and lateral aspects. The overall shape is noted, including the presence of scars. From the lateral aspect, it is possible to assess whether there has been chronic hyperinflation, which causes a 'barrel chest' appearance as seen in chronic asthma and cystic fibrosis. Harrison's sulcus is a depression along the length of the ninth ribs bilaterally that develops through the exaggerated action of the diaphragm during respiration. It is an acquired abnormality indicative of long-standing chronic respiratory insufficiency. There is a need to inspect from behind for scoliosis, as children with a long-standing lobar collapse or effusion may have reduced expansion on the affected side, leading to scoliosis. Scoliosis also arises from primary musculoskeletal diseases leading to restrictive lung disease. Developmental anomalies of the chest, such as pectus excavatum (depressed sternum) or pectus carinatum (pigeon chest), may also be noted.

## Work of respiration

The work of respiration is an important subjective observation. Difficulty in breathing will usually cause

**Box 12** Age-related respiratory rates indicative of a lower respiratory tract infection

| Age range | Definition of 'fast breathing' (breaths/minute) |
| --- | --- |
| Up to 2 months | >60 |
| 2–12 months | >50 |
| 1–5 years | >40 |

tachypnoea and tachycardia. The World Health Organization encourages the use of respiratory rate as an important physical sign of lower respiratory tract infections in children (Box 12). However tachypnoea is also seen in children with a blocked nose, fever, asthma or sepsis. In the developed world, an increase in the respiratory rate should be considered in combination with other signs and symptoms prior to making a diagnosis of pneumonia.

Chest wall recession (suprasternal, sternal, intercostal and subcostal) indicates increased work of breathing. Recession may be marked in situations of severe respiratory compromise, except where there is coexisting lung hyperinflation, when this important clinical sign may be masked. Increased work of respiration in the young infant may manifest as grunting, a reflex forced expiratory sound, and nasal flaring. In the older child the use of accessory muscles, including the sternomastoid, may be noted. Speech may be difficult if the work of respiration is increased acutely. The equivalent in infants is difficulty in feeding. The exhausted, breathless child with a 'silent chest' and little air movement into the lungs is a particularly worrying scenario.

## Pulse

Changes in both the rate and nature of the pulse are important signs of respiratory distress. Bounding pulses may indicate carbon dioxide retention, whereas significant airways obstruction may be accompanied by pulsus paradoxus. The latter is an exaggerated version of the normal diminution of pulse volume on inspiration. Although this may be measured as a reduction in the systolic blood pressure of more than 10 mmHg on inspiration, clinically it is often suspected purely by the examination of the radial pulse.

## Palpation and percussion

Expansion of lung zones is assessed by palpation. Palpable wheezing may be felt at the same time. Location of the apical impulse will help confirm mediastinal displacement or dextrocardia. If the apical impulse is difficult to locate, this may indicate hyperinflation. Percussion is difficult to elicit in the infant or small child. However, dullness to percussion may indicate a lobar collapse, consolidation or pleural effusion.

## Auscultation

Auscultation may be misleading in small children. Severe lung disease may be accompanied by an apparently normal examination on auscultation. The proximity of the main bronchi may mislead the unwary to diagnose bronchial breathing where none is present, or to confuse transmitted sounds from the upper airways with those emanating from lower airways. Wheezing is generally easy to identify, whereas both inspiratory and expiratory crepitations may be heard in many lung disorders. None is pathognomonic in relation to the aetiology of the lung disease. Routine application of whispering pectoriloquy is unhelpful in the majority of patients.

## Upper airways

The ears, nose and pharynx should be examined (except if severe upper airways obstruction is suspected). Nasal inflammation with mucus production may accompany respiratory tract disease, particularly infection or asthma.

## Abdominal palpation

Hepatomegaly may accompany lung disease. This may indicate heart failure in the infant with pulmonary oedema and, more commonly, follows downward displacement of the liver resulting from lung hyperexpansion. This is often encountered in infants with acute bronchiolitis.

## Peak flow measurements

Peak flow measurements are only reliable in the acute situation if the child has been used to performing them prior to the acute illness (Fig. 18). Children under the age of 5 rarely perform peak flow measurements effectively, so the technique must be carefully monitored if the results are to be believed.

## Oximetry

Oximetry is a valuable measurement of oxygenation. It does not record hypercarbia or hyperoxia, and is subject to movement artefact. Oxygenation is measured at skin or mucosal level, and erroneously low readings may be obtained when the peripheral perfusion is poor.

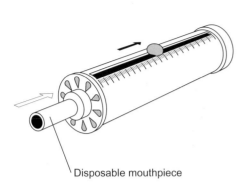
a

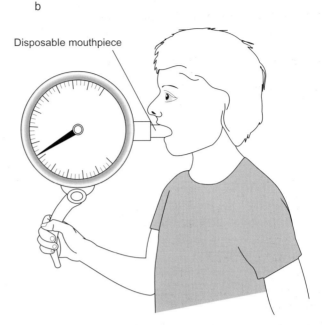
b

Disposable mouthpiece

Disposable mouthpiece

**Fig. 18** Peak flow meters. (a) Young children (5–7 years). (b) Children aged 7 years and over.

## Assessment of regular medication

In children receiving regular medication it is vital to check the type, dose and nature of the medication and the method of administration before altering management. Many medications, particularly anti-asthma medications, are given incorrectly or suboptimally.

## 3.4 Infections

### Learning objectives

You should:

- know the clinical features and management of the common respiratory illnesses of childhood

- be able to interpret the common radiological changes seen with lower respiratory tract infections

Respiratory tract infections are very common and are responsible for a significant morbidity in all paediatric age groups. The majority of cases have a viral aetiology, presenting and are treated in primary care.

## Upper respiratory tract infections

The nose and pharynx are the most common sites of infection. The classic triad of symptoms includes *fever*, *rhinorrhoea* and a *painful throat*. Many viruses are implicated, and include rhinoviruses, influenza, parainfluenza, RSV, adenoviruses, echoviruses and Coxsackie viruses. Antibiotics are of no benefit and therapy should be directed at ensuring an adequate fluid intake, appropriate analgesia, and antipyretic measures to reduce the possibility of febrile convulsions. Common sequelae include secondary bacterial infection and the spread of infection via the short eustachian tube to the middle ear, causing otitis media.

## Otitis media

Otitis media is common in the preschool child. Many cases are viral in aetiology, although bacterial agents include *Streptococcus*, *Haemophilus* and *Moraxella* species. The child is usually systemically unwell with a pronounced fever. Clinical signs include a bulging reddened tympanic membrane, which may perforate, releasing pus. Auroscopic examination is particularly uncomfortable. Many cases will resolve spontaneously, although as up to 50% may be due to *Strep. pneumoniae*, a 5–7-day course of a β-lactam or macrolide antibiotic is appropriate. This practice may have reduced previously common complications such as mastoiditis and meningitis.

## Tonsillopharyngitis

Tonsillopharyngitis is accompanied by pharyngeal erythema and a purulent discharge from the tonsils. *Streptococcus pyogenes*, *Haemophilus*, mycoplasma and viruses are the usual cause. Early use of penicillin has been partly responsible for the reduction in the incidence of rheumatic fever and poststreptococcal glomerulonephritis. Recurrent tonsillitis is an indication for tonsillectomy. Occasionally this clinical problem may indicate an immunodeficient state, particularly with immunoglobulin A deficiency.

## Laryngotracheobronchitis (croup)

Laryngotracheobronchitis is a viral infection involving parainfluenza viruses, rhinoviruses and respiratory syncytial viruses (RSV). A prodromal period occurs prior to the onset of a harsh barking cough and coarse stridor. The child may become tired and irritable, but is not usually systemically unwell. Although usually self-limiting, severe attacks, especially in children with underlying laryngeal narrowing, may result in severe obstruction requiring intubation to maintain a patent airway. The clinical course often fluctuates, with nocturnal exacerbations of stridor and cough. Croup can be frighteningly unpredictable. Younger children have narrower, more collapsible airways and may be more severely affected. Although the majority of patients will improve spontaneously, simple therapies such as temperature control and inhaled or rectal steroids have been shown to be of some benefit, although increasing the ambient humidity has not. Admission to hospital is based on the degree of respiratory distress.

## Epiglottitis

Epiglottitis, an acute bacterial infection usually with *Haemophilus influenzae* type b, is now rare as a result of Hib vaccination. Although it superficially resembles severe croup, epiglottitis presents suddenly with a high fever, the absence of a prodrome, soft stridor, and often dysphagia. The child appears toxic, is most comfortable sitting upright with an extended neck, is often drooling, and has signs of respiratory distress, including a soft stridor, tachypnoea and marked suprasternal recession. There is a serious risk of total upper airway obstruction if the child becomes upset following examination of the airway. Treatment centres on the maintenance of an adequate airway. Oxygen and nebulised epinephrine (adrenaline) by face-mask with the child sitting on a parent's lap in quiet surroundings not far from resuscitation equipment is ideal. This usually allows enough time for the most experienced physician with skills in paediatric intubation to arrive and perform tracheal intubation, preferably under controlled conditions in theatre. Intensive supportive care is generally required for about 2–4 days before the epiglottic swelling subsides sufficiently for extubation to be attempted.

Intravenous antibiotics, particularly third-generation cephalosporins, have largely superseded the use of chloramphenicol in this condition.

## Lower respiratory tract infections

### Bronchiolitis

Bronchiolitis is usually caused by RSV, although occasionally other viral agents may be responsible. It is common during winter months and largely affects those infants below the age of 1 year. Children with predisposing cardiorespiratory abnormalities, such as chronic lung disease and cystic fibrosis, are more severely affected. The diagnosis is made on clinical grounds, although RSV can be identified within a few hours by rapid immunofluorescence on a specimen of nasopharyngeal aspirate (NPA).

**Clinical features**
Infants may present with apnoea, though the majority also have mild fever, a dry staccato 'spluttering' cough, marked tachypnoea, recession and intermittent cyanosis. Widespread inspiratory crepitations and occasional wheezes may be heard. Feeds are often refused and dehydration may ensue. Partial bronchiolar obstruction causes hyperinflation, which in turn may depress the liver, resulting in apparent hepatomegaly.

**Chest radiograph**
Bilateral hyperinflation with variable, patchy areas of atelectasis is seen.

**Management**
Management involves general supportive care, including oxygen and adequate hydration, often necessitating intravenous fluids. Antibiotics are of no benefit unless a secondary bacterial infection develops. Some infants may need mechanical ventilation. Adjunctive therapies, including inhaled steroids, $\beta_2$-adrenoceptor agonists and the guanosine analogue antiviral agent ribavirin have not consistently been shown to improve the outcome. Following bronchiolitis, some infants develop increased bronchial sensitivity and develop recurrent wheezing during other intercurrent infections and on contact with aeroallergens.

### Pertussis

Pertussis is a notifiable bacterial infection caused by *Bordetella pertussis* and appears in epidemics. The natural history is biphasic: an early coryzal phase with rhinorrhoea and cough lasts 7–10 days, and is followed by the spasmodic phase, which may last for up to 3 months ('100-day cough'). Most cases are diagnosed during this second phase. Paroxysms of coughing typically involve repeated expiratory coughs followed by an inspiratory gasping 'whoop'. The latter may be absent, particularly in small children. The paroxysms may be associated with marked facial suffusion, vomiting, apnoea in infants, and syncope owing to hypoxia. The disease is probably mediated by the host's inflammatory response.

### Clinical features

Typical coughing spasms are associated with signs of hypoxia, an associated bronchopneumonia or lung collapse. Subconjunctival haemorrhages or periorbital petechiae/bruising are evident in those with protracted, severe bouts of coughing.

### Chest radiograph

Perihilar bronchial wall thickening and areas of segmental collapse and coexisting hyperinflation are common.

### Treatment

General supportive care is vital, and should include oxygen during paroxysms. The severity and frequency of both the spasm and the apnoeic episodes may be reduced using inhaled steroids or, at times, β₂-agonists such as salbutamol. A macrolide antibiotic such as erythromycin or clarithromycin has been traditionally prescribed to reduce the duration of infectivity, although it does not alter the course of the disease.

**Prophylaxis.** A vaccine is routinely available.

## Pneumonia

Viral, bacterial and atypical organisms may cause pneumonia. RSV may be one of the most common viral aetiological agents in infants, whereas bacterial causes include streptococci, staphylococci and *Haemophilus* species. Pneumonia caused by *Mycoplasma* species is becoming increasingly common in all age groups, and not just in the older child. In addition to these common infecting organisms, immunocompromised children may develop pneumonia with other rare, 'atypical' agents, such as *Pneumocystis*, *Aspergillus*, measles and varicella viruses.

### Clinical features

The respiratory rate is almost always increased. Coughing may not be a feature until later in the illness, when it may become troublesome and productive. Many children swallow their sputum rather than expectorate. Fever is usual, and cyanosis is seen in those with extensive pulmonary disease and when ventilation–perfusion mismatch arises. Other signs of respiratory distress or

**Table 19** Radiographic features of consolidation and collapse

|  | Consolidation | Collapse |
|---|---|---|
| Lobar opacification | Increased | Dense but contracted |
| Horizontal fissure | Horizontal | Shifted upwards |
| Bronchogram | May be visible | None |
| Lung volume | No loss | Loss |
| Mediastinal/ structural shift | None | To affected side |

**Table 20** Signs of consolidation and collapse

|  | Consolidation | Collapse |
|---|---|---|
| Lung/chest expansion | Reduced lung expansion (ipsilateral) | Reduced chest movement (ipsilateral) |
| Trachea | Central/no mediastinal shift | Deviated to affected side |
| Percussion note | Dull | Dull |
| Tactile vocal fremitus | Increased | Absent |
| Whispering pectoriloquy | Increased | Absent |
| Bronchial breathing | Ipsilateral | May or may not be present |
| Breath sounds | Reduced plus inspiratory crepitations | Reduced breath sounds |

respiratory failure may be associated with extensive consolidation or collapse. It must be emphasised that these clinical signs may be *absent*, and normal auscultation does not exclude the diagnosis. If in doubt, and despite a paucity of clinical signs, a chest X-ray is indicated in any child with suspected pneumonia. Atypical infections may result in minimal signs, but the child may be hypoxic with marked radiological abnormalities out of proportion to the apparent degree of illness. Consolidation is characteristic of pneumonia and may be difficult to differentiate from collapse. Radiographic features of consolidation and collapse are described in Table 19 and Figure 19, and the signs in Table 20.

### Pathophysiology

With consolidation, the lung parenchyma is filled with inflammatory exudate. This allows sound to travel more efficiently, hence bronchial breathing and increased tactile vocal fremitus (TVF) and whispering pectoriloquy (WP) develop. Resolution of this appearance ensues with liquefaction and the production of sputum. This results in crepitations within the alveoli and small airways. Collapse results from complete obstruction of

a Consolidation

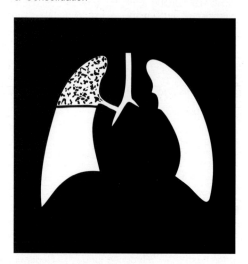

b Collapse

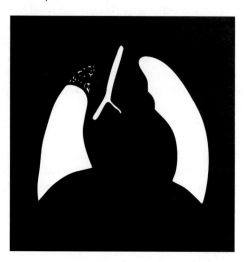

**Fig. 19** Radiographic features of pneumonic consolidation and collapse. (a) Consolidation with increased opacification but no loss in lung volume and a clearly visible air bronchogram. (b) Increased opacification in collapse is associated with ipsilateral deviation of the trachea and upward shift of the horizontal fissure.

the airway, with resorption of the air distal to the obstruction. This impedes the passage of sound, thus explaining the above clinical findings. There is subsequent loss of volume in that lung.

### Chest radiograph
Increased shadowing occurs either in a widespread pattern (bronchopneumonia) or in an anatomical pattern (lobar pneumonia). Consolidation affecting the lower lobes impinges on and partially obscures the hemidiaphragm. Middle and lingular lobe disease will partially obscure the heart border. Often a bronchogram is seen, indicating a patent bronchus overlying solid lung tissue. Increased radiographic opacification associated with collapse is not accompanied by a bronchogram but by loss of lung volume. Pneumonia may be complicated by general debility, febrile convulsions, septicaemia and air leaks. Pulmonary cysts (*pneumatocoeles*) are seen in staphylococcal pneumonia, whereas all pneumonias can cavitate and produce *lung abscesses*. Similarly, associated pleural effusions are possible, and these may occasionally become infected, producing a pus-filled *empyema*. Chronic lower respiratory tract infection following pneumonia or pertussis may result in damaged, dilated pus-filled bronchi, termed *bronchiectasis*. This complication is more common in those with underlying problems, e.g. immunodeficiency.

### Treatment
Supportive care with oxygen therapy to avoid hypoxia, and adequate but not excessive hydration, is important. A high fever, toxicity and consolidation on chest X-ray may imply a bacterial rather than a viral infection.

Where indicated, antibiotics may include amoxycillin plus clavulinic acid or a cephalosporin, together with a macrolide such as erythromycin or clarithromycin in order to cover mycoplasma. Antibiotics should be given for 10 days and, whenever possible, adjusted according to the results of sputum cultures. Chest physiotherapy and attention to hydration are also very important.

## Tuberculosis

Tuberculosis (TB), caused by the acid-fast bacillus *Mycobacterium tuberculosis*, is a relatively uncommon infection in children in the UK, but remains a potential and increasing problem in some areas and in at-risk groups. These include Asian immigrant families, lower socioeconomic groups and those with immunodeficiencies, particularly cell-mediated immunodeficiency and HIV infection (Box 13).

### Clinical features
Airborne infection is the most common route, with the infective focus becoming established in the periphery of

---

**Box 13** Presentation of tuberculosis in childhood

Incidental finding in asymptomatic child
On contact screening
Symptomatic pulmonary tuberculosis
Extrapulmonary manifestations
Rarely at birth after in utero transfer (congenital tuberculosis).

the lung. This focus, also called the *Ghon focus*, then usually involves the regional lymphatics and nodes to form the primary complex. Most patients with TB remain asymptomatic. Others develop fever, lethargy and weight loss. Post-primary spread may occur, with rupture of the focus into the airways, causing cough with productive sputum that is infectious. Failure to produce a primary complex, with rapid spread throughout the lung, produces *miliary* TB. Rarely, rupture of the focus into the airways precipitates tuberculous bronchopneumonia. Regional lymphadenopathy may obstruct a bronchus, resulting in a distal bacterial lobar pneumonia that fails to resolve with conventional antibiotics.

### Chest radiograph

Evidence of a primary complex may be noted based on a calcified peripheral lesion together with hilar lymphadenopathy. Miliary tuberculosis results in a classic widespread reticulonodular appearance.

### Extrapulmonary manifestations

Haematogenous spread is rare. Although this is usually rapid, it may occur months after the primary infection. Spread to the central nervous system causes meningitis which, despite being insidious in onset, is accompanied by a significant mortality and neurological morbidity. Spread to the bones, joints and kidneys is more common than to the peritoneum, tonsils and eyes.

### Treatment

Most regimens for pulmonary TB suggest combination therapy, including rifampicin, isoniazid and pyrazinamide for 2 months, with the two former agents being continued for a further 4 months. Alternative regimens are used for extrapulmonary and resistant disease.

### Screening

Screening using sensitivity to the intradermal injection of tuberculoprotein is the basis of the Mantoux and Heaf tests. Infection will manifest as a reaction to the protein. A false-negative result may occur if the test is performed very early in the infection or in the presence of a defective immune system. Concurrent steroid therapy will reduce the response. A chest X-ray is necessary in those with a positive response who have not been previously vaccinated.

## Pneumocystis carinii *pneumonitis*

*Pneumocystis carinii* pneumonitis affects those who are immunodeficient due to either disease or therapy. Currently, it is the presenting feature of HIV infection in 15–30% of infants. This organism proliferates in the alveoli, causing a pneumonitis. Cough with worsening respiratory distress and hypoxia is the main clinical feature, and spreading perihilar infiltrates are the radiological hallmark. High-dose co-trimoxazole is used in acute infections. Lower doses are used as chemoprophylaxis in children at risk, i.e. those receiving immunocytotoxic therapy for acute leukaemia. Pentamidine is used for those who do not respond to co-trimoxazole.

## 3.5 Asthma

### Learning objectives

You should:

- know the features of life-threatening asthma and how it is managed

- be able to demonstrate the use of the peak flow meter

- understand the differences between the inhaler devices available for paediatric use and know which is the most appropriate in a given situation

## Epidemiology

Although the diagnostic category of 'asthma' has broadened and the overall prevalence increased, the actual incidence is also increasing. Asthma is twice as common in boys as in girls, and shows geographical and socioeconomic variations. However, there is little difference between urban and rural populations. There are several potential precipitating factors, including a genetic predisposition (especially if the maternal family is affected), maternal smoking during pregnancy, parental smoking during infancy, indoor aeroallergens (e.g. cat fur and house dust mite) and viral infections, especially with RSV. Environmental pollutants may precipitate asthmatic episodes but do not seem to be causally linked to the development of childhood asthma.

## Pathophysiology

The pathophysiology of asthma is complex. Inflammatory cells, including eosinophils, are present in the airway lining. These, together with mast cells, are instrumental in producing bronchial hyper-responsiveness to various allergens. They secrete various cytokines such as leukotrienes, which propagate chronic inflammation of the airways associated with hypersecretion of mucus and oedema. Therefore, the asthmatic child has oedematous airways that readily bronchoconstrict to various stimuli.

**Box 14** Life-threatening asthma in children

**Features**
Inability to speak or drink, exhaustion
Cyanosis (oxygen saturation <85% in air)
Drowsiness, bounding pulses (>140 bpm), tremor/'flap',
  irritability (caused by hypercarbia)
Palpable pulsus paradoxus
'Silent chest', indicating insufficient air entry to allow
  identifiable breath sounds and use of accessory
  muscles
Inability to produce recordable peak flow (PF) record or
  PF <50% of expected for height.

**Management**
Reassurance and oxygen therapy
Give salbutamol and ipratropium bromide nebulised
  with oxygen – can be repeated 1–4-hourly until
  improvement
Oral or IV steroids

*If no improvement, give intravenous salbutamol or
aminophylline and admit to intensive care.*
Ventilatory support may be required
Regularly assess for infection, pneumothorax and
  electrolyte abnormalities (e.g. hypokalaemia caused by
  bronchodilators)

**Box 15** Evaluation of a child with chronic asthma

What is the frequency of acute episodes?
What is the frequency of symptoms such as nocturnal
  cough?
How often is medication required?
How many days of school have been missed?
Is there an exercise limitation, e.g. inability to compete
  in sport at school?
Has growth been affected under controlled asthma
  and/or steroid excess?
Is there a chest wall deformity?
What is the pattern of peak flow measurements, e.g.
  reduction in early morning values?

## Acute asthma

Acute asthma is potentially life threatening (Box 14). Precipitants include allergens and infections. Usually there is a rapid worsening of respiratory function associated with coughing and dyspnoea. Tachypnoea is common, and wheezing usually indicates bronchospasm. Clinically, there is a reduction in peak flow caused by airway obstruction and hyperinflation of the lungs. A marked increase in the work of breathing is associated with hypoxia and, eventually, respiratory failure with hypercarbia is established.

### Severe life-threatening asthma attacks

Many attacks may be aborted by appropriate therapy instituted at home using prearranged treatment plans. All acute attacks must be considered as potentially serious, and prompt treatment is a priority.

## Chronic asthma

The spectrum of childhood asthma is wide. Some infants cough or are intermittently wheezy only in response to viral illnesses. These children are believed to demonstrate airway hyper-responsiveness. Others have more chronic symptoms. The most common is nocturnal coughing, or recurrent wheeze in association with exercise or allergen exposure. Chronic asthma is punctuated with acute episodes. Therapy with β-adrenergic agonists remains the mainstay rescue therapy for episodes of wheeze or cough associated with infection, exercise or allergy. However, the frequency of acute attacks may be reduced, together with chronic symptoms, using prophylactic therapy. These are targeted at the underlying airway inflammation, rather than just bronchospasm. Several types of prophylactic agent are available, but the most commonly used are inhaled steroids (e.g. budesonide, beclamethasone and fluticasone). Others, such as sodium cromoglycate and theophyllines, are seldom used for prophylaxis in childhood asthma because of their doubtful efficacy and high risk of side effects. In contrast, inhaled long-acting $\beta_2$-adrenergic agonists (e.g. salmeterol) are effective in the control of brittle asthma, and have recently begun to be used in combination with inhaled steroids, with encouraging results. As preventative therapy, these drugs are necessary on a regular basis. In addition, many authorities advocate a reduction in allergen exposure, particularly exposure to the house dust mite, a frequent problem in many asthmatic and non-asthmatic patients. Avoidance of other allergens may be advisable.

In those with allergic disease, upper airway (nasal) inflammation may coexist. This may necessitate the use of topical anti-inflammatory drugs acting on the nasal mucosa, including nasal steroids.

## Asthma treatment

### Drugs

The variety of potential medications and their delivery systems may appear confusing (Table 21). Indeed, failure to improve clinically may not indicate worsening disease or poor compliance, but rather inappropriately delivered treatment. This is particularly common in relation to the types of inhaled therapy. Most children will be adequately controlled on intermittent bron-

**Table 21** Drugs used in the treatment of asthma

| Indications | Drug | Side effects |
| --- | --- | --- |
| Acute bronchospasm | Salbutamol | Tachycardia, agitation |
| | Terbutaline | Tremor |
| | Salmeterol | Tachycardia, agitation |
| | Steroids | Short course during exacerbations results in no side effects |
| Prophylaxis | Inhaled: Beclomethasone Budesonide | Dysphonia Oral candidiasis, adrenal suppression, growth impairment |
| | Fluticasone | |

chodilators, either alone or in combination with a prophylactic inhaled steroid. Long-term oral steroids are avoided because of their unwanted side effects on linear growth.

## Delivery devices

The variety of delivery systems is wide. Rescue therapy is usually inhaled. Oral preparations of salbutamol have been largely replaced by the inhaled version for reasons of efficacy and reduced side effects. However, the oral preparations are often easier to administer to infants. There are four major types of inhaler device (Fig. 20):

- **Nebuliser.** This is a powered, often portable, pump that delivers a large dose of drug via a face–mask.
- **Large-volume spacer.** This commonly uses a plastic 'bubble' with a valve that allows slowing of aerosol

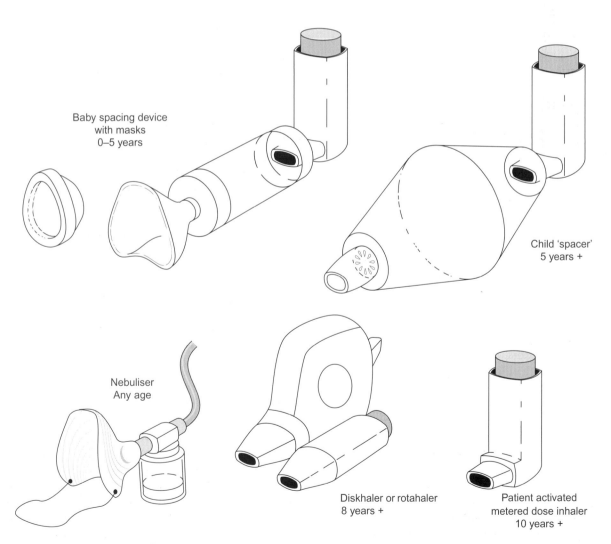

Baby spacing device with masks 0–5 years

Child 'spacer' 5 years +

Nebuliser Any age

Diskhaler or rotahaler 8 years +

Patient activated metered dose inhaler 10 years +

**Fig. 20** Drug delivery in asthma.

particles. The particles are inhaled once the child takes an inspiratory breath sufficient to open the valve. The spacer is used with a metered-dose inhaler and either a face-mask or a mouthpiece. Multiple doses may be administered.

- **Metered dose inhaler (MDI or 'puffer').** This device produces an aerosolised drug and requires a gas propellant. They are difficult to use without a spacing device, as actuation and inhalation require coordination and manual dexterity. The speed of particle release is too rapid for inhalation in most young children. Autohalers are metered-dose inhalers that are actuated on inspiration in an attempt to aid inhalation and improve drug delivery to the lower airway.
- **Dry powder devices.** These devices (e.g. turbohaler, diskhaler and rotahaler) deliver free drug in the form of a powder that is inhaled and not aerosolised. They allow inhalation at lower inspiratory flow rates. Although the need for coordinated activation and inhalation is less, they still require a substantial degree of manual dexterity.

### Device use

As a rough guide, the following devices are best used at the following ages. The indication for nebulisers has declined, and in the 0–5-year age group the use of a metered dose inhaler with a spacer and face-mask is recommended.

- Nebuliser: infancy to any age
- Large-volume spacer with face-mask plus metered dose inhaler: infancy to any age
- Dry powder devices: 8 years onwards
- Metered-dose inhalers without spacing device (including autohalers): 8–10 years and above.

### Inhalation technique

Regardless of the delivery device, it is imperative that both the device and the inhalation technique are monitored at clinic visits and prior to discharge from hospital for every patient. The optimal inhalation technique is as follows: the older child should stand (allows full use of the diaphragm) and tilt the jaw slightly upwards to ensure a maximal oropharyngeal airway. He should exhale completely and then make a firm seal with the lips around the spacing device mouthpiece. The metered-dose inhaler is activated by starting inhalation, and the child should inhale fully and then hold his breath for 5–10 seconds. If a spacer is used in an infant or younger child, it must be tilted to allow the valve to open. The chamber is 'primed' with one puff from the inhaler, and the child should then inhale and exhale four to five times through the device for each dose actuated.

Simple procedures such as washing the spacing device in a mild soap solution and allowing it to drip-dry will reduce electrostatic charge on the device and increase delivery of the drug into the lungs.

## Prognosis

Several studies would suggest that wheezing disorders in infants and older children are heterogeneous disorders with different outcomes. Most infants who wheeze in the first 1–2 years of life, often in association with viral infections, will stop wheezing after the age of 5–6 years. A parental (especially maternal) history of asthma, admission to hospital for a severe episode of wheezing or bronchiolitis, and a history of atopic eczema make it more likely for the child to wheeze persistently after the age of 6. The role of inhaled steroids for recurrent wheezy episodes in infancy and preschool children is debatable. Likewise, long-term inhaled steroids should only be used when an improvement occurs following a trial of such medication. The long-term side effects of inhaled steroids on the developing lung remains unclear. Nevertheless, up to 70% of asthmatic children may 'outgrow' their symptoms by late adolescence, with the remainder suffering variable degrees of recurrent wheeze or cough.

## 3.6 Cystic fibrosis

### Learning objectives

You should:

- understand the pathogenesis and the tests used for the diagnosis of cystic fibrosis
- know the natural history of the disease and its complications

## Genetics

Cystic fibrosis (CF) is the most common autosomal recessive inherited disorder in the UK, with a gene carriage rate of approximately 1 in 25 and an incidence of approximately 1 in 2500. The affected gene has been located on chromosome 7. It spans 27 exons and codes for a 1480 kDa peptide termed the cystic fibrosis transmembrane conductance regulator (CFTR). The protein comprises two areas that span the membrane, two nucleotide-binding areas and a regulatory domain. Several gene mutations have been recognised, the most common being ΔF508, where there is an absence of phenylalanine at position 508 in one of the nucleotide-binding areas.

## Pathophysiology

The CFTR controls electrolyte secretion and absorption in various organs. In the sweat gland, absence of this protein affects electrolyte reabsorption, hence the abnormal sweat test. In the lungs there is decreased chloride secretion and increased sodium reabsorption, resulting in viscous secretions and the production of a mucus that is difficult to clear. These secretions become colonised with various bacteria, in particularly those of the *Pseudomonas* species. The host response to this colonisation is chronic inflammation, which is believed to be a major cause of the lung damage. Viscid secretions elsewhere give rise to problems in the gastrointestinal, biliary and gonadal systems.

## Clinical presentation

Recurrent respiratory symptoms, including chronic cough and wheeze, are the classic presentation of CF. Other children may present following recurrent infections such as pneumonia, or after an atypical, prolonged or severe episode of acute bronchiolitis. Failure to thrive may pass unnoticed until such an infection occurs, or it may be a primary presenting feature of CF. Poor growth results from the combination of recurrent infection and malabsorption. Approximately 10% of patients present in the neonatal period with gastrointestinal disease, in particular meconium ileus. Thick tenacious meconium and a poorly developed large bowel result in gastrointestinal obstruction. Surgical resection of the affected gut or surgical removal of the meconium may be required. Rectal prolapse can occur as a result of the combination of chronic steatorrhoea and insufficient ischiorectal fossa fat failing to support the rectum. Some infants are diagnosed by screening techniques performed because of a family history. Rare presentations include nasal polyps, heat exhaustion, anaemia, short stature and electrolyte imbalance.

## Diagnosis

An abnormal sweat test is highly indicative of CF. Several methods may be used, but all aim to measure the concentration of electrolytes in sweat, particularly sodium and chloride, when levels exceed 70 mmol. The test requires 100 mg sweat for a valid result, but false-positive results may still occur. Other methods of diagnosis, including stool enzyme activity, are rarely used. The phenomenon of increased transnasal mucosal electrical potential has been advocated as a diagnostic tool. Molecular techniques to search for the most likely gene mutations are now widely employed for definitive diagnostic purposes and can be used antenatally.

**Table 22** Less common complications of cystic fibrosis

| System | Complication |
| --- | --- |
| Respiratory | Pneumothorax |
| | Haemoptysis |
| | Cor pulmonale |
| | Nasal polyps |
| Endocrine | Diabetes mellitus |
| | Pubertal delay |
| | Short stature |
| Male infertility | Absence of vas deferens |
| Psychosocial problems | |

## Complications of cystic fibrosis

Several organ systems are affected in CF. Major effects occur in the respiratory and gastrointestinal systems, but there are a number of less common complications (Table 22).

### *Respiratory effects*

The majority of CF sufferers develop chronic bacterial colonisation of their lower respiratory tract, a process encouraged by the combination of viscid secretions and reduced mucociliary clearance. A characteristic pattern of colonisation is usually observed, with *Staphylococcus aureus* and *Haemophilus influenzae* predominating in the infant and *Pseudomonas* species occurring with advancing age. The subsequent inflammatory host response results in eventual damage to the airways and marks the decline in respiratory function. Physiotherapy is the mainstay of therapy, with early prolonged use of antibiotics for respiratory infections. The need for prophylactic antibiotics in infancy and the use of combination intravenous and nebulised antibiotics when permanent colonisation by *Pseudomonas* sp. ensues is now recognised as the optimal treatment strategy. Bronchospasm may coexist as a result of the inflammatory process, or follow an allergic response to the fungus *Aspergillus*. Therefore, long-term bronchodilator treatment is usually required. As a result of host inflammatory cell and bacterial death, DNA is released in the mucus. Therapeutic administration of the recombinant DNAase enables this DNA to be enzymatically cleaved, resulting in thinner, less viscous mucus. Combined heart–lung transplants are performed in those with advanced disease.

#### Chest radiograph
Severe abnormalities are commonplace on X-ray examination, with areas of atelectasis alternating with opacities owing to sputum retention. Generalised bronchial wall thickening, lung overinflation and cyst formation occur as the intrapulmonary damage progresses (Fig.

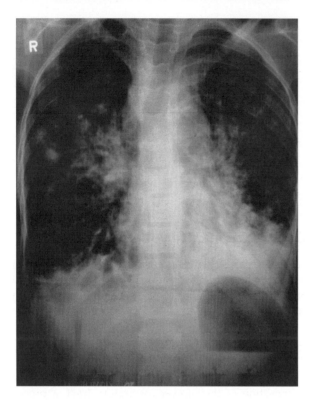

**Fig. 21** Chest X-ray showing chronic fibrosis, cystic and bronchiectatic changes in a child with severe cystic fibrosis.

21). Various scoring systems have been devised to allow quantification of these radiographic abnormalities.

### Gastrointestinal tract effects

Pancreatic insufficiency is common, leading to malabsorption, loss of fat-soluble vitamins and failure to thrive. Loss of ischiorectal fossa fat may result in rectal prolapse. Thick viscous gut secretions may cause meconium ileus in the neonatal period, presenting as gut obstruction shortly after birth. Antenatal perforation of the gut may occur. Rarely, a similar clinical picture with gastrointestinal obstruction may affect the older child, and is termed meconium ileus equivalent. Water-attracting radiographic media (Gastrografin) may successfully clear the obstruction, although surgery may be necessary.

Life-long pancreatic enzyme replacement is vital. Nutritional supplementation is often necessary to ensure growth, particularly as the energy requirements of these children are higher than normal. Fat-soluble vitamins should be given routinely to avoid vitamin deficiency states. These include hypophosphataemia and rickets (caused by vitamin D deficiency), cerebellar

ataxia and haemolytic anaemia (vitamin E deficiency), and coagulation defects (vitamin K deficiency). The last may, in turn, exacerbate any coagulopathy associated with liver dysfunction. Thick viscous bile may result in gallstones, biliary cirrhosis and hepatic impairment which, if severe, may necessitate liver transplantation.

## Prognosis

The prognosis in CF is variable, although generally many more children are living into adulthood. In the USA, studies suggest a median life expectancy of 30 years, but the rapid pace of change in the management of CF means that life expectancy should continue to improve.

## 3.7 Other respiratory disorders

### Learning objective

You should:

- know the clinical symptoms and the emergency management of a child with an acute aspiration

### Aspiration syndromes

Aspiration may occur at any age, although it is more common during infancy, when foodstuffs, particularly milk, are the most commonly aspirated materials. The right main bronchus is the most common site for a foreign body. Acute aspiration presents with a history of choking and coughing, classically in the toddler or young child who aspirates a small piece of food (e.g. peanut) or a toy. This may settle once the airway receptors have adjusted to the aspiration, only to recur if the child changes position. With significant airway obstruction, coughing will be associated with increasing distress, cyanosis and, unless relieved, will be followed by collapse. Nevertheless, many aspirations go unrecognised in the acute phase and present with consolidation that fails to improve on adequate therapy. Bronchoscopic removal of the foreign material is necessary, with antibiotic cover to prevent infection.

### Clinical features

Acute respiratory distress, wheezing and coughing are not always present. Partial airway obstruction may produce a 'ball-valve' effect, leading to progressive overinflation of the affected lung and tracheal and mediastinal shift away from the affected side. Poor air entry

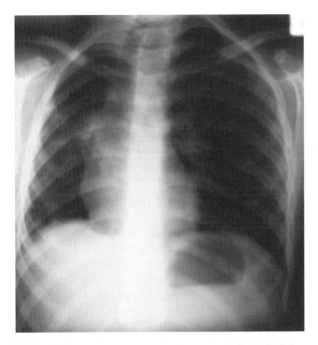

**Fig. 22** Chest X-ray taken in expiration showing overinflation of lung due to ball-valve effect of an aspirated foreign body.

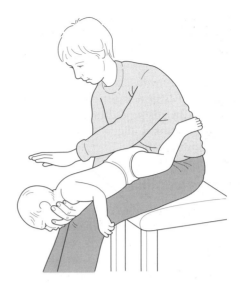

**Fig. 23** Back blows in a responsive infant.

will be detected in the affected lung, which is hyperresonant to percussion.

## Radiography

The classic abnormality in aspiration syndromes is over-inflation of the affected lung on an expiratory film (Fig. 22). An inspiratory film may appear normal if the aspirated material is not radio-opaque. Fluoroscopic screening may be helpful in establishing the diagnosis.

## Treatment

A choking child who is conscious should be encouraged to cough and helped by means of back blows plus chest thrusts in small infants (Fig. 23), or back blows plus abdominal thrusts (Heimlich manoeuvre) in older children (Fig. 24). If a foreign object is visible in the mouth this should be removed, but blind finger sweeps in an attempt to retrieve the foreign body are dangerous and contraindicated. Children who stop breathing and collapse should be given basic life support with rescue breaths and external cardiac compressions (see Section 4.6). Once the child is stable, the foreign body must be removed during bronchoscopy.

## Chronic aspiration

Chronic aspiration may present with recurrent respiratory symptoms or infections. It occurs in those with

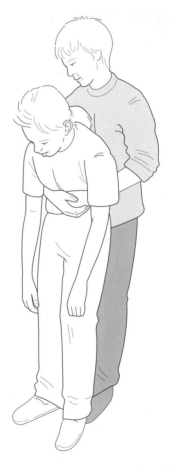

**Fig. 24** Heimlich manoeuvre in a responsive child.

abnormal anatomical connections, e.g. tracheo-oesophageal fistula (particularly 'H' type), those with poorly coordinated swallowing, e.g. cerebral palsy, or those with gastro-oesophageal reflux. The last may be managed medically with a combination of antacids and prokinetic drugs (e.g. domperidone), or surgically by fundoplication. In this procedure, the stomach is surgically wrapped around the base of the oesophagus, thereby preventing reflux.

## Fibrosing alveolitis

Fibrosing alveolitis is a rare disorder in childhood and may be an immune-mediated process or, in a minority of cases, caused by a genetic predisposition. The clinical features include progressive breathlessness and hypoxia. Widespread reticular shadowing is usually evident on the chest radiograph. Steroids may be beneficial in some patients.

## Lymphoid interstitial pneumonitis

Superficially resembling fibrosing alveolitis, lymphoid interstitial pneumonitis (LIP) is a feature of HIV infection, occurring in up to 40% of those vertically infected. The aetiology is uncertain, although Epstein–Barr virus has been implicated in some patients. Patients usually present with progressive dyspnoea, persistent coughing, clubbing and, occasionally, parotid gland enlargement. Abnormalities on X-ray examination include fine generalised reticular mottling, and this may precede clinical features. Both steroids and combination anti-retroviral drug therapy have been beneficial in some sufferers.

## Immune defects and the lung

Recurrent respiratory infections are common in those with immunodeficiency states, including the common IgA deficiency and minor defects such IgG subclass deficiency. Defective cell-mediated immunity may predispose to severe viral or fungal infections of the respiratory tract. Similarly, abnormalities of ciliary motility (dyskinesia) predispose to all types of respiratory infection. In Kartagener syndrome the ciliary defect is associated with recurrent sinusitis, bronchiectasis and situs inversus (including dextrocardia).

# Self-assessment: questions

## Multiple choice questions

1. Common features of bronchiolitis are:
   a. Stridor
   b. Apnoea
   c. Hepatomegaly
   d. Paroxysmal coughing
   e. Wheeze.

2. The following clinical findings are seen in lobar consolidation:
   a. Ipsilateral bronchial breathing
   b. Absent tactile vocal fremitus (TVF)
   c. Deviation of the trachea away from the affected side
   d. Hyperresonant percussion note
   e. Absent breath sounds.

3. Features suggestive of croup include:
   a. A fever of about 40°C or higher
   b. Wheeze
   c. Dysphagia
   d. Barking cough
   e. Variable stridor.

4. Pulmonary tuberculosis in childhood:
   a. Usually follows infection with *Mycobacterium bovis*
   b. Usually causes a severe bronchopneumonia
   c. May present with widespread reticular shadowing on the chest radiograph
   d. Is prevented by the Mantoux injection
   e. May be severe in those with cell-mediated immunodeficiency.

5. Pertussis infection:
   a. Causes atelectasis
   b. Is a notifiable infection
   c. Is optimally treated with ribavirin
   d. Is associated with subconjunctival haemorrhage
   e. May result in seizures.

6. Features indicative of severe life-threatening asthma include:
   a. Peak flow measurement less than 80% of normal
   b. Severe coughing
   c. Reduced respiratory rate
   d. Absent breath sounds
   e. Irritability.

7. Epidemiological factors of importance in asthma include:
   a. Parental smoking
   b. Previous respiratory syncytial virus infection
   c. Rural existence
   d. Affected mother
   e. Allergy to house dust mite.

8. An estimate of the chronicity of asthma symptoms involves:
   a. Monitoring diurnal peak flow measurements
   b. Number of school days missed
   c. Frequency of nocturnal cough
   d. Frequency of the use of rescue therapy
   e. Monitoring of height velocity.

9. Which of the following inhalation devices is appropriately paired with the correct age for use?
   a. Metered-dose inhaler at 2 years of age
   b. Turbohaler at 18 months of age
   c. Diskhaler at 3 years of age
   d. Autohaler at 3 years of age
   e. Spacing device plus metered-dose inhaler from birth.

10. The following statements are correct:
    a. Chronic undertreated asthma causes pectus excavatum deformity
    b. Chronic asthma is associated with clubbing
    c. Harrison's sulcus is a sign of acute obstructive airways disease
    d. Salbutamol is the ideal choice for prophylaxis of chronic asthma
    e. Barrel chest deformity is associated with chronic asthma.

11. Which of the following statements regarding the genetics of cystic fibrosis is correct?
    a. Gene carriage is approximately 1 : 2500
    b. Inheritance is autosomal recessive
    c. The gene is located on chromosome 6
    d. The gene product is an enzyme
    e. The most common mutation in UK sufferers is ΔF508.

12. Recognised clinical presentations of cystic fibrosis include:
    a. Rectal prolapse
    b. Haemorrhoids
    c. Meconium ileus

  d. Diabetes mellitus
  e. Liver failure.

13. Complications of cystic fibrosis include:
  a. Haemoptysis
  b. Pneumothorax
  c. Female infertility
  d. Precocious puberty
  e. Cor pulmonale.

14. With regard to cystic fibrosis, the following statements are correctly paired:
  a. Vitamin E and rickets
  b. Vitamin K and haemolytic anaemia
  c. Exocrine insufficiency and poor growth
  d. Vitamin A and steatorrhoea
  e. Vitamin D and cerebellar ataxia.

15. Correct statements regarding therapy for cystic fibrosis include:
  a. Physiotherapy is only indicated during acute respiratory infections
  b. Pancreatic supplements are needed even in the absence of steatorrhoea
  c. Glucose intolerance usually results in ketoacidosis
  d. Calorie intake must be increased above normal levels
  e. Nebulised antibiotics may be indicated when chronic *Pseudomonas* species colonisation occurs.

16. Aspiration in childhood:
  a. Commonly affects the left main bronchus
  b. Is common in neurologically impaired children
  c. May be silent
  d. Is a chronic complication of tracheo-oesophageal fistula
  e. Is best diagnosed on an inspiratory film.

17. Kartagener syndrome includes:
  a. Ciliary dysfunction
  b. Dextrocardia
  c. Gastro-oesophageal reflux
  d. IgA deficiency
  e. Clubbing.

18. Causes of clubbing include:
  a. Empyema
  b. Cystic fibrosis
  c. Fibrosing alveolitis
  d. Asthma
  e. Lymphoid interstitial pneumonitis.

## Case histories

### Case history 1

A 2-year-old child is admitted with an acute onset of coughing that started during a birthday party. He had been seen to choke while running around, having taken some peanuts from a bowl. Shortly afterwards, however, his coughing had settled and he had fallen asleep in his mother's arms.

1. List the clinical features that, on examination, may indicate acute aspiration.
2. List two useful investigations.
3. What is the treatment of choice for this aspiration?

### Case history 2

A 2-year-old boy undergoing chemotherapy for acute lymphoblastic leukaemia is admitted with a worsening cough and respiratory distress. His oximetric measurements reveal a saturation of 86% in 30% oxygen given by face-mask. His mother has been giving him vitamins, but has recently run out of co-trimoxazole.

1. List three useful respiratory investigations to aid in the diagnosis and management.
2. What is the most likely cause of the boy's symptoms?
3. What treatment is required?

## Short notes

Write short notes on the following:
1. The management of a 5-year-old girl referred with recurrent wheeze and nocturnal cough who has a strong family history of atopy and allergy.
2. The important features of an asthma inhaler device prior to prescribing such a device for an 8-year-old girl.
3. The management of the respiratory system in a 12-year-old child with severe cystic fibrosis.

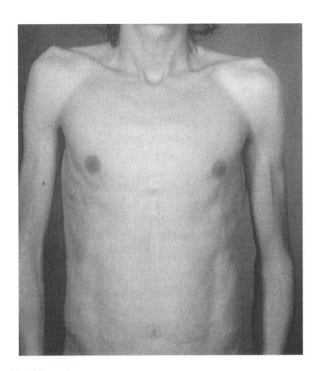

**Fig. 25**

## OSCE station

### OSCE 1
You are shown an 8-year-old child with cystic fibrosis and asked to examine the respiratory system (Fig. 25).

### OSCE 2
You are asked to demonstrate the use of a peak flow meter.

### OSCE 3
You are asked to demonstrate the use of an MDI with spacer.

# Self-assessment: answers

## Multiple choice answers

1. a. **False.** This is a feature of croup or other upper airways obstruction.
   b. **True.** It may be the presenting feature in very young infants.
   c. **True.** Usually occurs because of overinflation of the lungs.
   d. **False.** It is more of a feature of pertussis.
   e. **True.** As a result of airway oedema and mucus.

2. a. **True.** This is a classic feature of consolidation.
   b. **False.** TVF is increased.
   c. **False.** Tracheal deviation is a feature of loss of lung volume (i.e. collapse).
   d. **False.** This is a feature of pneumothorax.
   e. **False.** This is a feature of pleural effusion or lung segment collapse.

3. a. **False.** Toxicity and high fever are more likely with bacterial tracheitis or epiglottitis rather than croup.
   b. **False.** This is a feature of lower respiratory tract disorder.
   c. **False.** This is a feature of epiglottitis or foreign body aspiration.
   d. **True.** It is associated with viral prodromal illness.
   e. **True.** Variability is dependent upon humidity, temperature and diurnal variation.

4. a. **False.** The causative organism is *Mycobacterium tuberculosis*.
   b. **False.** It usually causes subclinical infection, revealed as a primary complex or Ghon focus on the chest X-ray.
   c. **True.** Miliary TB may present early as a result of rapid spread of infection.
   d. **False.** The Mantoux test reveals sensitivity to tuberculoprotein, i.e. evidence of infection.
   e. **True.** The most effective immune response to infection with *M. tuberculosis* is cell mediated, and if this is impaired the host is unable to contain the organism.

5. a. **True.** It causes whooping cough; a secondary pneumonia may ensue.
   b. **True.** There are approximately 30 notifiable diseases. The prime purpose of the notification system is speed in detecting possible outbreaks and epidemics.
   c. **False.** Ribavirin is occasionally used to treat bronchiolitis.
   d. **True.** Coughing spasms may cause subconjunctival bleeds.
   e. **True.** Hypoxic seizures may occur.

6. a. **False.** Peak flow less than 50% of predicted indicates severe asthma.
   b. **False.** Not an indication of severity.
   c. **False.** Rate is usually elevated unless the patient is semi-comatose.
   d. **True.** The 'silent' chest.
   e. **True.** It suggests carbon dioxide retention as a result of respiratory failure.

7. a. **True.** Asthma is a multifactorial disorder and the environment can act as a trigger point.
   b. **True.** Particularly in those who have had a lower respiratory tract infection in early childhood.
   c. **False.** There is no difference in prevalence between rural and urban areas.
   d. **True.** Multifactorial inheritance may be involved in this condition.
   e. **True.** Among the various triggers are pollution, house dust mites and pollen.

8. a. **True.** The 'morning dip' indicates poorly controlled asthma.
   b. **True.** Those with severe chronic asthma tend to stay away from school and are often unwell at home rather than admitted to hospital.
   c. **True.** This is an important symptom. Asthma may occur solely as a nocturnal phenomenon, and in some children cough rather than wheezing is the most prominent symptom.
   d. **True.** Those with chronic asthma are often able to predict an impending attack and seek relief.
   e. **True.** Chronically undertreated asthma causes short stature by reducing height velocity.

9. a. **False.** This device is inappropriate for a 2-year-old unless used with a spacer.
   b. **False.** Dry powders are only used in those over 4–5 years.

c. **False.** It requires too much dexterity for this age.

d. **False.** It is only useful for older ages.

e. **True.** It is easy to administer and use for all age groups, particularly for the youngest asthmatics.

10. a. **False.** This is a developmental anomaly.

b. **False.** Clubbing develops in chronic suppurative lung diseases such as cystic fibrosis or chronic interstitial lung disease, and is not a feature of reactive airway disease such as asthma.

c. **False.** This is a chronic sign.

d. **False.** Salbutamol is a rescue therapy used in the acute phase.

e. **True.** It is a sign of chronic overinflation.

11. a. **False.** Gene carriage is 1 : 25 in the UK.

b. **True.** If both parents are heterozygotes there is a 1 in 4 chance of the offspring being affected.

c. **False.** It is found on chromosome 7.

d. **False.** It is an ion channel (CF transmembrane conductance regulator).

e. **True.** This is a specific trinucleotide deletion that leads to the loss of phenylalanine from the protein encoded by the CF gene.

12. a. **True.** It is a consequence of malabsorption causing fat loss plus steatorrhoea.

b. **False.** This occurs in individuals with raised portal hypertension, e.g. cirrhosis, extrahepatic portal hypertension.

c. **True.** Approximately 10% present in the neonatal period with meconium ileus.

d. **False.** This is a late complication in 2%.

e. **False.** This is another late complication.

13. a. **True.** Progressive bronchiectasis leads to local hypoxia and an increase in the vasculature around the areas of bronchiectasis. These vessels are often dilated and rupture easily, resulting in haemoptysis.

b. **True.** Usually adolescents.

c. **False.** Male infertility can occur.

d. **False.** Pubertal delay occurs.

e. **True.** It is the result of pulmonary disease and its effects on pulmonary vasculature.

14. a. **False.** Vitamin E malabsorption is associated with cerebellar ataxia and haemolytic anaemia.

b. **False.** Vitamin K deficiency can cause coagulopathy.

c. **True.** Exocrine insufficiency results in malabsorption.

d. **False.** Vitamin A does not cause steatorrhoea. It is a fat-soluble vitamin, and in the presence of steatorrhoea (fat malabsorption) it may not be adequately absorbed.

e. **False.** Vitamin D deficiency may cause rickets.

15. a. **False.** Physiotherapy is necessary from the time of diagnosis.

b. **True.** Varying amounts are necessary to ensure adequate nutrition.

c. **False.** Ketoacidosis is rare.

d. **True.** Calories required are about 120% of normal.

e. **True.** Systemically administered antibiotics may not adequately penetrate the viscid secretions, and inhaled antibiotics may be required to attain sufficient antibacterial levels in the affected tissue.

16. a. **False.** It usually affects the right side.

b. **True.** Especially if there is pseudobulbar palsy, resulting in impaired coordination of swallowing.

c. **True.** It is revealed by repeated pneumonias.

d. **True.** Although not the typical presentation, recurrent aspiration may occur in certain types, notably the 'H' type fistula without oesophageal atresia.

e. **True.** But only if the aspirated material is either radio-opaque or causes infection. Expiratory films are better with foreign bodies, and demonstrate unilateral overinflation as a result of airway obstruction.

17. a. **True.** Kartagener is a subset of the immotile cilia syndrome.

b. **True.** It is felt that the normal rotation of the viscera depends on the functioning of embryonic cilia. Without ciliary movement, rotation becomes a chance occurrence: 50% have normal rotation and 50% have dextrorotation. Typically, dextrocardia (non-rotation of the heart) is accompanied by situs inversus totalis.

c. **False.** Gut motility, unlike ciliary motility, is unaffected.

d. **False.** Like gastro-oesophageal reflux, IgA deficiency is also associated with chronic lung disease, but not with Kartagener syndrome.

e. **True.** Clubbing occurs not as a component of the syndrome but as a result of the bronchiectasis that ensues because of ciliary dyskinesia.

18. a. **True.** The cause of clubbing is unknown, but it is thought to be the result of chronic hypoxia to the nail bed. It is therefore a feature of chronic hypoxic diseases such as central cyanotic conditions, chronic suppurative lung disease, and conditions where there is arteriovenous shunting, such as cirrhosis.
    b. **True.** It is probably a result of the chronic suppuration.
    c. **True.** Because of chronic hypoxia.
    d. **False.** Hypoxia is characterised by acute episodes rather than a chronic state.
    e. **True.** As a result of chronic hypoxia.

## Case history answers

### Case history 1

1. Clinical features include:

   - Any signs of respiratory distress, e.g. tachypnoea
   - Decreased air entry and reduced expansion on the side of aspiration
   - Evidence of tracheal deviation and lung collapse distal to any blockage
   - Crepitations or evidence of infection distal to blockage
   - Further coughing bouts as the child's position changes.

2. Expiratory chest radiograph, fluoroscopy and, very rarely, a bronchogram is necessary.
3. Bronchoscopy for removal of the foreign body, and the provision of antibiotic cover.

### Case history 2

1. Useful investigations include:

   - Chest radiograph: this will show perihilar shadowing
   - Arterial blood gas: to assess degree of hypoxia and hypocarbia resulting from impaired diffusion associated with hyperventilation, respectively
   - Bronchoalveolar lavage, to confirm the diagnosis microbiologically.

2. *Pneumocystis carinii* pneumonitis. This immunocompromised child has stopped his antibiotic prophylaxis (co-trimoxazole) given specifically to prevent *Pneumocystis* pneumonia.
3. High-dose co-trimoxazole or, rarely, pentamidine given intravenously. Once the acute infection has been treated the child needs to restart prophylaxis with oral co-trimoxazole until he is no longer immunocompromised.

## Short notes answers

1. The following points should be covered:
   a. Take a history to identify precipitating factors for wheeze and cough.
   b. Explore the degree of familial atopy and asthma.
   c. Discuss the use of skin tests etc.
   d. Assess any alternative diagnosis, e.g. cystic fibrosis.
   e. Assess severity of symptoms and degree of effect on life.
   f. Discuss allergen exposure and reduction, e.g. house dust mite, allergy to pets.
   g. Measure height, weight and teach peak flow measurement.
   h. Examine for evidence of acute or chronic respiratory disease.
   i. Demonstrate an age-appropriate device for rescue therapy and prophylaxis (if history suggests that prophylaxis is necessary).
   j. Provide monitoring diaries and written educational literature for child and parents.
   k. Construct emergency guidelines and ensure the parents are conversant with them.
   l. Involve general practitioner and specialist asthma nurse/health visitor in follow-up, particularly in monitoring compliance.
   m. Review side effects of the drugs being used.
   n. Review drug therapy along the following lines:

      Drug treatment is divided into the maintenance of therapy to control symptoms and the management of acute exacerbations. The two main classes of drug used are bronchodilators and drugs used to reduce bronchial inflammation and hyperactivity.
      The stepwise approach to chronic asthma (British Thoracic Society guidelines) are as follows:

      Step 1 $\beta_2$-agonist bronchodilator or ipratropium
      Step 2 $\beta_2$-agonist bronchodilator + inhaled steroids or cromoglycate
      Step 3 $\beta_2$-agonist bronchodilator + high-dose inhaled steroid (or add long-acting bronchodilator or leukotriene)
      Step 4 $\beta_2$-agonist bronchodilator + long-acting bronchodilator $\pm$ theophyllines or ipratropium $\pm$ leukotriene modulator $\pm$ alternate-day prednisolone
      Step 5 Review treatment every 3–6 months and see if you can step down but continue Step 2 agonist bronchodilator

   o. Review outcome – most children with a similar story will have intermittent symptoms, but there is a good chance that this will improve with age.

**Prognosis**

Will have intermittent symptoms, but there is a good chance that this will improve with age.

2. Important features include:

- Degree of complexity to operate
- Degree of manual dexterity of the child
- Degree of effort to inhale particles, i.e. flow rate required to operate device
- Single or multiple doses available?
- Ease of packing and social acceptability (necessary for compliance).

3. Respiratory management would include:

- Ensure adequate physiotherapy on a regular basis
- Treat infective exacerbations promptly
- Some authorities suggest regular courses of intravenous anti-pseudomonal therapy, e.g. every 3 months
- Nebulised anti-pseudomonal therapy if colonised
- Treat any tendency to asthma/bronchospasm: many need inhaled steroids
- Encourage exercise
- Ensure adequate nutrition
- Treat fungal infections
- Home oxygen therapy if necessary
- Consider other therapies, e.g. DNAase.

## OSCE answers

### OSCE 1

1. Remember to introduce yourself, and tell the child and parent what you are doing. Look around to see

if there us a sputum pot, inhaler, venous access, oxygen (nasal prongs or mask), medications etc.

Assess the following parameters:

General: height, weight, pulse rate, oedema, pallor, cyanosis, clubbing

Inspection: respiratory rate; accessory muscles of respiration; wasting; chest deformities or asymmetry; noisy breathing or wheeze; halitosis

Palpation: movement of chest wall, position of trachea and apical impulse; any palpable crepitus

Percussion: (may be difficult in small children)

Auscultation: listen for breath sounds: are they present equally on both sides? any additional sounds (crepitations, rhonchi and rubs)?

Others: beware of transmitted sounds in small children. When in doubt, ask them to cough and listen again. Check jugular venous pulse and liver size to assess for failure and downward displacement (indicates hyperinflated lung).

### OSCE 2 and 3

These are ideal 'demonstration' questions in an OSCE setting and you should be proficient in their application and use.

# 4 The cardiovascular system

**4.1** Introduction                                    73

**4.2** Clinical assessment                             73

**4.3** Congenital heart disease                        77

**4.4** Abnormalities of rhythm                         88

**4.5** Heart failure and acquired cardiac disease      89

**4.6** Cardiorespiratory arrest and resuscitation      91

Self-assessment: questions                              95

Self-assessment: answers                                99

## Overview

The most common group of structural malformations in children involves the heart. Major cardiac malformations occur in every 6–8/1000 live births and 10–20/1000 have some minor abnormality. Therefore, a basic understanding of the development of the heart aids the understanding of the various malformations and their clinical presentations. A simple history provides significant clues as to the nature of the defect. The physical examination of the cardiovascular system in the newborn period is different from that in older children, and you will need to familiarise yourself with the important landmarks and techniques. Diagnosis is aided by the chest X-ray and electrocardiogram (ECG), and you will need to recognise the changes peculiar to the common malformations. You will need to know the details of medical management of cardiorespiratory resuscitation, congestive cardiac failure and supraventricular tachycardia, and understand the basic principles of corrective surgical procedures

## 4.1 Introduction

### Normal anatomy

Figure 26 shows the normal position of the heart; it is this that determines the cardiac silhouette on the chest X-ray film. The right border is formed by the right atrium, with the superior and inferior venae cavae above and below, respectively. The left border is formed by the left ventricle below, the bulge from the pulmonary trunk in the middle, and the arch of the aorta above. The cardiac landmarks are dictated by the normal position of the heart in the thorax (Fig. 27).

## 4.2 Clinical assessment

### Learning objectives

You should:

- know the presenting features of congenital heart disease in children

- be able to examine the cardiovascular system and be able to make a diagnosis of the common cardiac conditions seen in childhood

- be able to appreciate the differences between normal and abnormal heart sounds

### Symptoms

Cardiac disease in childhood consists of structural abnormalities, diseases of the myocardium and arrhythmias. Structural abnormalities are often picked up incidentally with the chance finding of a murmur. Others produce abnormal strain on the pumping chambers and result in cardiac failure. Alternatively, congenital abnormalities involving incorrect connection of cardiac structures may result in *right-to-left* shunts with cyanosis.

### Heart failure

Symptoms attributable to heart failure can be divided into those caused by 'right heart failure' (RHF) and 'left heart failure' (LHF). RHF results in systemic venous congestion and presents with fluid retention. LHF results in pulmonary venous congestion, which presents with breathlessness and frequent lower respiratory tract infections (LRTI). In children, right and left heart failure are often present simultaneously.

Infants expend a considerable amount of energy during feeds. Those with heart failure become

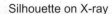

Silhouette on X-ray

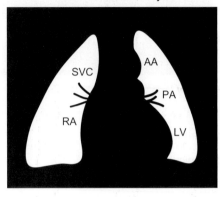

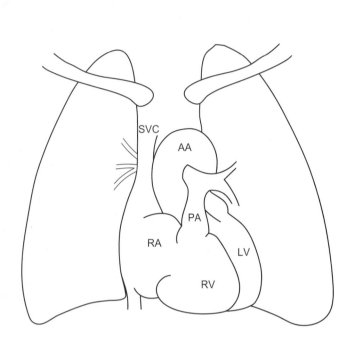

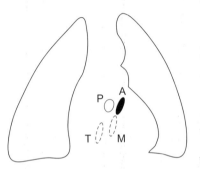

Position of cardiac valves

**Fig. 26** Normal cardiac position and silhouette on X-ray. SVC, superior vena cava; RA, right atrium; RV, right ventricle; PA, pulmonary artery; LV, left ventricle; AA, aortic artery; T, tricuspid valve; M, mitral valve; P, pulmonary valve; A, aortic valve.

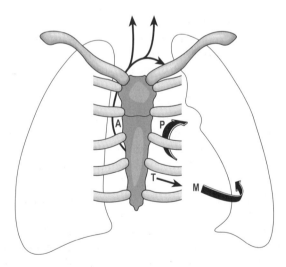

**Fig. 27** Normal cardiac landmarks relative to the sternum. A, aortic area, second right intercostal space; P, pulmonary area, second left intercostal space; T, tricuspid area, fourth left intercostal space; M, mitral area, fourth intercostal space, midclavicular line.

breathless with increased sweating during feeding. They are unable to suck for prolonged periods, and repeatedly 'come up for air' during feeds. An increased risk of LRTI may further exacerbate cardiac failure. Not only do these infants feed poorly, but much of their energy is channelled into maintaining an adequate cardiac output, and therefore they fail to thrive. Older children with heart failure have little reserve to cope with everyday or additional stress, and often deteriorate during exertion or an intercurrent illness.

## Cyanosis

As a result of shunting of blood from the right to the left side of the heart, venous blood meant for the pulmonary circulation is rerouted back into the systemic circulation, bypassing the lungs. As a result, there is a drop in the arterial blood oxygen concentration ($Po_2$) and tissue hypoxia ensues, clinically manifest as central cyanosis. The body compensates for progressive hypoxia by two mechanisms: an increase in heart rate (tachycardia) in order to increase cardiac output, and an increase in the circulating haemoglobin concentration (polycythaemia).

The cardiac reserve is, however, limited and tolerance to exertion is poor. Syncopal episodes may arise in those patients who develop sudden exacerbations of their hypoxic state.

## Lower respiratory tract infections

Patients with a history of recurrent LRTI may not always show signs of frank left heart failure, but the diagnosis is confirmed by the findings of a murmur, plethora and cardiomegaly on the chest X-ray film and an abnormal ECG.

## Arrhythmias

These are usually acute in onset and result in sudden 'palpitations', often associated with breathlessness. The blood pressure may drop during the arrhythmia, resulting in vomiting, 'funny turns' and syncope.

## Examination

This section provides you with the order of and techniques required to examine a child for cardiac abnormalities. Start the examination by assessing the child's general state of health and look for any dysmorphic features. Identify central cyanosis by inspecting the lips and tongue, and polycythaemia by the presence of a plethoric complexion and conjunctival congestion. Examine the nails for clubbing, anaemia and peripheral cyanosis. Work your way back to the heart, starting first with the peripheral pulses, then the blood pressure and finally the precordium.

## Pulses

In children, especially infants, the brachial artery is best used for the assessment of the pulse. This provides a good assessment of pulse rate, volume and character. The brachial (as opposed to the radial) artery is the same distance from the heart as the femoral arteries. Hence, with one hand feeling the right brachial pulse, check either femoral pulse for a palpable difference between the two. It is easier to appreciate a *brachiofemoral difference* based on a discrepancy in pulse volume rather than a delay in timing, especially in babies who have a heart rate above 100 bpm (Table 23).

A high-volume pulse is often a clue to the presence of a large left-to-right shunt, e.g. a patent ductus arteriosus. An easy way to assess this is to raise the child's arm above the head. In those with high-volume 'bounding' pulses the pulse remains easily palpable.

**Table 23** Change in pulse and blood pressure

| Age | Pulse (beats/minute) | Mean blood pressure (mmHg) |
| --- | --- | --- |
| Neonate | 120–160 | 60 |
| Infant | 90–110 | 75 |
| School age | 80–90 | 90 |
| Teenage | 60–80 | 100 |

## Jugular venous pressure

The jugular venous pressure (JVP) is difficult to assess in infants but can be seen in premature babies and in children aged 2 years or more. The JVP is best seen with the patient lying propped up at 45° with the head turned slightly to the opposite side, and can be accentuated by gentle pressure over the liver (hepatojugular reflux). The JVP is raised in RHF and fluid overload, when the upper level falls during inspiration. However, when the movement of the heart is restricted due to pericardial or pulmonary disease (cor pulmonale), the JVP, though elevated, will rise further on inspiration (Kussmaul sign).

## Blood pressure

To measure blood pressure (BP) the cuff size should be two-thirds that of the child's arm. In order not to miss a coarctation of the aorta, it is important to take the BP on both arms and either lower limb. In small babies, an easy method of measuring the systolic BP is to observe the pressure at which the limb turns pink on deflating the cuff ('flush' method). The variation in BP with age is shown in Table 23.

## Precordium

Examine the precordium for activity. Place your right hand over the precordium and locate the apical impulse. Normally this is in the fourth intercostal space in the midclavicular line or the anterior axillary line in infants. A 'buzzing' or 'whirring' sensation beneath your hand is indicative of transmitted tactile turbulence (a thrill). Using the hypothenar aspect of the hand placed vertically to the left of the sternum, feel for a right ventricular heave, which is suggestive of right ventricular (RV) hypertrophy. A laterally displaced, heaving apical impulse is indicative of left ventricular (LV) hypertrophy.

## Heart sounds

Using the bell of the stethoscope (unless you have a paediatric sized diaphragm), listen over the precordium

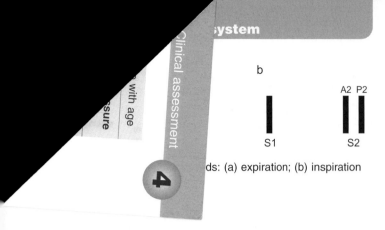

b

A2 P2

S1      S2

ds: (a) expiration; (b) inspiration

**Table 24** Grading system for systolic murmurs

| Grade | Nature | Thrill |
|-------|--------|--------|
| 1 | Barely audible | None |
| 2 | Soft, easily audible | None |
| 3 | Loud | None |
| 4 | Easily audible | Present |
| 5 | Loud, stethoscope barely on chest | Present |
| 6 | Heard away from chest wall | Present |

and initially concentrate on the heart sounds alone (Fig. 28). Listen for the first sound (S1) at the apex and lower left sternal edge (LSE). Concentrate on the second sound (S2). This normally has two components, but may on occasion be single. The first component results from closure of the aortic valve (A2), the second from closure of the pulmonary valve (P2). On inspiration, there is a fall in the intrathoracic pressure and more blood enters the right heart. This results in a delay in RV emptying, and the A2–P2 interval increases. On expiration, the split narrows and, particularly with a rapid heart rate, S2 may appear to be a single sound. If two components are clearly audible in all phases of respiration, assume there is wide fixed splitting of S2. Next concentrate on the intensity of the sound. Remember to auscultate over both aortic and pulmonary areas: if S2 is louder in the aortic area, then it is the aortic (earlier) component that is accentuated, and vice versa. If the child is crying, wait to auscultate until he or she pauses for breath.

## Added sounds

### Third sound
An extra third sound (S3) is said to reproduce the effect of a galloping horse, and is often heard in patients with heart failure. You can mimic this effect by drumming three fingers in succession on the tabletop.

### Clicks
Listen for additional sounds in between the two heart sounds. Clicks are momentary high-pitched sounds produced by the sudden opening of a stiff (usually stenotic) heart valve. They are generally produced by the pulmonary and aortic valves at the start of systole, heard immediately after the first heart sound, and are invariably followed by a murmur.

### Murmurs
Murmurs are sounds of a buzzing, whooshing or whirring nature and are caused by abnormal turbulence within the cardiac chambers or major vessels. Murmurs between S1 and S2 are systolic and are graded according to a simple system (Table 24). Diastolic murmurs

**Box 16** Features of innocent murmurs

Asymptomatic
Louder when there is fever, anaemia, exercise
Varies with respiration and posture
Systolic or continuous, never diastolic
Never palpable
No additional heart sounds

are never 'innocent' in aetiology, follow S2, and are not graded. The different types of murmur and their common causes are shown in Table 25.

*The majority of children with a cardiac murmur have an 'innocent' murmur.* These are present in up to 70% of neonates and 25–50% of older children. There are three main varieties. The *vibratory* (Still's) murmur, which as the name suggests sounds like the buzzing of a bee, is short midsystolic, heard over the precordium, diminishes on sitting up and disappears during puberty. The *pulmonary* murmur is a soft ejection systolic murmur heard in the pulmonary area and can be confused with pulmonary stenosis. The *venous hum* is a continuous blowing murmur which is usually heard below the clavicle and disappears on lying down. Differentiation between an innocent and a significant murmur can be difficult. If there is a doubt the child should be referred for evaluation (Box 16).

## Pulmonary sounds

It is important to listen to the lung fields for signs of infection and basal crepitations indicative of heart failure.

## Hepatomegaly

Hepatomegaly is a useful sign of heart failure, particularly as it is often difficult to assess jugular venous congestion and pedal oedema in children. Remember that the liver edge is normally palpable in small children 1–2 cm below the costal margin.

**Table 25** Murmurs and diagnoses

| Murmur | Phonocardiogram | Diagnosis |
|---|---|---|
| Ejection systolic | | Aortic stenosis, pulmonary stenosis, small ventricular septal defect |
| Late (ejection) systolic | | Coarctation of the aorta, mitral valve prolapse |
| Pansystolic | | Mitral incompetence, tricuspid incompetence, large ventricular septal defect, atrioventricular septal defect |
| Continuous | | Patent ductus arteriosus, collaterals (e.g. with coarctation), prosthetic shunts, arteriovenous fistulae |
| Early diastolic | | Aortic incompetence, pulmonary incompetence |
| Mid-diastolic | | Mitral stenosis |

## Confirmation of cyanosis: nitrogen washout test (100% oxygen)

The infant is assessed in 100% oxygen, where the nitrogen has been 'washed out'. The oxygen saturation and, preferably, the arterial $Po_2$ are measured before and after 100% oxygen. The $Po_2$ increases in those children with a respiratory or reversible cause for their cyanosis, but remains low when an intracardiac right-to-left shunt is present.

## Summary

Table 26 summarises the examination in cardiovascular disease.

## 4.3 Congenital heart disease

### Learning objectives

You should:

- know the signs, symptoms, diagnostic features and management of the common acyanotic diseases of childhood
- know the signs, symptoms, diagnostic features and management of the common cyanotic diseases of childhood

The major acyanotic and cyanotic congenital cardiac diseases (CHD) are listed in Table 27.

**Table 26** Summary of cardiovascular examination

| Examination | Information obtained |
|---|---|
| General | Wellbeing/unwell |
| | Failure to thrive |
| | Central cyanosis/plethora |
| | Clubbing |
| Pulses | Volume and rate |
| | Brachiofemoral difference |
| Blood pressure | Upper/lower limb differential |
| Precordium | Position/activity of apex |
| | Right ventricular heave |
| | Thrills |
| Heart sounds | S1 |
| | S2 |
| Added sounds | S3 |
| | Murmurs |
| | Clicks |
| Lung fields | Respiratory rate |
| | Crepitations |
| Liver size | Hepatomegaly |

## Frequency of specific congenital heart defects

Nine anomalies make up 90% of the cardiac abnormalities of childhood. About 10% will have complex lesions with more than one abnormality, and 10% will also have an associated non-cardiac abnormality. Little is known about the aetiology of these malformations, although the risk increases with some teratogenic drugs (e.g. phenytoin), infections (rubella, toxoplasmosis), and following a previously affected child (3% risk for subsequent sib-

**Table 27** Major acyanotic and cyanotic congenital heart diseases

| | Defects | (%) |
|---|---|---|
| **Acyanotic** | | |
| Left-to-right shunts | Ventricular septal defect (VSD) | 25–30 |
| | Atrial septal defect (ASD) | 6–8 |
| | Patent ductus arteriosus (PDA) | 6–8 |
| | Atrioventricular septal defect (AVSD) | 1–3 |
| Abnormal valves/ vessels | Pulmonary stenosis (PS) | 5–7 |
| | Aortic stenosis (AS) | 4–7 |
| | Coarctation of the aorta (CoA) | 5–7 |
| | *Mitral stenosis (MS)* | *1* |
| | *Ebstein's anomaly* | *1* |
| **Cyanotic** | | |
| Abnormal connections | Transposition of the great arteries (TGA) | 3–5 |
| | *Total anomalous pulmonary venous drainage (TAPVD)* | *1–3* |
| Obstructive lesions | Tetralogy of Fallot (TOF) | 5–7 |
| | Tricuspid atresia (TA) | 1–2 |
| | Pulmonary atresia (PA) | 1–3 |
| | Hypoplastic left heart (HyLH) | 1–3 |
| | *Hypoplastic right heart (HyRH)* | *1–3* |
| **Complex** | | |
| | *Truncus arteriosus (TA)* | *1–2* |
| | *Double outlet right or left ventricle* | *<1* |
| | *Single ventricle* | *<1* |

NB: Less common lesions are shown in italics.

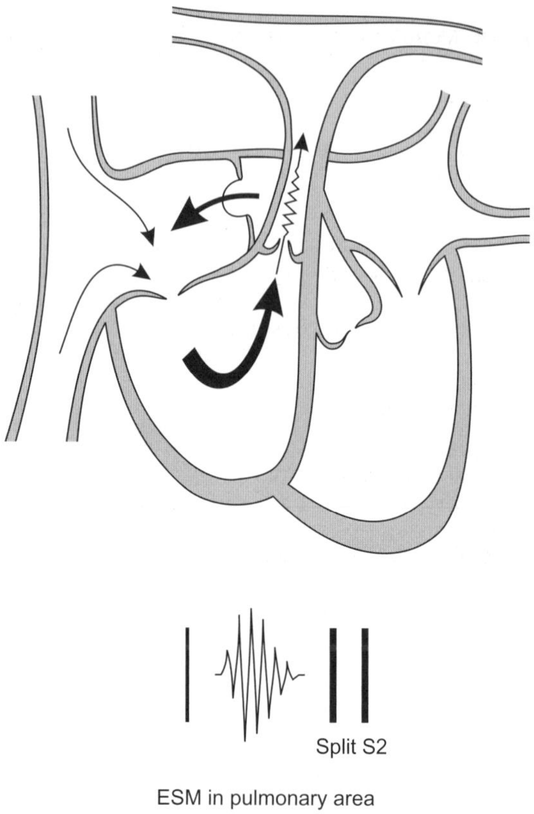

Split S2

ESM in pulmonary area

**Fig. 29** Atrial septal defect.

**Box 17** Chromosomal abnormalities and associated cardiac malformations

| | |
|---|---|
| Down syndrome (trisomy 21) | Atrioventricular septal defect, VSD |
| Edwards syndrome (trisomy 18) | Complex, PDA |
| Patau syndrome (trisomy 18) | Complex |
| Turner syndrome (XO) | CoA, AS (valvular) |
| Chromosome 22 microdeletion | Aortic arch abnormalities |

lings). Congenital heart disease (CHD) is also associated with major chromosomal abnormalities (Box 17).

## Acyanotic congenital heart disease

### Left-to-right shunts

#### Atrial septal defect
The more common ostium secundum atrial septal defects (ASD) are positioned at the site of the fossa ovalis and are generally isolated defects. Ostium primum ASDs are less common and arise in the lower part of the septum, where they can be associated with abnormalities of the atrioventricular valves. Indeed, they are more correctly classified as partial atrioventricular septal defects (AVSD). The pressure in the right atrium is lower than that in the left atrium. This results in shunting of oxygenated blood from the left to the right atrium, increasing blood flow by a factor of up to four times through the right side of the heart and pulmonary artery (Fig. 29). The typical clinical finding is that of a fixed, widely split second heart sound. Normally the second heart sound is made of the closure of the aortic valve (A2) followed by the pulmonary valve (P2). On inspiration, there is increased venous return to the right heart and the A2–P2 gap widens. In ASD, there is an excess of blood passing through the pulmonary valve, 'widening' the split. At the same time, the right ventricular stroke volume remains the same in inspiration or expiration, so the split is 'fixed'. The excess flow through the pulmonary valve produces an ejection systolic murmur (with no click) in the pulmonary area and a diastolic murmur in the tricuspid area. The common symptoms, signs and diagnostic features are shown in Box 18.

**Complications.** In early childhood, children with an ASD have low pulmonary vascular resistance and are asymptomatic. With increasing pulmonary vascular

**Box 18** ASD

**Symptoms**
None (most common)
Recurrent chest infections
Heart failure

**Signs**
Pink, normal pulses and normal blood pressure
Parasternal (right ventricular) lift
Wide and fixed split of the second heart sound
Ejection systolic murmur best heard third left intercostal
  space
Mid-diastolic murmur lower left sternal border
Arrhythmias (in adulthood)

**Investigations**
**ECG:** Peaked P wave – right atrial enlargment
Sinus rhythm with right axis deviation (ostium
  secundum)
Superior QRS axis, i.e left axis deviation (ostium
  primum)
May have right bundle branch block
**Chest X-ray** may show cardiomegaly with pulmonary
  plethora

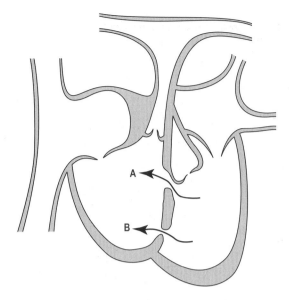

**Fig. 30** Ventricular septal defects: A, membranous; B, muscular.

resistance the right ventricular wall thickens and right-sided heart failure (RHF) develops during the second or third decade of life. Earlier symptoms are more likely with primum ASD (partial AVSD), which are complicated by left atrioventricular valve regurgitation, lower respiratory tract infections (LRTI) and failure to thrive. Nevertheless, it is rare to see complications of ASD, as almost all patients will undergo correction in childhood. If left untreated, complications arise during the third decade and include heart failure, especially during pregnancy, pulmonary hypertension and atrial dysrhythmias. Bacterial endocarditis is extremely rare with an ASD.

**Management.** Closure is recommended before school entry in all patients. Non-surgical catheter techniques utilising transdefect clamping devices have now become the first option for up to 80% of ASDs that have a sufficient rim of tissue surrounding the defect. Surgical repair is necessary in 20%, and involves direct suturing of small defects and the incorporation of an artificial patch (e.g. Dacron) in large defects.

### Ventricular septal defect

A ventricular septal defect (VSD; Fig. 30) is an abnormal interventricular connection. The defect may result from an incomplete fusion of the upper, membranous part of the septum (membranous VSD, 75%) or the lower muscular septum (20%). Both membranous and muscular VSD may vary in size, from $<0.5$ cm$^2$ to $>1.0$ cm$^2$, although muscular VSD are often multiple. Initially

blood flows under pressure from the left to the right ventricle across the VSD.

The age at presentation and the severity of symptoms depend on the size and therefore the degree of left–right shunting through the VSD. As shown in Box 19, small VSD ($<0.5$ cm$^2$) may be totally asymptomatic with no abnormal signs apart from an ejection or pansystolic (ESM, PSM) murmur at the left sternal edge (LSE). Large VSD ($>1.0$ cm$^2$) may result in heart failure, presenting with shortness of breath and excessive sweating on exertion or with feeds. These defects produce a significant left-to-right shunt, and a large-volume pulse is usually present. The apical beat is forceful and laterally displaced and a parasternal heave is present, signifying LV and RV hypertrophy, respectively. A thrill at the LSE is common. On auscultation, a loud P2 caused by pulmonary hypertension is often present (Fig. 31a). A third sound (S3) is heard in those in congestive cardiac failure (CCF). A 2–6/6 PSM all over the precordium, but best heard at the lower LSE, may be followed by a mid-diastolic murmur (MDM) at the apex caused by excessive flow across the mitral valve. Pulmonary crepitations and hepatomegaly are present in those patients in CCF.

**Complications.** Failure to thrive and LRTI are common with large defects. Bacterial endocarditis is a rare complication but generally occurs at the site of minimal turbulence, on the right of the interventricular wall. The excess pulmonary blood flow, which is under pressure, results in progressive reactive pathological changes in the pulmonary vasculature. Pulmonary arterial resistance increases and pulmonary hypertension develops. If left untreated, the progressive increase in pulmonary resistance can result in shunt reversal.

**Box 19** VSD

| Small VSD (<0.5 cm²) | Moderate VSD (0.5–1.0 cm²) | Large VSD (>1.0 cm²) |
|---|---|---|
| **Symptoms** | | |
| Generally asymptomatic. | None or recurrent chest infections | Heart failure, recurrent LRTIs and failure to thrive |
| **Signs** | | |
| Pink, normal pulses and BP | Pink, normal pulses and BP | Pink, normal pulses and BP |
| A thrill may be present | Thrill at LSE and LV impulse possible | Apical beat forceful and displaced parasternal |
| Normal heart sounds | Loud P2 best in the pulmonary area | heave, thrill LSE, loud P2, third heart sound |
| ESM (or PSM) at lower LSE | 2–6/6 PSM all over precordium | 2–6/6 PSM all over the precordium |
| | MDM | MDM |
| | Pulmonary crepitations, hepatomegaly | Pulmonary crepitations, hepatomegaly |
| **Investigations** | | |
| ECG: normal | LV hypertrophy, slight/moderate cardiomegaly | RV, LV hypertrophy |
| Chest X-ray: normal | Slight/moderate cardiomegaly, pulmonary plethora | Pulmonary plethora |

a                                                                 b

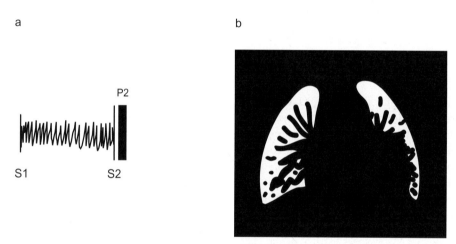

**Fig. 31** Findings in moderate-sized VSD. (a) Phonocardiogram shows a PSM at the LSE and a loud P2. (b) Chest X-ray film shows cardiomegaly and plethora.

The patient now becomes cyanosed and the shunt murmur disappears. This process is known as *Eisenmenger syndrome*.

**Management**. Up to 70% of small defects close spontaneously. Those with significant shunts develop heart failure and chest infections. These should be controlled (see below) and calorific intake maximised to prevent failure to thrive. Closure of the defect by patch repair under cardiac bypass surgery should be undertaken before school age, and certainly before pulmonary hypertension is established. Some selected VSDs may also be amenable to device closure by catheter techniques.

**Patent ductus arteriosus**

The ductus arteriosus constricts and closes in response to the rise in $P_{O_2}$, blood pH and prostacyclin levels after birth. If this mechanism fails or is reversed by prostaglandin $E_2$, the resulting connection allows blood to flow under pressure from the aorta into the pulmonary arteries. The patent ductus arteriosus (PDA) in the preterm infant is the result of a delay in closure. In a term infant, a PDA is the result of a deficiency in the structural framework of the vessel wall. Therefore, although 100% of premature babies born at 29 weeks of gestation will have a PDA, in the vast majority this closes spontaneously. In contrast, 6% of all term newborns have a persistent connection between the bifurcation of the pulmonary artery and the aortic arch, and in this group the PDA persists. Children with a PDA are often asymptomatic, with a murmur heard on examination (Fig. 32). Those with large shunts may present with symptoms and signs of excessive left-to-right shunting, as shown in Box 20.

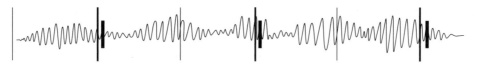

**Fig. 32** Patent ductus arteriosus. Continuous 'machinery' murmur.

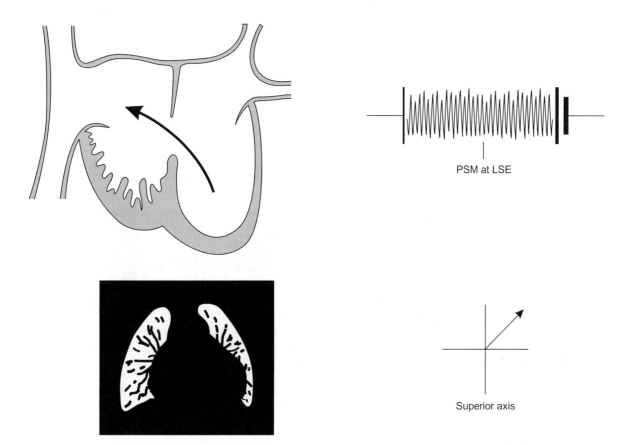

PSM at LSE

Superior axis

**Fig. 33** Atrioventricular septal defect.

**Complications**. Repeated lower pulmonary infections and CCF may result in failure to thrive. Subacute bacterial endocarditis and pulmonary hypertension are rare complications of a PDA.

**Management**. The CCF must be treated and conservative measures instituted to close a PDA, including fluid restriction, indomethacin and prostacyclin. Obliteration by the implantation of various 'umbrella/coil' devices during cardiac catheterisation is routine, though surgical ligation remains an important method of closure, especially in premature infants.

### Atrioventricular septal defect

In the atrioventricular septal defect (AVSD) the central portion of the heart (the 'endocardial cushion') fails to develop, resulting in a large defect straddling both the atria and ventricles and a single large (and incompetent)

atrioventricular (A–V) valve. The predominant flow is from LV to RA and, therefore, back to the lungs (Fig. 33). Dyspnoea, CCF and failure to thrive are common problems with an AVSD. A systolic thrill and PSM at the LSE are caused by A–V valve incompetence. The ECG reveals a superior axis and RV hypertrophy, whereas cardiomegaly and pulmonary plethora are seen on X-ray film. Pulmonary hypertension develops rapidly, and aggressive treatment of heart failure is necessary prior to surgical repair before 6–10 months of age. AVSD is classically associated with Down syndrome.

## Abnormal valves and vessels

### Pulmonary stenosis    (Fig. 34)

A constricted pulmonary valve ring impedes forward flow of desaturated blood into the lungs, resulting in a volume load on the right ventricle. Pulmonary stenosis (PS) is usually an isolated lesion, but can occur with other complex CHD and syndromes (e.g. Noonan). Children with PS often have no symptoms, although exercise intolerance and, at times RHF, may occur (Box 21). An ejection systolic murmur, sometimes preceded by an opening click as the stiff valve opens, follows the direction of blood flow and therefore radiates through to the back. The symptoms, signs, ECG and chest X-ray findings in PS are shown in Box 21.

**Complications.** PS is remarkably well tolerated and RHF is only seen in severe cases.

**Management.** Conservative pulmonary valvoplasty by balloon dilatation during cardiac catheter procedures is safe and effective. If necessary, this procedure may be repeated. Dysplastic valves and severe stenosis, especially if associated with calcification, require formal surgical pulmonary valvotomy. Pulmonary valve replacement is rarely necessary in children.

### Pulmonary incompetence
Pulmonary incompetence (PI) may be associated with a dysplastic valve and is common after operations on the RV outflow tract and balloon catheter dilatation

---

**Box 20** PDA

**Symptoms**
None (most common)
Recurrent chest infections
Heart failure with large shunts

**Signs**
None (most common)
Pink, normal or large volume, bounding/collapsing
  pulses
BP shows wide pulse pressure
Precordium is hyperdynamic with LV impulse at apex
Thrill at left infraclavicular area and second left
  intercostal space possible
Loud P2 with pulmonary hypertension
Third heart sound (S3) with CCF
Continuous 'waterwheel/machinery' murmur (Fig. 32)
  loudest at upper LSE, left infraclavicular area and back
Pulmonary crepitations and hepatomegaly with CCF

**Investigations**
**ECG.** Normal or shows LV hypertrophy
**Chest X-ray.** The film shows moderate cardiomegaly
  and pulmonary plethora.

---

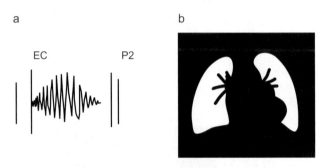

a                  b

EC        P2

**Fig. 34** Findings in pulmonary stenosis. (a) Phono-cardiogram shows an ejection click (EC), an ESM in the pulmonary area and soft P2. (b) Chest X-ray film shows a prominent pulmonary conus and an uplifted apex caused by RV hypertrophy.

---

**Box 21** Pulmonary and aortic stenosis

| Pulmonary stenosis | Aortic stenosis |
|---|---|
| **Symptoms** | |
| None (most common) | None (most common) |
| Recurrent chest infections | Exercise intolerance, dizzy or syncopal spells |
| Heart failure with large shunts | Angina, LV failure |
| | Sudden death |
| **Signs** | |
| None (most common) | None (most common) |
| Pink, normal pulses and BP | Pink, with a low volume pulse |
| Precordium normal (mild PS) | LV impulse at apex |
| Thrill at upper LSE and RV heave (severe PS) | Thrill in suprasternal notch |
| Ejection click follows the first heart sound (mild PS); | Opening ejection click heard with valvular stenosis |
|   no click and soft P2 (severe PS) |   aortic A2 is loud |
|   wide but variable splitting of S2 | |
| 2–4/6 ESM in the pulmonary area, radiating to back | 2–4/6 ESM in the aortic area, upper right sternal edge and neck |
| **Investigations** | |
| **ECG**. Normal or RV hypertrophy | LV hypertrophy |
| **Chest X-ray**. Prominent pulmonary conus, | Prominent aortic arch and cardiomegaly |
| RV hypertrophy | LV hypertrophy |

for pulmonary stenosis. It is well tolerated and patients are generally asymptomatic. A 2–3/6 early diastolic, 'decrescendo' murmur heard in the pulmonary area and radiating down the LSE may be the only abnormality on examination.

## Aortic stenosis

In the majority of patients aortic stenosis (AS) is caused by fusion of the valvular cusps (valvular AS). Subvalvular (subaortic) stenosis is caused by a fibrous shelf below the valve. Supravalvular stenosis is the least common abnormality, but may be associated with stenoses of other arteries and is a feature of Williams syndrome (mental retardation, elfin facies, hypercalcaemia). AS results in a restriction to forward blood flow into the aorta from the LV, and is either asymptomatic or results in exercise intolerance, syncopal attacks and, possibly, sudden death (see Box 21). Low-volume pulses may be associated with a harsh ESM (± thrill) in the aortic area that radiates to the neck.

**Complications**. These include angina, arrhythmias, LV failure and sudden death.

**Management**. Balloon valvoplasty is possible for moderate valvular stenosis. Surgery is required for dysplastic valves and aortic membranes.

## Aortic incompetence

Aortic incompetence (AI) is usually associated with a dysplastic and stenotic valve. It produces a large end-systolic volume in the LV. In order to compensate for this extra load the LV increases in size, producing a prominent apical impulse on examination.

The pulses are classically 'collapsing' in nature. A decrescendo early diastolic murmur is usually audible in the aortic area and along the LSE (i.e. radiates 'backwards', rather than up the aortic arch and into the neck).

## Coarctation of the aorta

Coarctation of the aorta (CoA) is a narrowing in the form of a discrete 'shelf' or a long constriction (Fig. 35). The narrowing may occur before (preductal) or after (postductal) the site of origin of the ductus arteriosus. In 95% of patients the coarctation is postductal, arising just beyond the origin of the left subclavian artery. This results in hypertension in both upper limbs. A preductal constriction preceding the origin of the left subclavian artery results in hypertension in the right upper limb alone. In children with untreated coarctation, collateral arteries generally develop by mid-childhood and augment the blood supply to the lower torso. Coarctation is often associated with a bicuspid aortic valve. It is the most common CHD in Turner syndrome.

**Symptoms**. In infancy, coarctation is usually preductal and the descending aorta is supplied by the PDA. When the PDA closes, these patients present in a criti-

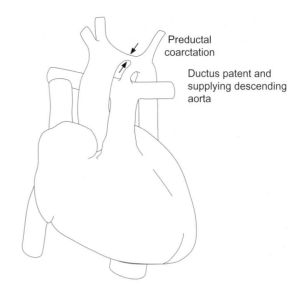

**Fig. 35** Coarctation of the aorta.

cal condition with severe CCF and poor perfusion to the lower trunk and limbs. Older patients are asymptomatic or develop dyspnoea and weakness after exercise. Those with hypertension may present with headaches, fainting attacks and dizzy spells.

**Signs**. The pulses in the lower limbs are weak compared with the right (or both) upper limbs, and brachiofemoral difference/delay is present. The BP is raised in the upper limbs and decreased in the legs. The apical impulse may be forceful, but heart sounds are usually normal. A late systolic murmur at the upper LSE radiating to the back and neck is common. Additional, continuous murmurs over the upper back and axillae are produced by turbulence in the collateral vessels.

**ECG**. LV failure is a late sign.

**Chest X-ray**. Cardiomegaly and plethora are observed in neonates. Prestenotic dilatation of the arch and LV prominence are seen in older children. Rib notching between the fourth and eighth ribs posteriorly is caused by intercostal collaterals and is only evident in older children who remain undiagnosed and untreated at the age of 6–7 years or more.

**Complications**. Hypertension and LHF are common. Coarctation of the aorta is also associated with aneurysms of the descending aorta and collateral vessels. Associated intracranial aneurysms may bleed, producing subarachnoid haemorrhage.

**Management**. Medical treatment of hypertension is required. Mild lesions are amenable to balloon dilatation. Infants presenting acutely in a critical condition require emergency surgical repair of the aorta. A discrete shelf can be excised and an end-to-end anastomosis performed in 40% of patients. Long segment lesions require more complex operations, involving the creation of a repair flap utilising the left subclavian artery or an additional artificial patch. Older children and those with re-coarctation may be treated with balloon dilatation, with or without a stent in those approaching adult size.

## Cyanotic congenital heart disease

### *Abnormal connections*

#### Transposition of the great arteries
Transposition of the great arteries (TGA) is the most common cyanotic lesion in neonates. The aorta arises

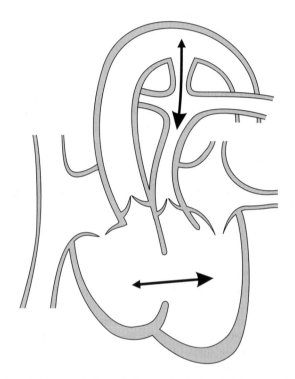

**Fig. 36** Transposition of the great arteries. In this example there is mixing, predominantly right to left, at the ventricular level (via VSD) and through the patent ductus arteriosus.

from the RV and the pulmonary artery from the LV. This results in two separate circulations 'in parallel', which is incompatible with life unless there is an additional right-to-left connection (Fig. 36). This is usually a PDA and/or a VSD. Neonates present with cyanosis, heart failure and sudden collapse in those where the circulation is almost entirely dependent on the ductus arteriosus, which closes after birth (Box 22). Although cyanosis, poor perfusion and signs of heart failure may be marked, murmurs may be unimpressive or absent. The chest X-ray may be normal or show moderate cardiomegaly with pulmonary plethora, especially in TGA with a VSD. The classic narrow mediastinum is the result of the aorta and pulmonary artery lying alongside each other and not at 90° to one another (Fig. 37). At the time when delayed surgery was the norm, a chest X-ray often showed a typical bell-clapper or

---

**Box 22** TGA

**Symptoms**
Severe cyanosis and tachypnoea in newborn period
Sudden collapse as ductus arteriosus closes
Heart failure in those with large VSDs

**Signs**
Central cyanosis
Tachycardia and marked tachypnoea
Hyperdynamic precordium
S2 is usually single as AV and PV are close together
Murmurs may be absent (especially without a VSD)
Pulmonary crepitations and hepatomegaly with CCF

**Investigations**
**ECG.** Normal or shows right sided dominance (no VSD); RV and LV hypertrophy with VSD
**Chest X-ray.** Moderate cardiomegaly, sometimes with narrow mediastinum, pulmonary plethora (especially with VSD).

---

a

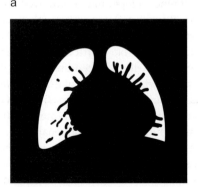

b

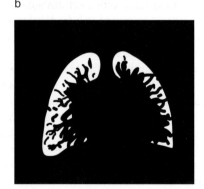

**Fig. 37** Chest radiograph in transposition of the great arteries. (a) In the absence of a VSD there is cardiomegaly, a narrow mediastinum and mild pulmonary plethora. (b) With a VSD there is cardiomegaly, a narrow mediastinum and marked plethora.

a

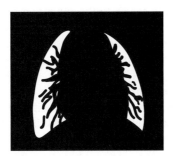

b

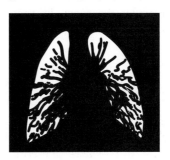

**Fig. 38** Anomalous pulmonary venous drainage on chest X-ray film. (a) Supra-diaphragmatic drainage results in cardiomegaly with a wide mediastinum and moderate pulmonary plethora. (b) Infradiaphragmatic drainage results in a small heart, overexpanded lungs and marked pulmonary plethora.

'egg-on-side' appearance. With early corrective surgery (switch operation) in the neonatal period and the presence of a normal thymic shadow (sail sign) in this age group, this radiological phenomenon is now rarely observed.

**Complications**. Patients with TGA are critically ill, in severe CCF, and require urgent operative intervention.

**Management**. This lesion is usually duct dependent and patients are generally unwell at presentation. They require oxygen, urgent treatment for heart failure and prostaglandin $E_2$ by infusion in order to reopen the ductus. Perforation of the atrial septum by a Rashkind balloon or blade septostomy allows mixing at atrial level and buys time before a definitive procedure is performed. Ideally, the great arteries (and coronaries) are reconnected to their appropriate ventricle ('switch operation'). This procedure is not possible after the first few months of life, when redirection of blood flow to the 'correct' ventricles can be established by means of an intra-atrial baffle or rerouting operation, based on the Mustard and Senning operations.

**Total anomalous pulmonary venous drainage**

Total anomalous pulmonary venous drainage (TAPVD) can be either supradiaphragmatic or infradiaphragmatic.

**Supradiaphragmatic drainage**. The pulmonary veins (PV) do not connect with the left atrium (LA) and return to the RA directly or via large mediastinal veins. Breathlessness is associated with signs of high-output CCF. Murmurs are often absent. Venous return is not obstructed and the mediastinum is congested, casting a wide shadow on X-ray film (cottage loaf/snowman appearance) (Fig. 38a). The ECG shows R axis deviation and RV hypertrophy.

**Infradiaphragmatic drainage**. The PVs aggregate behind the LA and return to the RA via a circuitous route beneath the diaphragm, where they become obstructed. A patent foramen ovale is required to

sustain life. Dyspnoea and recurrent chest infections are common symptoms, whereas cyanosis, tachypnoea, an RV heave and marked hepatomegaly are found on examination. Because of the obstructed venous return, the heart is small on X-ray (Fig. 38b). Pulmonary congestion results in marked plethora.

**Management**. Treatment of CCF, followed by surgical repair of the aberrant veins, is required.

## Obstructive lesions

### Tricuspid atresia

Tricuspid atresia (TA) prevents forward flow through the tricuspid valve and blood shunts right to left across the foramen ovale/ASD. A VSD is present in almost all cases and allows blood to flow from LV to RV and into the lungs. However, the VSD is often restrictive, and in these patients the circulation is maintained by the ductus arteriosus; closure of the ductus results in significant cyanosis and, at times, sudden collapse. Cyanosis is associated with a PSM in those with a VSD. LV hypertrophy with left axis deviation (superior axis) on ECG is characteristic of TA.

Emergency reopening of the ductus using prostaglandin precedes the insertion of a left–right shunt. The latter involves a prosthetic tube that connects the subclavian artery to the ipsilateral pulmonary artery (modified Blalock–Taussig shunt). This procedure may be repeated on the other side before a palliative operation is possible. These include Fontan-type procedures, which are indicated when just one functional ventricle is available (e.g. left ventricle in tricuspid or pulmonary atresia, and right ventricle in hypoplastic left heart syndrome). The Fontan circuit directs deoxygenated blood returning to the heart via the venae cavae directly into the lungs without the benefit of a pumping chamber. The forward flow of blood into the lungs is 'passive', depending solely on central venous pressure, and is therefore not applicable in those with raised pulmonary vascular resistance or pulmonary hypertension.

### Pulmonary atresia

In pulmonary atresia (PA) the atretic pulmonary outflow tract prevents forward flow into the lungs, and pulmonary blood flow is sustained in all cases by a PDA. Although not all infants with PA have a VSD, they are all duct dependent and will collapse as the PDA closes, or present with severe cyanosis, tachypnoea and a single S2 owing to the absence of the pulmonary component. The heart size is variable and pulmonary oligaemia marked on X-ray.

Those patients with a VSD are also duct dependent, but in addition may have collateral vessels that supply some parts of the lungs directly from the aorta. These create systemic pressure and result in patchy pulmonary congestion plus continuous murmurs audible over the back.

**Management**. Palliative Blalock–Taussig shunt(s) are necessary before a palliative Fontan-type procedure is feasible.

### Hypoplastic left heart syndrome

Hypoplastic left heart syndrome is the most common cardiac cause of death in neonates. The main left pumping chamber is severely underdeveloped, result-

ing in CCF in the first few weeks of life. Until recently this was a uniformly lethal condition, though a three-stage (Norwood) corrective procedure has shown good results and is considered in all except those with extreme hypoplasia.

### Tetralogy of Fallot

Tetralogy of Fallot (TOF; Fig. 39) is the commonest cyanotic CHD of childhood. It has four features:

- RV outflow tract (RVOT) obstruction
- RV hypertrophy (resulting from obstruction)
- A large VSD beneath the aortic outlet
- The aorta straddles both the left and the right ventricle (so-called 'overriding' aorta).

As a result, desaturated blood entering the right heart is shunted back into the systemic circulation (i.e. right to left). Twenty per cent of patients with TOF have a right-sided aortic arch; a few may have complete absence of the pulmonary valve. Children are commonly breathless on exertion, and to obtain symptomatic relief infants and toddlers will lie down, whereas older children assume a squatting position. Paroxysmal hypercyanotic episodes ('blue spells') classically arise in untreated young children aged 2 years or less, following defecation, crying or feeding. They are characterised by increasing irritability, prolonged crying, rapid deep respiratory movements and a dramatic exacerbation of cyanosis.

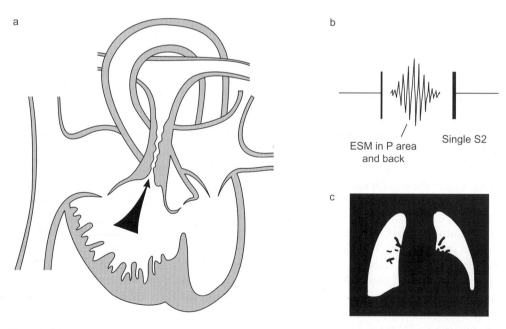

**Fig. 39** (a) Findings in Fallot's tetralogy. (b) Phonocardiogram shows an ESM in the pulmonary area and a single S2. (c) Chest radiograph shows absent pulmonary conus, RV hypertrophy and oligaemia.

At birth the RV outflow obstruction is usually not severe and cyanosis may not be obvious, but this becomes evident with increasing activity, often when crawling commences around 10 months of age. Progressive hypoxaemia results in compensatory polycythaemia. The clinical signs are typified by a single S2 and loud ESM at the upper LSE due to turbulence caused by the infundibular stenosis (Box 23). During hypercyanotic spells there is a significant increase in RVOT obstruction, blood flow through the outflow decreases, and the murmur disappears. The large VSD produces little turbulence and therefore does not produce a murmur.

**Box 23** Tetralogy of Fallot

**Symptoms**
Cyanosis and hypercyanotic spells
Exercise tolerance poor
Need to lie down/squat after exertion

**Signs**
Central cyanosis
Plethoric appearance
Hyperdynamic precordium with RV heave at LSE
Systolic thrill at the upper LSE in 50% of patients
S2 is single due to absent pulmonary component
Loud ESM at the upper LSE radiating to back

**Investigations**
**ECG**. R axis deviation and RV hypertrophy
**Chest X-ray** (Fig. 34). Small pulmonary conus, RV hypertrophy boot-shaped heart (*coeur en sabot*)
Pulmonary oligaemia

**Complications**. Progressive cyanosis is associated with failure to thrive. Hypercyanotic spells may be associated with syncopal attacks. Cerebral ischaemia and thromboses usually occur in the first 2 years of life, whereas cerebral abscesses develop in older children. Bacterial endocarditis and CCF are rare.

**Management**. Attempts to improve weight gain are essential. An adequate haemoglobin should be maintained, especially in patients with severe cyanosis and those with hypercyanotic spells. The latter require emergency treatment. The child should be placed in a knee-to-chest position ('simulated squatting') and given oxygen. Intravenous morphine may reduce the RVOT obstruction and is the first drug of choice, followed by sodium bicarbonate and intravenous propranolol. These children should then be maintained on regular oral propranolol until surgery. A palliative Blalock–Taussig shunt improves pulmonary blood flow. It is employed in severely cyanosed infants aged less than 6 months, those who are medically unfit for a major procedure, and those with hypercyanotic spells. The definitive repair involves total reconstruction of the RV outflow tract and closure of the VSD. It is increasingly the primary operation of choice, and can be performed without a prior Blalock–Taussig shunt in relatively healthy infants with favourable anatomy. The operative mortality is less than 5%.

## Summary

Table 28 summarises the findings in cyanotic heart disease.

**Table 28** Cyanotic CHD: clinical, ECG and chest X-ray findings

| Lesion | Murmur | ECG | Chest X-ray |
|---|---|---|---|
| **Presenting with CCF in the neonatal period** | | | |
| Transposition of the great arteries (TGA) (with VSD) | PSM | RV + LV hypertrophy | Egg-shaped cardiomegaly, marked plethora |
| Total anomalous pulmonary venous drainage (TAPVD) (obstructed) | – | RV hypertrophy | Small heart, plethora |
| Hypoplastic right heart | – | LV hypertrophy | Cardiomegaly, plethora |
| **Presenting without CCF in the neonatal period** | | | |
| TGA (no VSD) | – | RV dominance | Egg-shaped cardiomegaly, moderate plethora |
| Pulmonary atresia (PA) (with VSD) | PSM | LV hypertrophy | Moderate cardiomegaly, moderate plethora |
| PA (no VSD) | – | LV dominance | Cardiomegaly, oligaemia |
| Tricuspid atresia (TA) | ± PSM | Superior axis | Moderate cardiomegaly, oligaemia |
| **Presenting with CCF in infancy** | | | |
| TAPVD (unobstructed) | – | RV hypertrophy | Cottage loaf cardiomegaly, plethora |
| **Presenting without CCF in infancy** | | | |
| Fallot's tetralogy | ESM | RV hypertrophy | Boot-shaped cardiomegaly, oligaemia |

## 4.4 Abnormalities of rhythm

An electrocardiogram is a recording of the electrical activity of the heart on a moving strip of paper. Abnormalities may be within normal variation or may be indicative of disease (Table 29).

### Normal variations

**Sinus arrhythmia.** A normal accentuation of the heart rate with inspiration and the decrease with expiration.
**Ectopic beats.** These are common and disappear with exercise.
**Bradycardias.** Sinus bradycardia (<60 bpm) is a common finding in fit teenagers and during deep sleep.

## Bradyarrhythmias

### Heart block

#### First-degree block

In first-degree block the P–R interval is prolonged compared with the expected norm for age. Causes

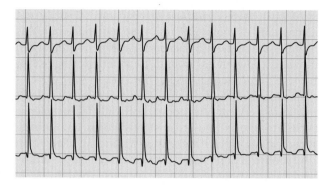

**Fig. 40** ECG showing supraventricular tachycardia.

include TGA, Ebstein's anomaly, digitalis, myocarditis and rheumatic carditis.

#### Second-degree block

The occasional p wave is not conducted to the ventricle. This may be consistent (Mobitz type I), or associated with progressive lengthening of the P–R interval until an action potential is not conducted (Wenckebach phenomenon).

#### Third-degree block

Complete heart block occurs when there is no association between the atrial (p) waves and ventricular depolarisation (QRS). It may be a congenital abnormality but is also associated with maternal systemic lupus erythematosus. If the AV node takes over as the pacemaker, the heart rate is around 60 bpm and the QRS retains a normal appearance. With an alternative ventricular pacemaker, the heart rate is 40 bpm or less and the QRS is wide and bizarre in shape.

#### Bradycardias

Pathological bradycardias are associated with raised intracranial pressure (in conjunction with hypertension), hypothyroidism, and occasionally myocarditis.

## Tachyarrhythmias

### Supraventricular tachyarrhythmias

Supraventricular tachycardia (SVT) involves a heart rate of about 180–300 bpm (Fig. 40). Patients may be asymptomatic, though they usually experience sweating, listlessness, lethargy and dizziness, and may become short of breath during an attack. Older children may report palpitations. Severe episodes may precipitate heart failure.

The p waves are absent on the ECG but the QRS complexes appear normal (Fig. 41). SVT result from an underlying Wolff–Parkinson–White syndrome (WPW) in 10% of patients and can only be diagnosed on a

| Table 29 Common ECG abnormalities | |
|---|---|
| **ECG finding** | **Diagnosis** |
| Peaked p wave | Right atrial hypertrophy |
| Broad, notched p waves | Left atrial hypertrophy |
| Tall R in $V_1$, deep S in $V_6$, R axis deviation | Right ventricular hypertrophy |
| Tall R in $V_6$, deep S in $V_1$, L axis deviation | Left ventricular hypertrophy |
| Broad QRS ( >0.1 s) | Bundle branch block |
| Flat QRS, T waves | Pericarditis |
| Long Q–T, depressed S–T, T wave | Hypokalaemia |
| Long P–R, wide QRS, peaked T wave | Hyperkalaemia |
| Long Q–T | Hypocalcaemia |
| Short Q–T | Hypercalcaemia |
| Bradycardia, small complexes, flat T wave | Hypothyroidism |
| Tachycardia, atrial fibrillation | Hyperthyroidism |
| Short Q–T, flat S–T, T waves, coupled beats | Digoxin toxicity |

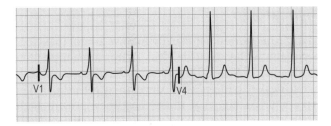

**Fig. 41** The QRS complex in Wolff–Parkinson–White syndrome, with a slurred δ wave and wide QRS.

**Table 30** Symptoms and signs of cardiac failure

| Symptoms | Signs |
| --- | --- |
| Poor feeding | Cold, clammy peripheries |
| Poor weight gain | Tachycardia |
| Cold sweats | Weak, thready pulse |
| Breathlessness | Gallop rhythm (53) |
| | Tachypnoea |
| | Wheezes and crepitations |
| | Hepatomegaly |
| | Periorbital, pedal, sacral oedema |

resting ECG. Abnormal conduction along an aberrant atrioventricular pathway bypasses the AV node and depolarises the ventricles earlier and via a different direction than the norm. This results in a shortened P–R interval (<0.12 s), an initial 'aberrant' depolarisation (producing the slurred δ wave), followed by normal ventricular conduction (resulting in a QRS superimposed on the δ wave).

Control of the SVT may be achieved by increasing the vagal (parasympathetic) stimulation to the heart by carotid sinus massage, Valsalva manoeuvre and, in infants, an ice pack applied to the face. Adenosine is effective but short acting. Digoxin and β-blockers may be necessary in refractory cases. If medical measures are not effective, mapping of the aberrant pathway followed by catheter ablation is the preferred option.

### Ventricular tachycardia

Ventricular tachycardia (VT) is rare but may be associated with severe aortic stenosis and post-cardiac arrest situations. VT results in a loss of cardiac output and necessitates emergency procedures to re-establish sinus rhythm, including intravenous lignocaine and cardioversion.

## 4.5 Heart failure and acquired cardiac disease

### Learning objectives

You should:

- appreciate the symptoms of congestive cardiac failure in infants and children

- how to assess for cardiac failure and treat the condition

- know the presenting features, diagnosis and management of the common cardiac infections seen in childhood

## Congestive cardiac failure

Congestive cardiac failure (CCF) is a clinical syndrome in which the heart is unable to pump enough blood to meet the body's needs and unable to 'clear' venous return. The symptoms and signs are discussed earlier in this chapter and are summarised in Table 30.

### Diagnosis

**ECG**. There are no ECG changes diagnostic of CCF.

**Chest X-ray**. Cardiomegaly, with or without pulmonary plethora, is a cardinal feature of CCF on the chest X-ray film.

**Echocardiogram**. The echocardiogram uses ultrasound waves to investigate the action of the heart as it beats. It demonstrates dilatation of the ventricular chambers, poor contractility of the ventricular walls, and a reduction in the volume of blood expelled with each contraction (i.e. the ejection fraction). The echocardiogram is also extremely useful in establishing the cause for the CCF (Box 24).

### General management

The patient should be propped upright and humidified oxygen delivered by face-mask. Attention should be paid to ensuring an adequate calorie intake and the avoidance of excess salt. An accurate fluid balance and daily measurement of body weight are mandatory. An underlying or exacerbating cause such as anaemia, infection, hypertension, arrhythmia or thyrotoxicosis should be treated.

**Drug treatment**
**Diuretics**. These alleviate cardiac failure by reducing fluid afterload on the heart. A loop diuretic, and in particular frusemide, is the drug of choice. They can be supplemented by an aldosterone antagonist (e.g. spironolactone), which is potassium saving.

**Afterload reduction**. This can be achieved by reducing the systemic vascular resistance by venous or arterial dilatation, or both. Angiotensin-converting enzyme inhibitors (ACEi) such as captopril and enalapril reduce the systemic resistance by the inhibition of angiotensin II and, after diuretics, are now the drugs of choice in heart failure. Like hydralazine and combined veno-arteriolar dilators (e.g. nitroprusside), they may cause hypotension. Venodilators, including nitroglycerides and nitrates, reduce venous congestion without improving cardiac contractility. Hydralazine acts by dilating the arteriolar bed, and also produces a tachycardia.

**Inotropic drugs.** These improve cardiac contractility and function. Digitalis glycosides, including digoxin, were previously widely used, often with a diuretic. A shortening of the Q–T interval and sagging of the S–T segment and T wave are often observed with therapeutic doses. Digoxin toxicity results in a prolongation of the P–R interval, sinus bradycardia, A–V block and supraventricular and, occasionally, ventricular ectopics, bigeminy and tachyarrhythmias. Toxicity is enhanced in patients with renal dysfunction, hypothyroidism, acidosis, severe hypoxia, hypokalaemia, hypercalcaemia, and with verapamil and amiodarone.

*Dopamine and dobutamine.* These inotropic drugs are given by intravenous infusion in situations when cardiac function is severely compromised. Unlike dopamine, dobutamine is virtually cardioselective and does not compromise renal circulation and function when used in high doses.

## Myocarditis

Myocarditis is rare but usually follows a viral infection, especially with Coxsackie virus B. It is a manifestation of rheumatic fever, diphtheria and some drugs (e.g. cytotoxics). Children who develop myocarditis may have a preceding viral illness and then present with signs of congestive heart failure. Cardiomegaly, pulmonary plethora and occasionally bilateral pulmonary effusions are evident on a chest X-ray film. The ECG shows S–T segment and T-wave depression.

## Pericarditis

Pericarditis in childhood is related to either infection or chemicals and is associated with myocarditis. Patients often develop a fever, heart failure and retrosternal pain. The last is exacerbated on lying flat and improves on leaning forward, thereby allowing the chest cage to fall away from the inflamed pericardium. A 'scratching' friction rub may be audible on examination, and if a pericardial effusion is present the heart sounds may appear muffled and distant. Pulsus paradoxus is detected on measuring the BP. 'Globular' cardiomegaly on the chest X-ray film is suggestive of an effusion, whereas low-voltage complexes throughout and S–T elevation in the chest leads are typical ECG changes in this condition. Treatment should include adequate rest, oxygen, anti-inflammatory agents such as non-steroidal analgesics, and steroids. Penicillin is added with rheumatic fever. Large effusions may cause acute heart failure ('tamponade') and require cardiocentesis.

## Bacterial endocarditis

Bacterial endocarditis is inflammation of the lining of the heart cavity and valves. It can be acute or subacute.

### Acute endocarditis
This is often caused by *Staphylococcus aureus* and occurs de novo in young infants with septicaemia but without pre-existing disease of the heart. The patient develops severe cardiac failure and the condition is fatal in more than 50%.

### Subacute endocarditis
Subacute endocarditis (SABE) occurs in children who have an underlying cardiovascular abnormality, usually comprising a structural defect with a significant pressure gradient within the heart. Although most children with congenital heart disease are at risk for SABE, this complication is particularly common in those with

a VSD and aortic stenosis. Children with indwelling central venous catheters and intracardiac prosthetic materials are particularly at risk. Infection follows a bacteraemia, which may be triggered by dental or surgical procedures. In patients with dental caries a bacteraemia may follow vigorous chewing or brushing of the teeth. Vegetations develop and may fragment, resulting in emboli travelling to the brain, spleen, kidneys and lungs. The causative organisms commonly include *Streptococcus viridans* (*albus*), β-haemolytic streptococci, *Staphylococcus aureus* and enterococci.

## Clinical manifestations

The patient presents with a fever, anorexia and general malaise. Examination confirms a raised temperature, a 'new' or additional murmur, splenomegaly in 70% of patients and evidence of microembolic disease. The last includes skin petechiae and haematuria. Finger clubbing, tender spots on the ends of the fingers (Osler's nodes), haemorrhages over the palms and soles (Janeway lesions) and splinter haemorrhages are rare in children with SABE. Pulmonary and central nervous system emboli are usually seen in patients with left-sided cardiac lesions and those with cyanotic CHD.

## Investigations

Confirmation of the organism is difficult and requires *repeated blood cultures*, e.g. four to six over the space of 24–48 hours. Arterial rather than venous cultures may provide a better yield. Echocardiography may confirm intracardiac and mural vegetations if they are >2 mm in diameter.

## Management

Heart failure requires urgent treatment. Intravenous high-dose β-lactam and aminoglycoside should be commenced, pending the results of blood cultures. Antibiotics are continued for 4 weeks and adjusted according to in vitro results on bacterial sensitivity. Antibiotic treatment is successful in 80–90% of all patients, though the prognosis varies with the infecting organism. Recovery occurs in 90% of patients with *Streptococcus viridans* infection and in 50% of those with *Staphylococcus aureus* infection. Operative intervention may be required for infected prostheses.

## Prevention of SABE

Good dental hygiene is of paramount importance. Antibacterial prophylaxis is required prior to all dental

**Box 25** Antibiotic prophylaxis is NOT required with

An isolated secundum ASD, 6 months after successful repair of an ASD, PDA or VSD
Mitral valve prolapse
Kawasaki disease with no residual valvular dysfunction
Rheumatic fever with no residual valvular dysfunction
Implanted pacemakers

procedures, major surgery and surgery on the upper airways, and instrumentation of the gastrointestinal and genitourinary tracts. Prophylaxis is not required in certain procedures such as endotracheal intubation, gastrointestinal endoscopy, caesarian section, circumcision, sterile skin biopsy, urethral catheterisation in non-infected individuals, cardiac catheterisation and the insertion of pacemakers. All children with a structural cardiac abnormality are at risk of SABE, except those listed in Box 25. At-risk patients should receive oral or intravenous/intramuscular antibiotics one or half an hour before the procedure, respectively, as listed in Table 31. Those with acquired valvular heart disease, hypertrophic cardiomyopathy, previous SABE and intracardiac prostheses are at particularly high risk of SABE, and a second antibiotic (usually gentamicin) is required for prophylaxis.

## 4.6 Cardiorespiratory arrest and resuscitation

### Learning objective

You should:
• know the steps for basic paediatric life support

In previously healthy but seriously compromised children cardiorespiratory collapse occurs when all other compensatory mechanisms fail. As a result it carries a dismal outcome, with approximately just 10% surviving this end-stage event, even if this occurs in a paediatric intensive care setting. Prevention, therefore, is the priority in all seriously ill children. Nevertheless, early and effective cardiopulmonary resuscitation (CPR) may help those where a chance for survival exists.

## Basic life support

The majority of cardiorespiratory arrests are secondary to hypoxic events, and asystole is significantly more common than ventricular fibrillation. Hence, the priority is to oxygenate the patient, then administer effective cardiac compressions. These are encompassed in the 'ABC' approach, addressing the **A**irway, **B**reathing and **C**irculation. The rescuer must ensure safety for himself and the patient, attempt to stimulate the patient and, if there is no response, call for help as soon as possible. He should then proceed to open the airway by slight head tilt and chin lift, followed by assessment of breathing by listening and looking at chest expansion for 10 seconds. If there is no spontaneous breathing, rescue breaths are administered. The rescuer's mouth is placed over the mouth and nose in infants, or the mouth alone while pinching the nose in older children, and at least two effective breaths given, confirmed by

adequate chest movement (Fig. 42). Assessment of cardiac output is determined by feeling a large pulse (brachial in infants, carotid in older children) for 10 seconds. In children, if there are no signs of circulation, external cardiac compressions are commenced by placing the heel of one hand over the midsternum and applying enough pressure to move the chest wall by about one-third to half the anterior–posterior diameter, at a rate of about 100 compressions per minute (Fig. 43). These are alternated with rescue breaths at a rate of 5 : 1 (see Section 2.5 and Table 14 for newborn resuscitation). Reassessment should be carried out every 60 seconds, and resuscitation discontinued if there are signs of life, help arrives, or the rescuer becomes exhausted (Fig. 44).

**Table 31** Antibiotic prophylaxis for endocarditis

| Procedure | Normal-risk patients | | High-risk patients |
|---|---|---|---|
| | First-line antibiotic | Penicillin allergy | |
| Dental, respiratory and oesophageal | Amoxycillin (O/IV/IM) | Macrolide (O) | |
| Other gastrointestinal genitourinary | Amoxycillin (IV) | Vancomycin (IV) | Amoxycillin OR vancomycin (IV) PLUS gentamicin (IV) |
| Infected soft tissue, bone/joint | Flucloxacillin (O) or third-generation cephalosporin (O) | Clindamycin (O) | Vancomycin (IV) |

O, oral route; IV, intravenous; IM, intramuscular.

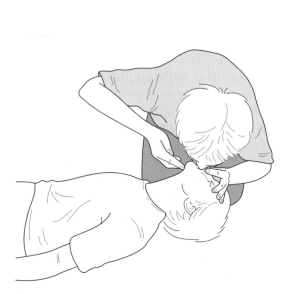

**Fig. 42** Rescue breaths in a child.

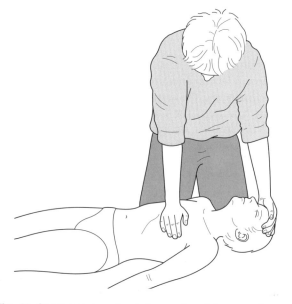

**Fig. 43** Chest compression between 1 and 8 years of age: one-hand technique.

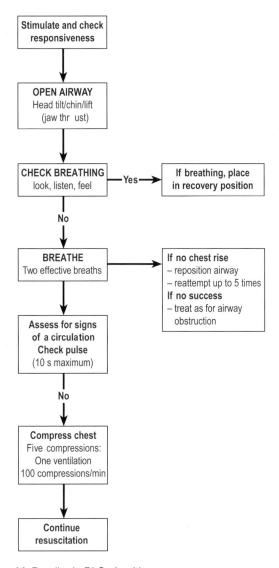

**Fig. 44** Paediatric BLS algorithm.

*Advanced life support*

In a hospital setting, or when trained help with appropriate equipment is available, resuscitation can proceed beyond the basic ABC. Again, safety must be ensured, followed by a call for help and the initiation of basic life support. An adequate airway may be established by means of airway adjuncts and ultimately endotracheal intubation (ETT). Breathing is assisted by ventilatory inflating bag devices with 100% oxygen, and external cardiac compressions provided as above. Intravenous access should be established as quickly as possible (although many drugs, such as epinephrine (adrenaline), lignocaine, atropine and naloxone, can be given down the ETT). The intraosseous route is now the preferred option if IV access is not available within 90 seconds. An ECG should be connected and the administration of drugs considered. Because the majority of collapsed children manifest asystole, the drug of choice is adrenaline (10 μg/kg) followed by a saline flush, and repeated every 3 minutes with continuous CPR (Fig. 45). Sodium bicarbonate is a second-line drug but should be considered where there has been prolonged CPR and the likelihood of a severe metabolic acidosis exists. Glucose

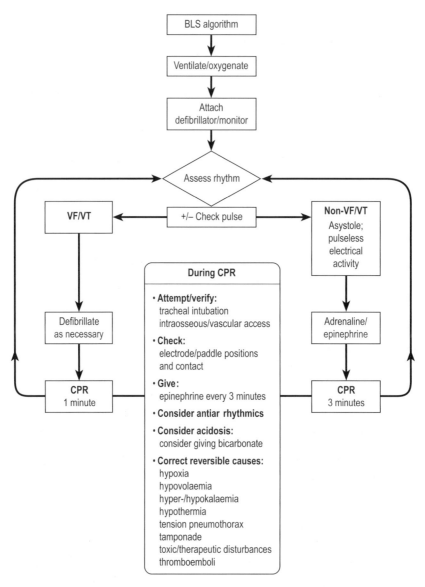

**Fig. 45** Management of cardiorespiratory arrest rhythms.

should not be forgotten, particularly in the neonate, and 5–10 mL/kg of 10% glucose should be given once hypoglycaemia is confirmed. Volume expanders such as normal saline (0.9%) and plasma substitutes are vital in shocked patients, and blood for haemorrhage. In those where the ECG confirms a shockable rhythm, i.e. ventricular fibrillation or pulseless ventricular tachycardia, DC shocks should be given and repeated at 60-second intervals, ensuring the safety of all the rescuers at all times (Fig. 45).

# Self-assessment: questions

## Multiple choice questions

1. The following describe the cardiac silhouette on X-ray:
   a. The right heart border is formed mainly by the right atrium
   b. The left border is formed mainly by the left atrium
   c. The left atrial appendage is prominent in children
   d. The thymic shadow may obscure the upper cardiac margins
   e. A right-sided aortic arch is always associated with other congenital heart defects.

2. The following statements are correct:
   a. Breathlessness is a manifestation of left heart failure
   b. Infants with congestive cardiac failure become more breathless on crying
   c. Cyanosis decreases on crying
   d. A good indicator of central cyanosis in infants is circumoral cyanosis
   e. A liver that is palpable 1 cm below the costal margin suggests right heart failure.

3. The following statements are true:
   a. Radiofemoral delay is a reliable sign of coarctation of the aorta in neonates
   b. A thrill is always indicative of a pathological murmur
   c. A parasternal lift suggests left ventricular hypertrophy
   d. A murmur originating from turbulence across the mitral valve is best heard at the left sternal edge
   e. The aortic component of the S2 follows the pulmonary component.

4. The following statements are true:
   a. Congenital heart disease occurs approximately once in every 100 live births
   b. Ventricular septal defect is the most common cardiac lesion in Down syndrome
   c. Coarctation of the aorta may be associated with hypertension
   d. Pulmonary stenosis requires surgical repair in almost all patients
   e. The nitrogen washout test amounts to placing a child in 100% oxygen.

5. The following congenital heart defects are examples of left-to-right shunts:
   a. Ventricular septal defect
   b. Tetralogy of Fallot
   c. Coarctation of the aorta
   d. Patent ductus arteriosus
   e. Aortopulmonary window.

6. The following complications are associated with left-to-right shunts:
   a. Lower respiratory tract infections
   b. Bacterial endocarditis
   c. Central cyanosis
   d. Syncopal attacks
   e. Systemic hypertension.

7. Congenital cardiac lesions that may result in failure to thrive include:
   a. Aortic stenosis
   b. Large ventricular septal defect
   c. Isolated, small muscular ventricular septal defect
   d. Atrial septal defects
   e. Moderate pulmonary stenosis.

8. In congenital heart disease, poorly palpable femoral pulses may be caused by:
   a. Hypercyanotic spells
   b. Coarctation of the aorta
   c. Arteritis
   d. Patent ductus arteriosus
   e. Aortic stenosis.

9. Blood flows predominantly from left to right in the following conditions:
   a. Atrial septal defect
   b. Fallot's tetralogy
   c. Ventricular septal defect
   d. Tricuspid atresia
   e. Duct-dependent congenital heart lesions.

10. Common complications of tetralogy of Fallot include:
    a. Failure to thrive
    b. Bacterial endocarditis
    c. Cerebral abscesses
    d. Cerebral thrombosis
    e. Congestive cardiac failure.

11. Cyanotic conditions usually presenting with symptoms at birth include:
    a. Pulmonary stenosis
    b. Tetralogy of Fallot
    c. Transposition of the great arteries with pulmonary stenosis
    d. Pulmonary atresia
    e. Tricuspid atresia.

12. The following operations may be used in cyanotic CHD:
    a. Senning procedure
    b. Rashkind balloon septostomy
    c. Aortic flap repair
    d. Blalock–Taussig shunt
    e. Fontan procedure.

13. The following are serious abnormalities:
    a. Multiple ventricular ectopics
    b. Sinus arrhythmia
    c. Atrial ectopic beats
    d. Complete A–V dissociation
    e. Bradycardia during sleep.

14. Supraventricular tachycardia:
    a. Can cause CCF in utero, resulting in hydrops fetalis
    b. Usually produces a heart rate of 120 bpm
    c. Is not usually associated with any symptoms
    d. Is increased by parasympathetic stimulation
    e. Can be treated using digoxin and propranolol.

15. The following associations are correct:
    a. Wide QRS and short P–R interval in Wolff–Parkinson–White syndrome
    b. Short Q–T, raised S–T in hypokalaemia
    c. Slow sinus rhythm and low-voltage complexes with hypothyroidism
    d. Coupled beats, S–T and T-wave depression with digoxin toxicity
    e. Short Q–T and hypocalcaemia.

16. The following associations are correct:
    a. Progressive prolongation of the P–R interval in Wenckebach block
    b. Ventricular tachycardia and increased blood pressure
    c. Flat QRS and T waves with pericarditis
    d. Atrial fibrillation and hyperthyroidism
    e. Tall R wave in $V_1$, deep S in $V_6$ in left ventricular hypertrophy.

17. Congestive cardiac failure (CCF) in childhood:
    a. Is rarely a manifestation of congenital heart disease
    b. Has particularly obvious symptoms during feeds in neonates
    c. Generally produces cardiomegaly and oligaemia as seen on the chest X-ray film
    d. May be the presenting abnormality in children with myocarditis
    e. Can be controlled with diuretics and digoxin in most cases.

18. First-line agents in the management of CCF include:
    a. Frusemide (furosemide)
    b. Oxygen
    c. Morphine
    d. Propranolol
    e. Digoxin.

19. Myocardial damage is associated with the following:
    a. Coxsackie virus B infection
    b. β-Haemolytic streptococcal infection
    c. Uraemia
    d. Diphtheria
    e. Cytotoxic agents, especially anthracyclines.

20. The manifestations of a pericardial effusion include:
    a. Pulmonary plethora on chest X-ray
    b. A fall in the jugular venous pressure on inspiration
    c. Pulsatile, tender hepatomegaly
    d. Pedal oedema but no ascites
    e. Globular cardiomegaly on chest X-ray.

## Case histories

### Case history 1

A 9-month-old infant presents with lethargy and failure to thrive. He had been admitted twice in the previous 3 months with chest infections. His mother had not noted any colour changes but was certain she could feel a 'vibration' beneath the chest wall.

How would you proceed to establish a diagnosis?

## Case history 2

An infant was well for the first 2 days of life, after which he became acutely unwell. He refused all feeds, was listless and breathless. On examination he was poorly perfused, tachycardic and tachypnoeic. A blood gas taken with the child in 100% oxygen showed a $P_{O_2}$ of 4.5 kPa.

How would you manage this child?

## Case history 3

A 5-year-old girl known to have a small VSD presents with fever of 10 days' duration. On examination she appears unwell and pale. Pedal oedema, a 3/6 pansystolic murmur heard best at the lower left sternal edge and basal pulmonary crepitations are detected. The splenic tip is just palpable.

What is the most likely diagnosis, and how would you investigate this child?

## Case history 4

A 2-year-old girl, previously operated on for Fallot's tetralogy at 10 days old, presents to the local district general hospital. You note a history of progressive lethargy over the past few weeks, as well as episodic attacks involving facial pallor and diminished exercise tolerance. The child looks cyanosed, and has a left-sided intercostal scar and a loud ejection systolic murmur in the pulmonary area.

1. What additional questions would you ask her parents?
2. What additional steps may you take to obtain further information?
3. What operation was performed on day 10 of life?

You organise some tests, which show a haemoglobin of 16.5 g/dL, haematocrit of 57%, oxygen saturation of 82% in air and marked oligaemia on the chest X-ray film.

4. What is the explanation for these results?

You admit the child for observation. During the next 24 hours the nurses reported that she remained lively, although she frequently became more 'blue' and had to stop and lie down while playing. On one occasion she became very pale and drowsy but responded to loud vocal stimulation.

5. What clinical complication should be considered at this point?
6. What is the physiological explanation for the intermittent decrease in oxygen saturations?
7. Why does the patient lie down while playing?
8. What further investigation is indicated?

You have organised transfer to the tertiary centre for next week but are called to see the child as an emergency on the second night. You find that she is unrousable, extremely pale, with weak pulses and no audible murmurs.

9. What is the explanation for this acute deterioration?
10. What action would you take?

## Short notes

Write short notes on the following:

1. Criteria to decide whether a heart murmur is likely to be functional (innocent) or related to an underlying structural abnormality.
2. The natural history of a moderately sized ventricular septal defect that is left unrepaired.
3. The management of heart failure.
4. The causes of cardiomyopathy.

## Viva voce question

What is the rationale for antibiotics as prophylaxis against bacterial endocarditis in children with congenital heart disease?

## OSCE questions

### OSCE 1

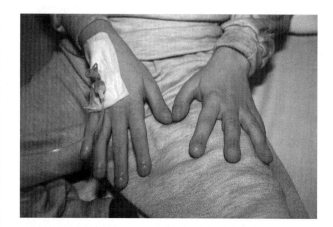

**Fig. 46**

1. What abnormality is shown in Figure 46?
2. Where might you observe similar abnormalities?
3. Name two causes for this abnormality.

### OSCE 2

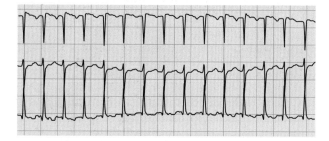

**Fig. 47**

a. What is the heart rate, and what does this ECG (Fig. 47) show?
b. What clinical manoeuvres may revert this rhythm to normal?

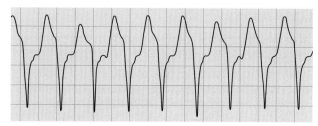

**Fig. 48**

a. What does this ECG (Fig. 48) show?
b. What immediate treatment is indicated?

# Self-assessment: answers

## Multiple choice answers

1. a. **True**. The right atrial border with a short section of superior vena cava above and inferior vena cava below.
   b. **False**. It is the left ventricle.
   c. **False**. This is inconspicuous in children.
   d. **True**. Classically it appears as an overlying 'sail' shadow.
   e. **False**. This can be associated with CHD (e.g. Fallot's tetralogy), but is also a normal variant.

2. a. **True**. Other symptoms are lethargy, excessive sweating and poor feeding.
   b. **True**. Crying, like feeding, increases the work of the heart.
   c. **False**. Cyanosis, like breathlessness, increases on crying.
   d. **False**. Central cyanosis is manifest by a bluish discoloration of the lips and mucous membranes.
   e. **False**. This is a common finding in normal children.

3. a. **False**. Brachial rather than radial artery should be used. In neonates, the heart rate is too rapid to detect 'delay' and a difference in pulse volume and BP is more important.
   b. **True**. Innocent murmurs are not accompanied by a thrill.
   c. **False**. It suggests right ventricular hypertrophy.
   d. **False**. Mitral murmurs are best heard over the apical impulse.
   e. **False**. Closure of the pulmonary valve is delayed compared with the aortic valve so that A2 preceeds P2.

4. a. **True**. It is roughly 8 in 1000 live births.
   b. **False**. Atrioventricular septal defects (AVSD).
   c. **True**. It affects both limbs or the right upper limb.
   d. **False**. Many are mild, requiring no intervention; the majority can be improved by balloon valvoplasty.
   e. **True**. Nitrogen is effectively 'washed out' in an environment consisting of 100% oxygen.

5. a. **True**. Blood flows from left to right ventricle.
   b. **False**. Right-to-left flow, resulting in cyanosis.
   c. **False**. No shunt present with simple coarctation.
   d. **True**.
   e. **True**. This is a connection between the aorta and pulmonary trunk.

6. a. **True**. Infections occur secondary to increased pulmonary plethora.
   b. **True**. Endocarditis may complicate VSDs where left-to-right shunts exist.
   c. **False**. Central cyanosis is associated with right-to-left shunt.
   d. **False**. Right-to-left shunts and arrhythmias give rise to syncopal attacks.
   e. **False**. Though pulmonary hypertension is a late feature of severe left-to-right shunting.

7. a. **False**. Aortic stenosis is asymptomatic or presents with exercise intolerance, arrhythmias and, occasionally, sudden death.
   b. **True**. Large VSDs present with heart failure in infancy, resulting in failure to thrive.
   c. **False**. It only occurs with large, multiple lesions.
   d. **False**. ASDs generally produce minimal haemodynamic constraints on the heart, and are therefore not usually associated with failure to thrive.
   e. **False**. Though it may occur with critical pulmonary stenosis.

8. a. **True**. In tetralogy of Fallot.
   b. **True**. This is the classic association.
   c. **True**. Arteritis involving the lower aorta and distal branches will result in poorly palpable femoral pulses.
   d. **False**. PDA gives rise to bounding pulses.
   e. **False**. Femoral pulses are generally palpable with aortic stenosis.

9. a. **True**. Almost always occurs.
   b. **False**. This is a cyanotic condition, therefore deoxygenated blood must bypass the lungs by shunting right to left across the VSD.
   c. **True**. Except if pulmonary hypertension develops with shunt reversal (Eisenmenger syndrome).

d. **False**. This is cyanotic CHD.

e. **False**. These are cyanotic conditions with right-to-left shunting at atrial level (tricuspid, pulmonary atresia) or ventricular level (TGA).

10. a. **True**. As with most cyanotic conditions.
    b. **True**. Occurs in unoperated patients on the right ventricular infundibulum or valves; after correction, patients will require antibiotic prophylaxis for dental and certain surgical procedures.
    c. **True**. From septic emboli secondary to endocarditis.
    d. **True**. Secondary to polycythaemia.
    e. **False**. Heart failure is not usually a feature of tetralogy of Fallot.

11. a. **False**. This is an acyanotic condition.
    b. **False**. These develop symptoms later in life.
    c. **True**. This presents with cyanosis, heart failure and sudden collapse in the newborn period.
    d. **True**. Presents with cyanosis in the newborn.
    e. **True**. Presents with cyanosis in the newborn.

12. a. **True**. For transposition of the great arteries.
    b. **True**. It is used for duct-dependent lesions.
    c. **False**. This is used to repair coarctation.
    d. **True**. This improves blood fiow to the lungs.
    e. **True**. This connects the right atrium to the pulmonary arteries.

13. a. **True**. Ventricular ectopics, especially when they occur in runs, are associated with significantly decreased cardiac output.
    b. **False**. This is a normal finding.
    c. **False**. Atrial ectopics are usually isolated phenomena and are not associated with altered cardiac function.
    d. **True**. This is third-degree heart block.
    e. **False**. This is a normal finding.

14. a. **True**. It is a relatively common cause of hydrops fetalis.
    b. **False**. The heart rate is more than 180 bpm.
    c. **False**. Symptoms include breathlessness, tiredness, syncope, palpitations.
    d. **False**. This will slow an SVT.
    e. **True**. As well as flecainide.

15. a. **True**. Together with a $\delta$ wave, these are classic features of the WPW syndrome.
    b. **False**. Long Q–T and depressed S–T occur in hyperkalaemia.
    c. **True**. Classic ECG findings in hypothyroidism.

d. **True**. As well as other dysrrhythmias.

e. **False**. Hypocalcaemia is associated with a long Q–T.

16. a. **True**. In Wenckebach secondary block the P–R interval increases progressively until a QRS potential does not materialise and a beat is dropped.
    b. **False**. There is a loss in cardiac output and BP falls.
    c. **True**. Small voltage complexes are typical of pericarditis.
    d. **True**. Hyperthyroidism is associated with rapid arrhythmias, including atrial fibrillation.
    e. **False**. These occur in RV hypertrophy; LV hypertrophy produces tall R in $V_6$ (>20 mm), deep S in $V_1$ (>20 mm).

17. a. **False**. CCF is common in many cyanotic, duct-dependent conditions and those involving an excessive left-to-right shunt (e.g. VSD).
    b. **True**. This is when they are required to exert maximum effort.
    c. **False**. It produces cardiomegaly and pulmonary plethora.
    d. **True**. Sometimes with associated arrhythmias.
    e. **True**. Though angiotensin-converting enzyme (ACE) inhibitors may be used as well.

18. a. **True**. Frusemide primarily reduces afterload on the heart.
    b. **True**.
    c. **False**. However, it may be used with caution in those in severe distress (NB: it may cause respiratory depression).
    d. **False**. It may precipitate CCF.
    e. **True**. Although still available, its use in childhood is becoming less popular.

19. a. **True**. The virus causes infective myocarditis.
    b. **True**. It gives rise to rheumatic fever.
    c. **True**. This causes chemical myocarditis.
    d. **True**. Toxic myocardiopathy occurs in 15% of patients with diphtheria and is responsible for around 55% of deaths, usually because of secondary arrhythmias.
    e. **True**. Anthracyclines (e.g. doxorubicin, daunorubicin) can result in dose-dependent myocardial damage, loss of myocardial cells and progressive cardiomyopathy.

20. a. **True**. Plethora is secondary to restriction to venous return from the lungs.
    b. **False**. There is a rise in the JVP on inspiration.

c. **True**. It is caused by restriction to venous return and subsequent venous congestion in the lower body.
d. **False**. Both pedal oedema and ascites occur.
e. **True**. Uniform cardiomegaly is typical of a pericardial effusion on X-ray.

## Case history answers

### Case history 1

The history is suggestive of an acyanotic congenital cardiac defect associated with increased pulmonary blood flow and a significant left-to-right shunt. The first stage would be to complete a thorough history and examination, concentrating on symptoms and signs of heart failure and looking for bounding pulses, precordial heaves, a thrill, murmur, pulmonary crepitations and hepatomegaly. An ECG should be ordered to look for signs of ventricular hypertrophy, and a chest X-ray to establish whether the child has cardiomegaly and pulmonary plethora. A provisional diagnosis can now be made. This should be confirmed by echocardiography, which should reveal both the structural abnormality and the extent of the intracardiac shunt. Further information regarding the abnormality and the shunt, as well as intracardiac pressures and oxygen saturation, can be obtained during cardiac angiography, using catheter techniques. The last is particularly useful when investigating a patient prior to consideration for corrective cardiac surgery.

### Case history 2

The history is highly suggestive of a duct-dependent congenital heart condition; the collapse has been precipitated by closure of the ductus arteriosus, resulting in cyanosis and serious compromise of the cardiac output. The possible diagnoses at this age would include transposition of the great arteries, tricuspid and pulmonary atresias, and complex congenital heart disease.

Regardless of the diagnosis, the infant is severely hypoxic and shocked. Therefore, the management should include resuscitation with oxygen and fluids in order to re-establish a reasonable BP. An attempt should be made to reopen the duct with prostaglandin $E_2$, and respiratory support should be considered. An ECG and chest X-ray should be ordered, a referral to a paediatric cardiac centre organised, and arrangements made for an urgent echocardiogram.

### Case history 3

This child has probably developed subacute bacterial endocarditis. Embolic signs of SABE, including lesions on the hands (splinter haemorrhages, Janeway spots), retina (Roth spots) and kidneys (haematuria), should be looked for. She requires immediate admission to hospital, treatment of the heart failure and urgent investigation. It is important to confirm the microbiological diagnosis and repeated blood cultures should be taken, preferably during a temperature 'spike'. Arterial rather than venous samples are more likely to provide positive cultures. An ECG is required to exclude associated arrhythmias, a chest X-ray to assess cardiomegaly and plethora, and an echocardiogram to look for intracardiac vegetations and assess cardiac damage (e.g. heart valves) and ventricular function.

### Case history 4

1. You need to know whether she has had any faints or whether she squats while playing. You require the precise details of the original operation. You need to know if she is on any regular medication. You require details of the tertiary cardiac centre, her consultant etc.
2. Contact the tertiary centre for all relevant details.
3. A left sided Blalock–Taussig (B–T) shunt.
4. Progressive hypoxia has resulted in a compensatory increase in circulating red cells, resulting in polycythaemia with an increased haemoglobin. The X-ray examination confirms poor blood flow into the lungs, suggesting that the patient is outgrowing her palliative B–T shunt, which is no longer adequate.
5. The patient is having hypercyanotic spells.
6. Progressive right ventricular outlet tract (RVOT) obstruction has resulted in right ventricular hypertrophy and a progressive rise in RV pressure. Eventually the RV pressure has equalled – and later surpassed – the LV pressure, and blood is now shunting from right to left across the VSD along the reversed pressure gradient. As a consequence, deoxygenated blood is passing directly into the systemic circulation and bypassing the lungs. Acute exacerbations in the RVOT obstruction lead to sudden cyanotic spells, which manifest as acute pallor/dusky attacks.
7. Hypercyanotic spells are associated with profound hypoxia, which prohibits physical exertion. In some cases the situation is severe enough to result in syncope. Squatting or lying down increases the systemic vascular resistance and hence the LV pressure. This action also decreases venous return

to the right heart and, in so doing, may decrease the shunt across the VSD and reduce the degree of cyanosis.

8. This story should prompt a further re-evaluation of the patient with an echocardiography and, possibly, cardiac angiography, with a view to planning an urgent corrective surgical procedure.

9. Total obstruction of the RVOT has resulted in no blood flow across the pulmonary infundibulum and valvular area, and hence the disappearance of the murmur. This has led to profound hypoxia, culminating in syncope.

10. Such severe attacks may be aborted with intravenous morphine and propranolol, which reduce the muscular obstruction in the RVOT. The patient should be given oxygen, stabilised, and transferred urgently to the tertiary centre.

## Short notes answers

1. The criteria can be divided into the following areas.

    **History**. An innocent murmur would have complete absence of symptoms. Symptoms indicative of an abnormality include:

    • Breathlessness
    • Excessive fatigue, malaise
    • Poor exercise tolerance, poor feeding
    • Colour changes
    • Recurrent chest infections
    • Failure to thrive
    • Palpitations.

    **Examination**. In an innocent murmur there would be no clinical signs apart from the murmur. The murmur:

    • Would be systolic, normal heart sounds
    • Would be soft, occasionally shrill; never >3/6; no thrill
    • Would have little radiation
    • Would be heard over precordium and/or neck (not back)
    • Changes with position of the head and neck
    • Decreases on lying down and with pressure on the ipsilateral jugular vein
    • May be exacerbated by exertion.

    **Investigations**. ECG, chest X-ray, echocardiogram examinations are all normal in an innocent murmur.

    **Follow-up**. No abnormal symptoms/signs develop. The murmur often disappears with time.

2. A moderate VSD is associated with a left-to-right shunt. This increases pulmonary blood flow. If not repaired, this results in the establishment of pulmonary arterial hypertension over a period of years. During this time the child is likely to develop several lower respiratory tract infections and worsening heart failure. The excessive energy expenditure in maintaining cardiac output results in failure to thrive. Depending on the severity of the shunt, irreversible pulmonary hypertension will develop by the second or third decade. This will eventually lead to systemic and suprasystemic pressures in the right ventricle and the left-to-right shunt reverses (Eisenmenger syndrome). The patient would become cyanosed and the condition no longer operable. Death from pulmonary hypertension and heart failure would be inevitable.

3. The management of cardiac failure includes the following (NB: measures appropriate to an intensive setting are shown in italics):

    General advice

    • Improve calorie intake
    • Avoid excessive salt in diet
    • Sit/sleep upright
    • Treat infections.

    Improve oxygenation

    • Correct anaemia
    • *Give oxygen.*

    Inotropic support

    • Digoxin
    • *Dopamine, dobutamine.*

    Load reduction

    • Diuretics: frusemide (furosemide), spironolactone
    • Vasodilators: hydralazine, *nitrates, nitroprusside.*

4. The causes of cardiomyopathy include:

    • Idiopathic
    • Post infection (especially viral)
    • Drugs (e.g. cytotoxics)
    • Inborn errors of metabolism (e.g. glycogen storage disease).

## Viva voce answer

Children with a structural abnormality of the heart, an endocardial scar or intracardiac prosthetic material are at risk of developing bacterial overgrowth at the abnormal site. This takes the form of adherent vegetations, which may result in local damage and valvular dysfunction and carries the risk of distant embolic disease. The risk of bacterial organisms 'lodging' on these sites is particularly great during a bacteraemic episode. Therefore, any procedure known to result in bacteraemia, such as dental procedures, gastrointestinal, urogenital and other surgical procedures, should be covered with antibiotics. Thereby, organisms released into the circulation are killed before they can establish a focus of endocarditis. The organisms involved are usually staphylococcal, streptococcal and coliform species, and therefore prophylaxis generally involves a penicillin and an aminoglycoside antibiotic.

## OSCE answers

### OSCE 1
1. Finger clubbing with peripheral cyanosis
2. The toes

3. a. Any cause of cyanotic congenital heart disease, e.g. tetralogy of Fallot, pulmonary atresia
   b. Cystic fibrosis

### OSCE 2
Figure 47

a. 280–300 bpm
   supraventricular tachycardia
   (sinus tachycardia)
b. Valsalva manouvre, diving reflex, ice-cold immersion, carotid sinus massage (eyeball pressure)

Figure 48

a. Wide QRS complex ventricular tachycardia (VT)
b. Electrical defibrillation (cardioversion)

# 5

# The digestive system

**5.1** Introduction     105

**5.2** Abdominal pain     106

**5.3** Vomiting     107

**5.4** Constipation     108

**5.5** Diarrhoea     108

**5.6** Genetic/inflammatory disorders     111

**5.7** Disorders of the liver, pancreas and peritoneum     114

Self-assessment: questions     117

Self-assessment: answers     120

## Overview

This chapter covers the basic examination of the abdomen and reviews common presenting symptoms in childhood and infancy, such as abdominal pain, vomiting and reflux. You should have a good understanding of the common infections of the gastrointestinal tract, and in particular you need to be able to assess for dehydration in a child with diarrhoea and know how to correct rehydration. Some chronic and inflammatory gastrointestinal disorders that can lead to malabsorption and failure to thrive, such as coeliac disease, are common, whereas others such as Crohn's disease and ulcerative colitis are relatively uncommon. Nevertheless, these conditions contribute significantly to the workload of a general paediatric unit and are covered in some detail. Finally, this chapter reviews the more common disorders of the liver, and especially the various hepatic infections.

## 5.1 Introduction

### Normal features and assessment

The normal function of the gastrointestinal tract is dependent on the balance achieved by the normal motility of the gut, the sphincter tone, exocrine secretion, the integrity of the absorptive surfaces and humoral control. These functions begin in utero, when amniotic fluid is swallowed by the fetus. The gut undergoes rapid maturation at birth as it adjusts to the onset of intermittent oral feeding and colonisation by microflora. The coordinated swallowing movements develop in the first couple of months, and the infant begins to show an interest in solid foods at about 4 months. The earliest stools after birth consist of meconium. As the baby begins to feed, green-brown transition stools replace meconium. Subsequently, there can be a wide variation in the consistency and frequency of the stools, influenced in part by the kind of food and milk being ingested. A protuberant abdomen is common in infants and toddlers and is related to the lordotic stance adopted at that age. It is common to find a palpable liver (up to 2 cm) and a soft spleen tip. As the abdominal musculature is underdeveloped at this age, the vertebral column and abdominal aortic pulsations are easily felt. It is also normal to be able to feel stools in the left lower quadrant in the descending and sigmoid colon.

### Examination of the gastrointestinal tract

During the examination of the gastrointestinal tract in children it is important to look for systemic signs of dysfunction. These include anaemia, jaundice, clubbing, dependent oedema, distended veins and state of hydration. Remove all clothes so that the pelvic region is clearly visible, otherwise you can easily miss torsion of the testis or an incarcerated hernia! Inspection of the abdomen is often a clue to the presence of organ enlargement or a mass, with the umbilicus often pushed away from the distending mass. A child's abdomen is soft, and vigorous palpation can miss a soft but enlarged liver or spleen. It is better to start palpating with the edge of the index finger, lower down in the right inguinal fossa, and dipping the extended fingers during expiration. Children do not localise pain very well and careful examination is required to identify regions of tenderness or guarding. Hernial orifices, the scrotum and anal regions must be examined and, when required, a rectal examination is performed.

## 5.2 Abdominal pain

### Acute abdominal pain

In children, acute abdominal pain is a common problem. A carefully elicited history and physical examination is often sufficient to distinguish surgical from medical conditions. Most of the conditions mentioned in Figure 49 are described elsewhere in the book and will not be discussed further.

### Recurrent abdominal pain

Recurrent abdominal pain is a common problem affecting 10% of children. No cause is found in 90% of cases, and in the rest a urinary bacterial infection or constipation is often the cause. It is essential to identify those with an organic condition promptly. This enables specific management of physical disease and confident counselling of those with a functional problem. In most cases, a careful history and examination may lead to a diagnosis. The periodicity of the complaint, localisation of pain to the periumbilical or hypochondrial regions, absence of coexistent symptoms and intervening good health suggest the absence of an organic cause. Furthermore, the absence of nocturnal symptoms is generally a reassuring sign. Usually a blood count, urine culture and urinalysis are sufficient in the way of investigation. Those with more severe symptoms should be seen during an attack and may require further investigations, as outlined in Table 32.

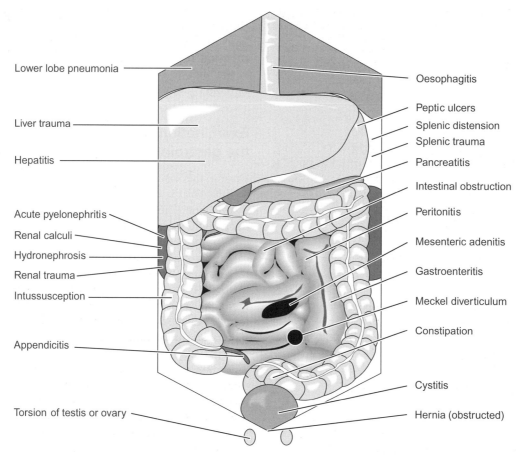

**Fig. 49** Causes of acute abdominal pain.

**Table 32** Causes of recurrent abdominal pain in children

| Disorder | Characteristics | Identifying features |
|---|---|---|
| **Intolerance** | | |
| Lactose intolerance | Bloating, flatulence, diarrhoea | Hydrogen breath test, reducing substances in stool, stool pH |
| Excessive fructose or sorbitol ingestion | Bloating, diarrhoea | Large intake of fruit, fruit juices or sorbitol-containing sweets |
| **Inflammatory** | | |
| Acid peptic disease | Pain related to meals relieved by antacids | Endoscopy, upper GI contrast X-rays, pH study |
| Cholecystitis | Right upper quadrant pain | Ultrasound of the abdomen |
| Pancreatitis | Persistent boring pain, may radiate to the back | Serum amylase, lipase, ultrasound |
| **Infection** | | |
| Parasite infection | Diarrhoea, bloating | Stool evaluation, test for *Giardia* sp. |
| **Metabolic/genetic** | | |
| Diabetic ketoacidosis | Acidosis, dehydration | Blood sugar, ketones |
| Sickle crisis | Anaemia | Haematological evaluation |
| Gilbert syndrome | Jaundice | Serum bilirubin |
| Acute intermittent porphyria | Severe pain precipitated by drugs, infection, fasting | Urine porphyrins |
| **Surgical** | | |
| Hernia | Dull abdominal wall pain | Physical examination, computed tomography (CT) scan |
| Cholelithiasis | May worsen with meals | Ultrasound of the abdomen |
| Renal calculi | Severe, intermittent colic | Ultrasound and plain abdominal X-rays |
| **Others** | | |
| Constipation | Difficult, infrequent firm stool | Examination, PR, plain abdominal X-ray |
| Henoch–Schönlein purpura | Systemic symptoms | Clinical diagnosis, urinalysis |
| Abdominal migraine | Nausea, family history | Typical history; normal examination |
| Abdominal epilepsy | May have prodrome | EEG |
| Lead poisoning | Constipation, anaemia | Serum lead level, haemoglobin |

## 5.3 Vomiting

### Learning objectives

You should:

* know the common causes for vomiting in young children
* be able to diagnose and manage a child with gastro-oesophageal reflux

Vomiting is a common symptom in childhood. Although the cause is often benign, it can result in a great deal of distress. The aetiology is age related. Healthy infants often *posset* or regurgitate feeds. This may happen many times a day and the infant is usually content, though possibly hungry. This may be quite distressing to the parent, as apart from all other considerations it makes all the clothes smell of vomit. Vomiting is coordinated by the medullary vomiting centre, which is influenced by the chemoreceptor trigger zone and higher CNS centres. Therefore, many systemic conditions may precipitate vomiting. These include causes of raised intracranial pressure, inborn errors of metabolism, systemic acidosis, medications and chemotherapy. Infections, either systemic or localised (otitis media, cystitis, meningitis), can also present initially with vomiting. The common gastrointestinal causes of vomiting include infections, obstruction or motility problems (Box 26).

### Gastro-oesophageal reflux

When the lower oesophageal sphincter is not competent, excessive and passive reflux of the gastric contents may cause significant symptoms. Vomiting or regurgitation has its onset usually within the first week of life and abates by the age of 2 years as the child attains a more upright posture. Bleeding due to the associated oesophagitis results in iron-deficiency anaemia and, rarely, haematemesis. Aspiration pneumonia occurs in infancy and can lead to chronic coughing, wheezing and recurrent pneumonia in childhood. In mild cases, a diagnosis is often made by a response to therapy. More complex cases are confirmed by barium oesophagography under fluoroscopic control, endoscopy, gastric scintiscans, or by continuous monitoring of the distal

---

**Box 26** Causes of acute vomiting

**Gastrointestinal causes**

| | |
|---|---|
| Intestinal obstruction | bile-stained with upper GI obstruction; abdominal distension with lower GI obstruction |
| Oesophagitis | bloodstained vomitus |
| Pyloric stenosis | projectile vomiting |
| Gastroenteritis | often with diarrhoea ± dehydration |

**CNS causes**

| | |
|---|---|
| Raised intracranial pressure | |
| Infections | meningitis, encephalitis |
| Tumours | |

**Others**
Urinary tract infections
Inborn errors of metabolism
Cyclical vomiting

---

oesophageal pH. In most children, simple measures are often effective. Appropriate management includes increased time spent in a baby chair, nursing in the prone position with the head-end elevated, thickening of feeds, antacids, addition of an alginate preparation (e.g. Gaviscon), prokinetic agents (e.g. domperidone) and, if indicated by pH studies, a histamine $H_2$ receptor antagonist or omeprazole. Where there is danger of an oesophageal stricture forming, surgical intervention in the form of a Nissen fundoplication may be necessary.

## Peptic ulceration

Acute ulcers occur in the stomach and are usually a result of stress or drugs such as non-steroidal anti-inflammatories (NSAIDs) or steroids. Chronic ulcers tend to occur in the duodenum and are associated with *Helicobacter pylori* (*H. pylori*) infection. Diagnosis is usually made on endoscopy, and *H. pylori* can be detected on biopsy or a rapid urease test. Omeprazole or ranitidine promotes ulcer healing, and a 6-week course of antibiotics such as amoxicillin, clarithromycin and metronidazole helps to eradicate *H. pylori*.

## 5.4 Constipation

### Learning objectives

You should:

- know the common causes of constipation in a young child

- be able to offer advice to the mother of a child with constipation

The definition of constipation is relative. Many children may only have a soft stool once every 2–3 days, which is passed without difficulty. Only when the stool is hard and there are problems in passing it should a diagnosis of constipation be made. A nursing infant may have infrequent stools. True constipation in the neonatal period is usually secondary to Hirschsprung disease, neurological or spinal disease, intestinal obstruction, drugs or hypothyroidism. In the majority of children constipation is functional in origin. Ineffective colonic peristalsis, also seen with opiate use and hypothyroidism, will result in defective rectal filling. The resultant stasis leads to the excessive drying of stool and a failure to initiate reflexes from the rectum that normally trigger evacuation. This process is controlled by pressor receptors in the rectal muscles. Consequently, disorders of the spine and of the nerves and muscles that coordinate the action of the rectal muscles and control the anal sphincter may contribute to faecal retention. Constipation tends to be self-perpetuating. Hard and large stools in the rectum become more painful and difficult to evacuate, especially if compounded by the presence of an anal fissure. Distension of the rectum and colon decreases the sensitivity of the defecation reflex and the effectiveness of peristalsis. Finally, watery colonic contents may percolate around hard stool and be passed unperceived by the child. This involuntary *encopresis* or soiling may be mistaken for diarrhoea. Although constipation in itself causes no long-term systemic effects, it can have a marked emotional effect on the family. In those with functional problems, treatment is divided into four phases: education about the problem; disimpaction, usually with a phosphate enema or stool softeners; prevention of the reaccumulation of stools, usually achieved with dietary control and laxatives; and reconditioning to normal bowel habits. The last may have to wait until an anal fissure has healed, and needs to be positively reinforced by using star charts or small rewards.

## 5.5 Diarrhoea

### Learning objectives

You should:

- know the common causes of diarrhoea in childhood

- be able to assess and manage a child with dehydration

# Acute diarrhoea

Worldwide there are an estimated one billion episodes of and 3.3 million deaths due to diarrhoea each year among children aged less than 5 years. In the developed world gastroenteritis is common and usually mild, but should not be underestimated. The common aetiological agents and their basic pathogenetic mechanisms are described in Table 33. The mechanisms of diarrhoea differ with the infective agent. The organism may:

- Invade the mucosa, causing inflammation of the lamina
- Produce cytotoxins that disrupt cell function and protein synthesis
- Secrete an enterotoxin that alters cellular salt and water balance yet leaves the cell morphology undisturbed
- Adhere to the mucosal surface, disrupting normal cell function.

About 75% of fluid ingested, which includes the gastric, pancreaticobiliary and intestinal secretions, is reabsorbed by the small intestine and about 24% by the large intestine. Primary absorption of water in the small intestine is done in the *tip* cells of the microvilli. This is an active process using sodium–glucose and sodium–amino acid transporters. Sodium and chloride ions are exchanged actively for hydrogen and bicarbonate ions, maintaining both electroneutrality and pH homeostasis. An active intracellular pump then pumps the excess sodium into the bloodstream and the chloride back into the lumen.

## Osmotic diarrhoea

As shown in Figure 50, rotavirus invades and destroys the mature villus tip cells. This leads to an increased migration of immature cells from the crypt that are unable to carry on the absorptive process, and an *osmotic diarrhoea* results. The cells are restored in 48–72 hours and

**Table 33** Infective causes of acute diarrhoea in childhood

| Pathogen | Enterotoxin | Cytotoxin | Invasive | Adhesive | Symptoms | Antimicrobial therapy[a] |
|---|---|---|---|---|---|---|
| *Escherichia coli* | | | | | | |
| Enterotoxicogenic | ST, LT | | | + | WD | |
| Enteropathogenic | | | | | WD | Cotrimoxazole |
| Enteroinvasive | | | +++ | | D | Ciprofloxacin |
| | | | | | | Azithromycin |
| | | | | | | Ceftriaxone |
| Enterohaemorrhagic | | +++ | | D | | |
| Enteroaggregative | ++ | ++ | | + | WD | |
| Enteroadhesive | | | | +++ | WD | |
| *Shigella* species | Shiga | | +++ | | WD, D | Cotrimoxazole |
| | | | | | | Ciprofloxacin |
| | | | | | | Azithromycin |
| *Salmonella* species | + | + | ++ | | WD, D | Cefotaxime |
| | | | | | | Cotrimoxazole |
| | | | | | | Azithromycin |
| *Vibrio cholerae* | A and B | | | | WD | Doxycycline |
| | | | | | | Cotrimoxazole |
| | | | | | | Ciprofloxacin |
| *Campylobacter jejuni* | + | | ++ | | WD, D | Erythromycin (macrolides) |
| | | | | | | Ciprofloxacin |
| | | | | | | Azithromycin |
| *Clostridium difficile* | A and B | | ++ | | PMC | Metronidazole |
| | | | | | | Vancomycin[c] |
| Rotavirus | | Cytotoxic | | | WD | – |
| *Entamoeba histolytica* | | | +++ | | D | Metronidazole |
| *Giardia lamblia* | | | | +++ | | Metronidazole |
| *Cryptosporidium* sp. | ? | Cytotoxic | | | | Paromomycin[b] |

ST, stable toxin; LT, labile toxin; WD, watery diarrhoea; D, blood and mucus, dysentery; PMC, pseudomembranous colitis, bloody diarrhoea, usually antibiotic related.
[a] Only some of the antibiotics that can be used are mentioned. In most instances there are specific indications for using antibiotics, e.g. injudicious use of antibiotics in *Salmonella* infections may actually prolong excretion.
[b] Only for use in those with AIDS.

## Osmotic diarrhoea

## Secretory diarrhoea

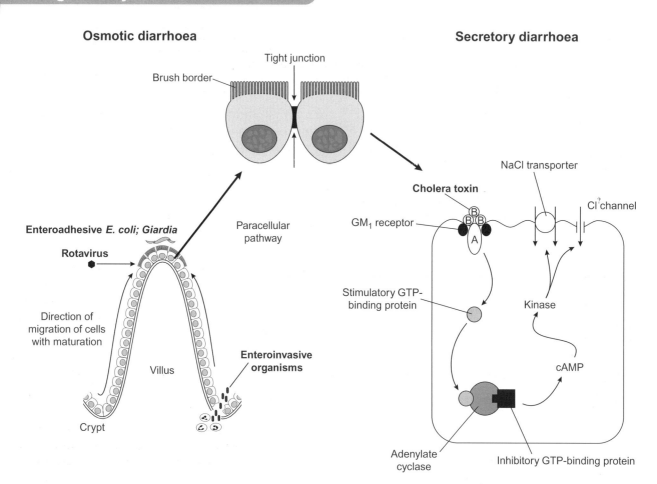

**Fig. 50** Mechanisms of acute diarrhoea.

the diarrhoea resolves. Pathogens such as *Giardia* and enteroadhesive *Escherichia coli* can adhere to the brush border, blunting the microvilli and decreasing their absorptive capacity, and invasive pathogens can destroy the villus cells, causing an inflammatory exudate.

### Secretory diarrhoea

Secretory diarrhoeas occur with enterotoxin-producing organisms. Figure 50 illustrates the binding of cholera toxin subunit B to the glycolipid (GM$_1$) receptor. Subunit A penetrates the cell, and by increasing cyclic AMP (cAMP), inhibits the sodium/chloride ion pump and stimulates the chloride channel. As water follows the sodium ion gradient, this results in secretion of water and electrolytes into the intestinal lumen. The toxins produced by enterotoxicogenic *E. coli* behave in a similar fashion.

### Site of action

In general, enterotoxin-producing agents infect the small intestine, invasive and cytotoxin-producing organisms favour the large intestine, and those with enteroadhesive function are seen at both sites.

### Dehydration

The result of any of these mechanisms is the net loss of fluid and electrolytes from the body, which is more severe in secretory diarrhoeas. It can place a severe stress on infants, who have a higher percentage of body water, a higher metabolic rate and a larger surface-to-volume ratio. The assessment of dehydration relies upon a series of clinical signs that reflect changes in body tissues and circulatory status (Table 34).

In general, mild and moderate dehydration can be corrected using oral rehydration solutions, which contain glucose or sucrose with sodium chloride. Malnourished children often have chronic deficits of electrolytes and depleted energy reserves. The WHO ORS (oral rehydration solution) therefore has a significantly higher electrolyte content than the solutions commonly used in the UK (Table 35). The solutions vary in composition and often come as powders that require reconstitution. In such cases, careful instructions must be given to the parents to ensure that the solution is made up as recommended. Where such commercial formulations are not available, cheap local ingredients such as boiled rice water with added salt (to taste as

**Table 34** Assessment of dehydration

| | Dehydration (loss in body weight, %) | | |
| --- | --- | --- | --- |
| | Mild (<5%) | Moderate (5–9%) | Severe (>10%) |
| Heart rate | Normal | Increased | Tachycardia/bradycardia in prearrest situation |
| Blood pressure | Normal | Normal or reduced | Greatly reduced |
| Skin | Normal | Decreased turgor | Decreased turgor |
| Fontanelle | Normal | Normal/slightly depressed | Sunken |
| Mucous membrane | Slightly dry | Dry | Dry |
| Extremities | Perfused | Delayed capillary refill | Cool, mottled |
| Mental status | Normal | Normal or lethargic | Lethargy, coma |
| Urine output | Slightly decreased | Decreased | Absent |
| Thirst | Slightly increased | Increased | Greatly increased |

**Table 35** Oral rehydration therapy

| Composition | UK (mmol/L) | World Health Organization (mmol/L) |
| --- | --- | --- |
| Sodium ions | 30–50 | 90 |
| Potassium ions | 20 | 20 |
| Chloride ions | 30–50 | 80 |
| Citrate | 10 | 10 |
| Glucose | 200 | 100 |
| Osmolality | 200–265 | 310 |

salty as tears) can be used. The deficit is generally given over a 4–6-hour period, and at that time a gradual reintroduction of normal diet can be started while still providing replacement fluids. In some cases of moderate dehydration and in those with severe dehydration, it is best to use intravenous rehydration. Where the child is in shock, 10–20% of the deficit may be replaced by bolus infusion of crystalloid or colloid solutions. Acidosis may accompany dehydration, and although rehydration will correct this to an extent, if it is severe enough to cause air hunger, sodium bicarbonate can be added to the infusion. Serum electrolytes need to be monitored, as dehydration can be associated with hypo- and hypernatraemia. Antibiotics are used only in specific instances (e.g. *Vibrio cholerae*), and *antidiarrhoeal and antiemetic agents are not recommended*. In most cases early feeding will actually enhance the ability of the intestine to regenerate, and there is little to recommend the use of dilute or low-lactose-containing formulae on a routine basis to 'decrease the osmotic load'.

## Chronic diarrhoea

Persistent diarrhoea in an otherwise thriving child is not an unusual complaint. Chronic non-specific diarrhoea (CNSD), or so-called toddler's diarrhoea, occurs between 1 and 5 years of age. Typically, watery stools are produced four to ten times a day and often contain undigested food particles. The child remains otherwise well. The most likely explanation for this is an exaggerated gastrocolic reflex. Therapy is directed at reassuring anxious parents, decreasing the amount of fluid and fruit juice ingested, and increasing the fibre and fat content of the diet.

### Postinfectious diarrhoea

Postinfectious diarrhoea is caused by brush border damage. This leads to secondary, reversible disaccharidase deficiencies, and the diarrhoea persists because of secondary cow's milk or lactose intolerance. This may be aggravated in children allergic to cow's milk protein or soy protein substitutes, which are often used in such cases. A change to more easily tolerated foods (such as starch-based compounds) is usually all that is required. Rarely some children may have congenital lactase or sucrase–isomaltase deficiency or galactose–glucose malabsorption; these are characterised by diarrhoea from birth, and the child will require lifelong abstinence from foods containing the offending sugars.

## 5.6 Genetic/inflammatory disorders

### Learning objectives

You should:

- appreciate the different clinical presentations of coeliac disease, Crohn's disease and ulcerative colitis

- be familiar with the different diagnostic tests required to make a diagnosis of coeliac disease, Crohn's disease or ulcerative colitis

There are several gastrointestinal disorders of uncertain aetiology that may involve a genetic susceptibility and immune-mediated pathogenesis.

## Gluten-sensitive enteropathy (coeliac disease)

Gluten-sensitive enteropathy or coeliac disease (CD) is a permanent inability to tolerate dietary wheat or rye gluten. The susceptibility to developing coeliac disease is probably inherited, and the incidence is 1 in 2000 in the UK and as high as 1 in 300 in western Ireland. However, the wide range of phenotypes, from active to silent disease, suggests that early dietary and environmental factors play a role as well. CD is an immunologically mediated small-intestinal enteropathy that results in progressive flattening of the villi and malabsorption. The majority of children present before the age of 2 years, with progressive growth failure dating from the time gluten-containing solids were introduced into the diet. Symptoms include greasy, bulky, foul-smelling stools and vomiting. The child becomes irritable, anorexic, anaemic and hypotonic, with a protuberant abdomen and wasted buttocks. The condition is suspected by the presence of anaemia, which may be microcytic or macrocytic because of iron and folate deficiencies, as well as the presence of antigliadin, antiendomysial and tissue transglutaminase antibodies in the serum. Confirmation of the diagnosis is by an intestinal biopsy (Fig. 51) and the therapeutic response to a gluten-free diet. The therapy is withdrawal of wheat, rye, oats and barley, as these contain gluten, and the introduction of rice and maize-based cereals. Although some children will tolerate gluten in their diet at a later age, there is concern that those who are not on a gluten-free diet are at an increased risk of developing small bowel malignancies, especially lymphoma. Dietary restrictions are therefore best recommended lifelong, though compliance may be an issue in the turbulent teens.

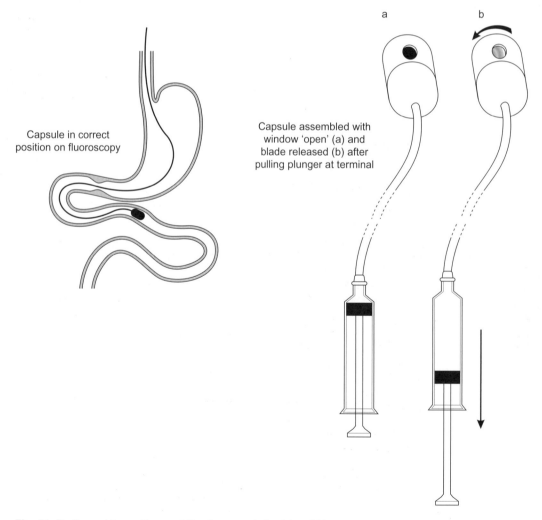

Capsule in correct position on fluoroscopy

Capsule assembled with window 'open' (a) and blade released (b) after pulling plunger at terminal

**Fig. 51** Radiographic position and Crosby capsule for jejunal biopsy.

## Crohn's disease (regional enteritis)

Although the aetiology of Crohn's disease remains unknown, there has been a dramatic increase in its prevalence, with approximately 10–20 per 100 000 children affected in the UK. Although a genetic predisposition is likely, current research is focused on abnormalities in the intestinal mucosal immune system, which is thought to be dysregulated by the faecal stream. The initial lesion is a localised ulcer over a lymphoid follicle. These ulcers then coalesce and inflammation spreads to deeper tissue. Characteristically, there is segmental involvement with 'skip areas' and the bowel wall becomes thickened. Loops of bowel may become adherent, and fistulae can develop and progress into chronic abscesses. Later in the course of the disease deep fissures may form, leading to the classic 'cobblestone' appearance of the mucosa (Fig. 52) as well as the development of strictures. In children, 50–60% have involvement of the terminal ileum and variable segments of the colon, 30–35% have small bowel involvement only, and approximately 10–15% have disease limited to the large bowel. The common clinical features are listed in Box 27. The onset is often insidious and subtle, and this may lead to a considerable delay in diagnosis. Diffuse mucosal involvement will result in a protein-losing enteropathy, malabsorption and malnutrition. There is currently no cure for Crohn's disease, which follows a waxing–waning course. The goal of therapy is to induce and maintain a remission of active disease, and also to correct malnutrition and promote growth. Energetic nutritional programmes based on elemental diets correct the growth failure and induce remission of active disease. Apart from psychosocial and nutritional support, drugs such as corticosteroids, 5-aminosalicylates, metronidazole and immunomodulatory agents are often used for acute episodes. Ultimately, the majority of children will require surgery to deal with complications such as strictures and fistulae.

## Ulcerative colitis

As with Crohn's disease, the aetiology of ulcerative colitis remains unknown, though the incidence of disease has not changed appreciably. Current hypotheses include a genetic predisposition with an altered immunological response within the intestinal mucosa. Unlike Crohn's disease, the inflammation is continuous and is usually restricted to the colonic mucosa. Macroscopically, the mucosa is friable and granular, and ulceration may be present in association with a bloody mucopurulent exudate. The ulceration is often patchy and may be interspersed with areas of regenerating epithelium, resulting in a pseudopolyp formation. Pancolitis is most common (62%), whereas disease of the left colon (22%) or rectum (15%) occurs less often. Occasionally there is an inflammatory reaction in the distal ileum, called 'backwash ileitis'. The most common presenting symptom, therefore, is *diarrhoea* mixed with *mucus* and *blood* and accompanied by tenesmus and abdominal pain. Attacks are graded as mild, moderate or severe, depending on the stool

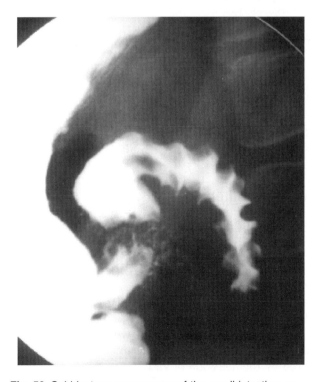

**Fig. 52** Cobblestone appearance of the small intestine on barium radiography in Crohn's disease.

---

**Box 27** Features of Crohn's disease

**Intestinal symptoms**
  Abdominal pain – colicky, intermittent
  Diarrhoea – with or without blood
  Growth failure
  Oral and/or perianal ulcers

**Extraintestinal symptoms**
  Fever
  Arthritis
  Uveitis
  Erythema nodosum
  Pyoderma gangrenosum

**Diagnosis**
  Barium follow-through:
    Narrowing structures
    Fissuring (rose-thorn ulcers)
    Mucosal irregularities (cobblestoning)
  Intestinal biopsy

**Table 36** Comparison of Crohn's disease and ulcerative colitis

| Characteristic | Crohn's disease | Ulcerative colitis |
|---|---|---|
| Rectal bleeding | Occasional | Common |
| Abdominal mass | Common | Not present |
| Rectal disease | Occasional | Nearly universal |
| Ileal involvement | Common | Occasional (backwash ileitis) |
| Perianal disease | Common | Unusual |
| Strictures | Common | Unusual |
| Fistulae | Common | Unusual |
| Skip lesions | Common | Unusual |
| Transmural involvement | Common | Unusual |
| Crypt abscesses | Unusual | Common |
| Granulomas | Common | Unusual |
| Risk for colonic cancer | Slightly increased | Greatly increased |

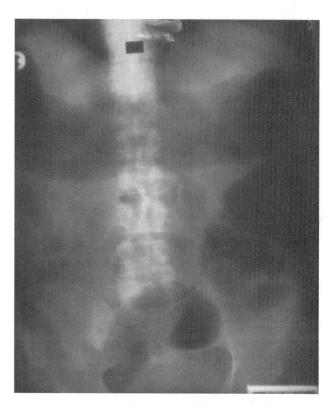

**Fig. 53** Plain X-ray of the abdomen showing a toxic megacolon in a patient with ulcerative colitis.

frequency, abdominal tenderness, fever, and the degree of anaemia and hypoalbuminaemia. In 5–10% of cases the disease may present with fulminating colitis and toxic megacolon. On examination, the only positive findings may be minimal abdominal tenderness, although in severe disease the child may be pyrexial, dehydrated, anaemic and profoundly toxic. Growth retardation is seen in only 20% of those with ulcerative colitis, though other extraintestinal manifestations seen in Crohn's disease are also features of ulcerative colitis. Table 36 lists the common distinguishing features between Crohn's disease and ulcerative colitis. Investigations should include an abdominal roentgenogram to exclude a toxic megacolon (Fig. 53), and stool cultures for infective agents that may mimic ulcerative colitis (e.g. *Shigella*, *Salmonella* and *Campylobacter* species). Colonoscopy with multiple mucosal biopsies is required to confirm the diagnosis. Childhood disease tends to run a more complicated course than that in adults, with an increased likelihood of pancolonic involvement, proximal extension of initially localised disease and colectomy. Mild disease can often be kept under control with sulfasalazine. Acute attacks are treated with topical corticosteroid preparations, including enemas, foams or suppositories. More extensive disease requires oral or systemic corticosteroids under careful supervision. Extensive refractory colitis may be an indication for immunosuppressant therapy with azathioprine or cyclosporin A. Some children may ultimately require a restorative proctocolectomy with an ileal reservoir.

## 5.7 Disorders of the liver, pancreas and peritoneum

### Learning objectives

You should:

- know the natural history of the common viral infections of the liver in childhood
- be able to clinically assess a child for signs of liver cell failure

### Infectious hepatitis

An increasing number of hepatotropic viruses are being identified using advanced molecular techniques (Table 37). Many other viruses, such as herpes simplex, cytomegalovirus (CMV), Epstein–Barr virus (EBV), HIV, varicella, enteroviruses, adenovirus and arboviruses, can also cause hepatitis as a component of multisystem disease.

In general, children infected with hepatitis viruses are usually asymptomatic or anicteric. Infection is recognised by the detection of viral antibodies in the serum at a later date. Symptomatic children present with nausea and vomiting, and on examination they are

**Table 37** Hepatic viruses

| Virus | Classification | Transmission | Chronicity | Vaccine | Interferon therapy |
|---|---|---|---|---|---|
| A (HAV) | Picornavirus | Faeco–oral | No | Yes | No |
| B (HBV) | Hepadnavirus | Parenteral, perinatal, sexual | Common | Yes | Yes |
| C (HCV) | Flavivirus-like | Parenteral, rarely perinatal and sexual | Common | No | Yes |
| D (HDV)[a] | Satellite virus | Parenteral, perinatal, rarely sexual | Common | No | Yes |
| E (HEV) | Calcivirus | Faeco–oral | No | No | No |
| G (HGV) A–C | Flavivirus | Parenteral | Probably | No | No |

[a] Only occurs with HBV infection.

found to be icteric, with a tender, enlarged liver. Elevated liver enzymes and serum bilirubin and detection of viral antigen, RNA or antibody confirm the diagnosis. In most cases, supportive care is all that is required (i.e. hydration and analgesia) as the infection runs its course. However, in some children the disease is complicated by acute liver failure. This is characterised by encephalopathy and coagulopathy, and fulminant liver failure may ensue. Such critically ill children often have multiorgan failure and require management in an intensive care unit. The degree of clinical symptoms is a reflection of the intensity of the immune response to the virus. In HBV infection, those with clinical hepatitis usually clear the virus. Carrier status is more commonly seen in younger children, who often have subclinical or anicteric hepatitis.

## Chronic hepatitis

Chronic hepatitis is a continuing inflammatory disorder of the liver with the potential to progress to cirrhosis, continue unchanged, or resolve with or without treatment. The disease entity is arbitrarily defined into three major pathological categories: chronic persistent, chronic active, and the rarer chronic lobular hepatitis. The aetiology includes viral infections (HBV, HCV), autoimmune disease, Wilson disease, drugs and inflammatory bowel disease. Percutaneous liver biopsy is essential to differentiate between the various conditions. Chronic active hepatitis tends to progress towards cirrhosis, and if associated with HBV infection carries the risk of hepatocellular carcinoma. Immunosuppressant therapy can provide symptomatic relief and delay the onset of cirrhosis in those with autoimmune chronic hepatitis, and α-interferon has been used with a degree of success in chronic carriers of HBV and HCV.

## Wilson's disease (hepatolenticular degeneration)

Wilson's disease is an autosomal recessive condition characterised by a defect in the transport and storage of copper. Excess copper is not excreted by the biliary system nor taken up by the copper transport protein caeruloplasmin, but is deposited into the tissues instead. Progressive liver damage ensues. Subsequently, with deposition of copper in the basal ganglia, extrapyramidal symptoms may appear and a Kayser–Fleischer ring is seen in the cornea, along with sunflower cataracts. Renal tubular damage and haemolytic anaemia may further complicate matters. Investigations include plasma caeruloplasmin levels (usually low), liver biopsy with copper estimation, and studies of urinary copper excretion. Early diagnosis before irreversible tissue damage occurs allows for a good response to treatment with penicillamine. Genetic counselling and screening should be offered to all siblings.

## Cirrhosis

Cirrhosis is the irreversible end stage of liver injury. Pathologically, structurally abnormal nodules surrounded by prominent fibrous tissue replace the liver architecture, and the diagnosis can therefore only be confirmed on biopsy. The clinical features are those of chronic hepatocellular failure and portal hypertension. The liver is usually small (enlarged in biliary cirrhosis) and the spleen is often palpable. Collateral veins may be present on the abdomen, with portal blood being deviated via the paraumbilical veins to the umbilicus and radiating from the umbilicus to the systemic circulation. Jaundice and ascites may also be present. Cutaneous features include spider angiomata (naevi), palmar erythema and clubbing. Those with compensated cirrhosis may be asymptomatic. Signs of decompensation include the development of dependent oedema, ascites, hepatic encephalopathy, septicaemia and/or peritonitis, and alimentary bleeding from oesophageal or rectal varices secondary to portal hypertension. An aetiological diagnosis must be sought and the histological diagnosis confirmed. Treatment is supportive. Nutritional supplementation should take into account fat malabsorption and resultant vitamin A, D, K and E deficiency. In end-stage cirrhosis only a liver transplant will be of long-term benefit.

## Portal hypertension

Portal hypertension usually presents with intestinal bleeding and splenomegaly. The majority of cases are caused by thrombosis of the portal vein (extrahepatic), either idiopathic or secondary to sepsis of the umbilical vein and portal system in infancy. Hepatic cirrhosis and congenital hepatic fibrosis may also cause portal hypertension. The exact cause needs to be established by selective angiography of the coeliac axis and a liver biopsy. In portal venous thrombosis, long-term management is conservative for as long as possible, with ligation of varices where necessary. There is a tendency for bleeding from oesophageal varices to improve with age. Splenorenal shunts are technically difficult and rarely successful before the age of 10 years.

### Reye syndrome

Reye syndrome is a relatively rare, heterogeneous condition characterised by an acute derangement of liver and brain function. The principal abnormality is a severe self-limiting disturbance of the hepatic mitochondrial architecture, with decreased mitochondrial enzyme activity, lasting up to 6 days. The reasons for the mitochondrial dysfunction are unknown. However, the use of aspirin and viral infections have been causally linked. It seems prudent, therefore, to avoid the use of aspirin in children with viral infections. The clinical picture is characterised by refractory vomiting, reduced consciousness and convulsions. Low blood glucose, elevated plasma ammonia, high liver transaminases and prolonged coagulation are the hallmarks of the condition. Management must be in an intensive care unit with facilities for ventilation and control of raised intracranial pressure. Reye syndrome is associated with a high mortality rate, and many survivors are handicapped for life.

## Pancreatitis

Viral infections, drugs, biliary microlithiasis and blunt abdominal injuries account for the majority of cases of acute pancreatitis seen in children. It is characterised by abdominal pain, persistent vomiting and fever. The pain is epigastric and does not always radiate to the back. The abdomen may be distended and quite tender, and a mass (pancreatic pseudocyst) may be palpable. Diagnosis is based on ultrasonography and raised serum amylase and lipase. Medical management aims to restore fluid–electrolyte homeostasis and relieve pain. The prognosis is excellent in uncomplicated cases but poor in those with acute haemorrhagic pancreatitis.

## Peritonitis

Peritonitis can be a result of infectious, autoimmune, chemical or neoplastic processes. Infectious peritonitis is either primary or secondary in origin. Primary peritonitis tends to occur in children with ascites resulting from either nephrotic syndrome or cirrhosis. The causative agents are often encapsulated bacteria, such as pneumococci and *Haemophilus influenzae*. The onset may be sudden or insidious, and is characterised by fever, abdominal pain and a toxic appearance. Abdominal palpation may reveal rebound tenderness and rigidity, with absent bowel sounds. When in doubt, the diagnosis needs to be confirmed by paracentesis and culture of the peritoneal fluid. In primary peritonitis, only a single organism should be isolated. The presence of multiple organisms is suggestive of secondary peritonitis and is an indication for a laparotomy to localise a possible intestinal perforation. The management is primarily antibiotics, fluids and bowel rest (nil orally, nasogastric drainage). Surgery is only required for those in whom a perforated viscus is suspected.

# Self-assessment: questions

## Multiple choice questions

1. Persistent diarrhoea following acute viral gastroenteritis may be due to:
   a. Inappropriate use of antibiotics
   b. Use of oral rehydration solutions
   c. Acquired lactose intolerance
   d. Persistent rotavirus infection
   e. Immunodeficiency.

2. Ulceration of the buccal mucosa is classically seen in:
   a. Vincent angina
   b. Herpes simplex infection
   c. Herpangina
   d. Oral candidiasis
   e. Prodromal measles.

3. A 4-month-old infant presents with recurrent chest infections and failure to thrive. The possible diagnoses are:
   a. Cricopharyngeal incoordination
   b. Achalasia cardia
   c. Gastro-oesophageal reflux
   d. Tracheoesophageal fistula
   e. Coeliac disease.

4. With regard to intestinal polyps:
   a. The majority can be detected on rectal examination
   b. The commonest presentation is painless rectal bleeding
   c. The polyps seen in Peutz–Jegher syndrome are premalignant
   d. The polyps seen in Gardner syndrome are benign
   e. Non-familial juvenile colonic polyps usually occur as solitary lesions.

5. The following are causes of secretory diarrhoea:
   a. *Vibrio cholerae*
   b. Neuroblastoma
   c. Enteropathogenic *Escherichia coli*
   d. Rotavirus
   e. Coeliac disease.

6. Features of Crohn's disease include:
   a. Abdominal mass
   b. Non-caseating granulomas
   c. Crypt abscesses
   d. Strictures
   e. Increased risk of colonic cancer.

7. Typical features of ulcerative colitis include:
   a. Rectal bleeding
   b. Abdominal mass
   c. Fistulae
   d. Increased risk of colonic cancer
   e. Involvement of the terminal ileum.

8. A 6-year-old child presents with painful, bloody mucous diarrhoea and has bilateral swollen tender knee joints. The differential diagnoses include:
   a. Shigellosis
   b. Ulcerative colitis
   c. Tuberculosis
   d. Crohn's disease
   e. *Campylobacter* infection.

9. With regard to the digestion of carbohydrates:
   a. Disaccharidases are located on the intestinal brush border
   b. Lactose intolerance is detected by testing the stool for reducing substances
   c. Monosaccharides are directly absorbed in the duodenum
   d. Disaccharide intolerance is a component of toddler's diarrhoea
   e. Salivary and pancreatic amylases break down starch to glucose and maltose.

10. In normal digestive function:
    a. Iron is converted to the ferric form in the stomach
    b. The soluble iron compound is mainly absorbed passively in the duodenum
    c. Malabsorption of D-xylose suggests a proximal intestinal mucosal lesion
    d. Calcium is absorbed actively in the lower intestine
    e. The hormone secretin stimulates the secretion of pancreatic enzymes.

11. The following describe lipid absorption:
    a. It is dependent on the presence of bile salts
    b. Digestion of triglycerides by lipase begins in the duodenum
    c. Chylomicron formation facilitates absorption by the villi
    d. Medium-chain fatty acids are directly absorbed in the stomach
    e. Unused bile salts are excreted, imparting to the faeces their characteristic colour.

12. Complications of the short bowel syndrome include:
    a. Megaloblastic anaemia
    b. Ileal bacterial overgrowth
    c. Gastric hypersecretion
    d. Failure to thrive
    e. Osmotic diarrhoea.

## Case histories

### Case history 1

A 5-year-old boy is brought to you with a history of three episodes of bloody stools, 1 month apart.
Discuss your approach to making a diagnosis in this patient.

### Case history 2

A 2-year-old girl presents with a history of passing 10–15 watery stools and has vomited at least four times in the last 24 hours. She appears distressed but otherwise cooperative, and drinks thirstily from a glass of fruit juice but then vomits. The nurse informs you that her pulse is 96 bpm, temperature 37.9°C and blood pressure 100/60 mmHg.
Discuss the management of this child.

### Case history 3

While on night rounds, you see a child newly diagnosed with ulcerative colitis admitted for colonoscopy the following morning. The parents draw you aside and say that although their son has responded well to the treatment they are unsure of the prognosis.
Explain how you will proceed to tackle this situation.

### Case history 4: Total 20 marks

A 2-year-old girl was brought to paediatric A&E in summer with a low-grade fever and a 2-day history of occasional vomiting and profuse diarrhoea.

1. What is the most likely diagnosis, and the most common group of causative agents?

The child was reasonably alert, active and had a wet nappy, and the casualty officer decides to send her home after a full examination.

2. What advice should the casualty officer give to the mother at this point in time?

Despite the casualty officer's advice, the child's symptoms continue to deteriorate and she is brought back to A&E after a further 36 hours. She is now miserable and lethargic. The paediatric registrar is called to review the child and suspects that she may be dehydrated.

3. What symptoms might be suggestive of dehydration at this stage?
4. What clinical signs would be indicative of dehydration?

Indeed, the clinical assessment confirms 5–10% dehydration and the registrar arranges for her admission to the paediatric ward.

5. Outline the key points in the management (investigations and treatment) of this child at this stage.

## Short notes

Write short notes on short bowel syndrome.

## OSCE questions

### OSCE 1

A 7-year-old child presented with a 6-month history of irritability, poor weight gain and loose stools. A biopsy was taken during the course of his investigation (Fig. 54).

a. Where was the biopsy taken from?
b. What procedure was employed to obtain the biopsy?
c. What does the biopsy show?
d. What is the most likely diagnosis?
e. How would you treat this patient?

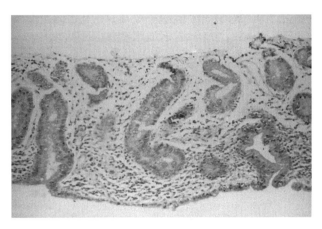

**Fig. 54**

### OSCE 2

A dynamic X-ray study was performed in a child who plotted on the third centile for weight and required repeated hospital admissions (Fig. 55).

a. What radiological study was carried out?
b. What three abnormalities does it show?
c. What is the most likely diagnosis?
d. Name two complications of this condition.

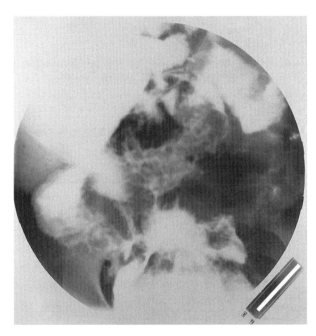

**Fig. 55**

# Self-assessment: answers

## Multiple choice answers

1. a. **True**. Classically due to disruption of the normal homeostatic gut flora.
   b. **False**. These are used to treat the diarrhoea.
   c. **True**. This is usually transient but may last a few weeks.
   d. **False**.
   e. **False**. The immunosuppressed may be unable to clear the infection in the usual way.

2. a. **True**.
   b. **True**. It is caused by anaerobic infection of the gingival tissues.
   c. **True**. The causative agent is Coxsackie virus A.
   d. **False**. It causes 'thrush' – small white flecks.
   e. **False**. Measles causes an enanthem – sandy, grainy flecks on the buccal mucosa called Koplik spots.

3. a. **True**. This is an oesophageal motility disorder that presents with symptoms similar to those of gastro-oesophageal reflux.
   b. **True**. This is an oesophageal motility disorder with obstruction occurring at the gastro-oesophageal junction.
   c. **True**. The acid contents of the stomach are aspirated into the lungs.
   d. **True**. Only the H type will present at this age.
   e. **False**. Failure to thrive occurs later as gluten-containing solids are introduced and respiratory disease is not a feature.

4. a. **True**.
   b. **True**. Mostly seen during or immediately after a bowel movement.
   c. **False**. This is an autosomal dominant condition with mucocutaneous pigmentation and polyposis. Although the polyps themselves are not premalignant, there is an increased risk of intestinal or extraintestinal cancer.
   d. **False**. This is an autosomal dominant condition with multiple intestinal polyps and tumours of the soft tissue and bone, pigmented fundi and extracolonic cancers. The intestinal polyps are premalignant.
   e. **False**. More than half of the children affected have more than one polyp, though multiple polyps are rare.

5. a. **True**. It produces a secretory toxin.
   b. **True**. It is caused by the production of vasoactive intestinal peptide (VIP).
   c. **False**. Enterotoxicogenic *E. coli* produces secretory diarrhoea via ST and LT toxins.
   d. **False**. Rotavirus produces osmotic diarrhoea.
   e. **False**. Diarrhoea results from malabsorption.

6. a. **True**. Mass results from inflammation and formation of adhesions.
   b. **True**.
   c. **False**. This is a feature of ulcerative colitis.
   d. **True**. Transmural inflammation leads to partial small-bowel obstruction.
   e. **True**. As in all inflammatory bowel disease.

7. a. **True**. Bleeding is often from localised rectal ulceration (proctitis).
   b. **False**. This is a feature of Crohn's disease.
   c. **False**. This is a feature of Crohn's disease.
   d. **True**. This is a feature of all inflammatory bowel diseases.
   e. **False**. This is a typical feature of a Crohn's disease; 'backwash' ileitis is rare in UC.

8. a. **True**. It is also known as Reiter syndrome.
   b. **True**. Arthritis may become chronic in nature.
   c. **False**. Although tuberculous intestinal ulcerations can occur and so can arthritis, they do not occur together.
   d. **True**. Usually pauciarticular, with occasional spondylitis.
   e. **True**. It can cause a reactive, self-limiting arthritis.

9. a. **True**. They occur in the 'tip' cells located on the top of the microvilli.
   b. **True**. Clinitest detects reducing sugars as found in lactose intolerance
   c. **True**. Because they do not need to be broken down.
   d. **False**. This is a probably a motility disorder.
   e. **True**. Glucose is absorbed and maltose is further hydrolysed by glucosidase.

10. a. **False**. It is converted into the soluble ferrous form.
    b. **False**. It is actively absorbed.
    c. **True**. It is a pentose that is minimally metabolised and is almost entirely absorbed by the upper small intestine.

d. **False**. Active absorption occurs in the upper small intestine.

e. **False**. It stimulates secretion of bicarbonate ions and pancreatic fluid.

11. a. **True**. Bile salts form micelles with lipids, ensuring the efficient transportation of their hydrolysed products to the absorptive epithelium.

b. **True**. This lipase is secreted by the pancreas into the duodenum.

c. **True**. Chylomicron contains a complex of triglycerides and cholesterol that can be directly transported into the lymph.

d. **False**. Medium-chain triglycerides do not require emulsification or micelle formation, and are directly absorbed in the small intestine.

e. **False**. Bile salts are mainly absorbed (enterohepatic circulation); bile pigments provide the characteristic colour.

12. a. **True**. It is caused by folate malabsorption.

b. **True**. This results from stasis.

c. **True**. Hypergastrinaemia occurs but is usually not a clinical problem.

d. **True**. Failure to thrive is caused by a combination of chronic diarrhoea and malabsorption.

e. **True**. The inability to absorb normally secreted intestinal contents through loss of absorptive surface results in osmotic diarrhoea.

## Case history answers

### Case history 1

In this child we can exclude a bacterial enteritis, as this presents acutely. An intussusception is unlikely to be recurrent. There are several possible conditions.

**Anal fissure**. Is there a history of constipation? Is defecation painful? Is there an anal tag, and is an anal fissure visible on inspection? Does the blood coat an otherwise normal stool?

**Colonic polyps**. Is there a family history of similar problems or bowel cancer (familial polyposis syndrome)? Is there unusual pigmentation of the skin (Peutz–Jegher and Gardner syndromes)? In the majority a rectal examination is sufficient to detect a polyp, though fibreoptic colonoscopy must be performed to look for other polyps.

**Inflammatory bowel disease**. Usually ulcerative colitis presents with blood and mucus in the stools. The diagnosis is based on history and confirmed on colonoscopic biopsy.

**Meckel diverticulum**. This is discussed in Chapter 12.

**Henoch–Schönlein purpura**. This is discussed in Chapter 11.

**Sexual abuse**. This is obviously a diagnosis of exclusion. Clues are provided by bruising and tearing around the anal sphincter and the presence of any form of sexually transmitted disease.

### Case history 2

The child has mild-to-moderate dehydration. You need to ascertain when she last passed urine. She should be admitted and started on oral rehydration: 150 mL/kg body weight should be prescribed over 24 hours. The first 50 mL/kg should be given alone over the first 4–6 hours. On re-evaluation, the child should have passed urine at this point and be better hydrated. If so, then additional feeds (either milk or solids) are allowed if she desires it. If dehydration persists, intravenous fluids are required. The fluid should be offered as frequent small feeds and the parent reassured that the vomiting will lessen as the hydration improves. Neither antiemetics nor antidiarrhoeals are to be encouraged. A serum urea and packed cell volume (PCV) will confirm the state of hydration. Serum electrolytes need to be checked to confirm that the child has not developed hypo- or hypernatraemia. The stool can be examined for pathogens. In this age group, with this kind of presentation, the causative agent is often rotavirus. If the child is well hydrated at 24 hours, the oral rehydration fluid should be continued intermittently with feeds. The parents should be reassured that the diarrhoea will decrease over the next few days. A small number of children are unable to digest milk or milk-containing products immediately after the diarrhoea and may require alternative food products, such as lactose-free or soy-based formulae for 2–3 weeks before the reintroduction of a normal diet.

### Case history 3

An answer can be divided into several parts.

**The setting**. This is a child with a chronic disease that follows a relapsing pattern with potential serious sequelae. Information like this preferably needs to be discussed in a quiet corner where the parents are comfortable, and not on an open ward. It is also beneficial to have a member of the nursing staff present when you talk to the parents, so they are able to reinforce what you have said.

**Pacing**. You need to know what the parents understand about the situation and the disease process.

**Information**. Provide the information they require. Do not overburden them with too much information or jargon. Explain that 90% of patients with ulcerative colitis will experience one or more relapses after initial treatment. Most will lead a normal life despite chronic disease, but about a fifth will be chronically incapacitated. The prognosis is linked to the extent of involvement, and those with isolated distal colitis have the best outcome. Whereas most will be managed on a combination of medical and supportive measures, a proportion of patients (30%) will require surgery, and often a colostomy for the control of symptoms. Explain the symptoms of fulminant colitis and that it is a medical emergency requiring urgent admission. As there is a risk (albeit small) of developing a malignancy, regular surveillance of the colonic mucosa needs to be carried out using colonoscopy and biopsy.

**Respond to feelings**. Be prepared for statements such as 'we didn't know that', or 'no-one told us that', as the parents may well be in a state of denial. If they are overtly anxious, you may need to inform the members of the team looking after the child about their doubts and concerns.

## Case history 4

| | | Score |
|---|---|---|
| 1 | Gastroenteritis | 1 |
| | Probably viral, e.g. rotavirus | 1 |
| | | (2) |
| 2 | Oral rehydration | 0.5 |
| | Light diet | 0.5 |
| | Control temperature | 0.5 |
| | Point out signs of possible dehydration | 0.5 |
| | | (2) |
| 3 | Decreased activity | 0.5 |
| | Lethargy | 0.5 |
| | Confusion | 0.5 |
| | Decreased skin temperature | 0.5 |
| | Poor colour | 0.5 |
| | Fewer wet nappies | 0.5 |
| | | (3) |
| 4 | Tachycardia | 1 |
| | Poor skin perfusion | 0.5 |
| | Prolonged capillary return | 0.5 |
| | Cool peripheries/increased temperature gap | 0.5 |
| | Thready pulses | 0.5 |
| | Oliguria | 0.5 |
| | Confusion, decreased conscious level | 0.5 |
| | Hypotension | 1 |
| | | (5) |
| 5 | Set up intravenous infusion | 2 |
| | Check electrolytes, glucose | 1 |
| | Check blood gas (and acid–base status) | 1 |
| | Blood culture | 1 |

| | | |
|---|---|---|
| Give maintenance fluids + 10% for dehydration | | 1 |
| Give as dextrose/saline mixture | | 1 |
| Control fever | | 1 |
| | | (8) |

*No marks for antibiotics, antiemetics, antidiarrhoeal agents*
*0.5 for CBC or CRP*
Total 20

## Short notes answer

The short bowel syndrome occurs when there is a congenital or acquired loss or shortening of the bowel and a resultant decrease in its absorptive surface. Malabsorption results in vitamin $B_{12}$ deficiency (and hence the megaloblastic anaemia), failure to thrive and an osmotic diarrhoea. An alteration in the intestinal milieu leading to changes in pH results in bacterial overgrowth, and occasionally can lead to oversecretion of gastrin. The latter results in gastric hypersecretion. Treatment entails nutritional supplementation, at times utilising total parenteral nutrition via an indwelling central venous catheter. Vitamin and trace element supplementation is also required. Gastric acidity is controlled with $H_2$ antagonists, and overgrowth of bowel microorganisms with the judicious use of antibiotics.

## OSCE answers

### OSCE 1
a. Jejunum
b. Closed biopsy using Crosby capsule
c. Total villous atrophy with submucosal inflammation
d. Coeliac disease
e. Correct deficiencies, e.g. iron, folate, and a strict gluten-free diet.

### OSCE 2
a. Contrast (barium) meal and follow-through
b. Rose thorn ulcers, skip lesions, cobblestone mucosa
c. Crohn's disease
d. Malabsorption with deficiency states (iron, folate, vitamin $B_{12}$)
   Fistulation (and short bowel syndrome)
   Stricture formation
   Gastrointestinal perforation
   Gastrointestinal bleeding
   Gastrointestinal and peritoneal abscess formation
   Malignant change

# 6 Neuromuscular disease

**6.1** Introduction 123

**6.2** Examination 123

**6.3** Congenital abnormalities 124

**6.4** Handicap 127

**6.5** Infections 128

**6.6** Seizures and headaches 130

**6.7** The spinal cord and peripheral nerves 134

**6.8** Neuromuscular disorders 135

Self-assessment: questions 137

Self-assessment: answers 141

## Overview

Despite general apprehension among undergraduates relating to the neurological examination of children, if approached logically this is really quite a straightforward exercise. Indeed, students would be expected to perform a basic examination of the cranial and peripheral nerves, both common cases in clinical examinations. Students should also appreciate and be able to manage the more common neurological problems, including congenital defects, headaches, infections, seizure disorders, handicap and other chronic neuromuscular diseases. Ultimately, children with such conditions and their carers are faced with a host of diverse problems and require a coordinated multidisciplinary approach if their management is to be effective.

## 6.1 Introduction

The average medical student is filled with dread at the prospect of having to examine the nervous system in a child. This is unnecessary; this system, though complex, is concerned with clearly defined functions, and a logical, systematic approach will result in a realistic appreciation of the basic problem(s) facing the neuro-logically abnormal child. Certainly, the undergraduate is not expected to be conversant with rare neurodegenerative conditions, but must be able to discuss the problems relating to cerebral palsy, epilepsy and similar conditions that, ultimately, make up a significant proportion of the paediatric workload.

## 6.2 Examination

### Learning objective

You should:

- be able to carry out a clinical examination of the nervous system in a child

### General examination

If the examination is presented as a game, most children will cooperate sufficiently to enable a good assessment of the nervous system. Observation of the child while playing and interacting with parents and siblings is of paramount importance. The head shape should be noted and head circumference measured. Mannerisms, movements and posturing must be observed in the light of the child's chronological age. Particular attention to neurocutaneous stigmata, hepatosplenomegaly and dysmorphic features should form a routine part of the general examination.

### The cranial nerves

The first cranial nerve is rarely examined in children and requires the use of standard smelling agents. A cursory assessment is possible by asking direct questions about the child's sense of smell. The second nerve is tested individually by covering one eye and asking the older child to read picture cards (acuity), checking visual fields using an interesting small toy with the child focusing on your nose, and by fundoscopy. Nerves III, IV and VI are tested together by steadying the child's head while asking him to follow with his eyes a bright object traversing a large 'H'. The sensory modality of the fifth nerve is checked by asking the child to close his eyes and say 'yes' every time you touch the three divisions

**Table 38** Cranial nerve assessment in infants

| Nerve | Test |
|-------|------|
| I | Not tested |
| II | Blinks to bright light; appears to fix/follow (3+ months); fundoscopy |
| III–VI | Assess highlights on pupils for squint, abnormal position of globe |
| V | Corneal reflexes; sucking movements |
| VII | Facial asymmetry especially while crying |
| VIII | Startles to sound; quietens with soothing; tuneful babbling |
| IX–X | Gag reflex |
| XI | Not tested |
| XII | Tongue movements |

**Table 39** Grading of muscle power

| Power | Observation |
|-------|-------------|
| 0 | No power |
| 1 | Barely perceptible power |
| 2 | Movement with gravity removed (i.e. horizontally) |
| 3 | Movement just overcomes gravity |
| 4 | Movement against gravity and some resistance |
| 5 | Normal power |

(ophthalmic, maxillary and mandibular). The corneal reflex test is unpleasant and limited to comatose children and very small infants. If the motor component of the fifth nerve is intact, the child should be able to push his jaw laterally against your hand. Facial asymmetry with loss of nasolabial folds and drawing of the face to the normal side on smiling/grimacing is indicative of a seventh-nerve palsy. The child should normally be able to bury his eyelashes, blow out the cheeks and open/close the mouth tightly. Weakness throughout one side suggests a seventh-nerve lower motor neuron lesion; preservation of the forehead creases implies an upper motor neuron lesion. The eighth nerve is checked by direct questions relating to hearing and a distraction test in children aged 6–18 months. Nerves IX to X are functioning normally if the uvula rises symmetrically when the child says 'aah'. An intact eleventh nerve allows the child to raise his shoulders and push his head against resistance. The 12th nerve is assessed by asking the child to protrude and waggle the tongue from side to side. An accurate examination of the cranial nerves is possible, even in young infants (Table 38).

## Motor examination

Initially, it is essential to establish whether the child experiences any pain in any joints or limbs, and the examination must be conducted carefully.

**Muscle tone** is assessed by observing posture and moving joints through their range of movement. Hypotonic neonates assume a frog-leg position, whereas older children are floppy. Spasticity is characterised by increased tone that relaxes suddenly (clasp-knife) and is often associated with clonus. Rigidity implies constant resistance to passive movement.

**Power** is appreciated by inviting the child to perform specific functions against resistance, and is graded from 0 to 5 (Table 39).

**Reflexes** are assessed by using a rigid finger in neonates and a small hammer in older children, after demonstrating that the exercise is painless. Plantar reflexes are not downgoing until the child is walking.

**Mobility and gait** (crawling, walking etc.) must be documented. Abnormal movements include slow twisting movements (dystonia), writhing actions (athetosis) and rapid involuntary jerks (chorea).

**Speech** is commonly affected in motor disorders, including cerebellar abnormalities. The latter manifests as staccato speech, hypotonia, pendular nystagmus and reflexes, poor coordination, dysdiadochokinesia and an intention tremor.

## Sensory examination

Sensory assessment requires considerable concentration on the part of the child and often proves the most difficult part of the neurological examination. A piece of cotton wool and a sterile needle are used to assess *touch* and *pain* sensation. The process must be carefully explained to the child, who is then asked to close his eyes and indicate each time there has been contact with the skin. The two sides must be compared simultaneously according to dermatomes. *Vibration* sense is tested with a tuning fork, *temperature* by using warm and cold objects and *joint position* by asking the child to identify positions of the thumbs and big toes with the eyes closed.

## 6.3 Congenital abnormalities

### Learning objectives

You should:

• know the common developmental anomalies of the nervous system seen in childhood

• be able to perform a relevant clinical examination of a child with hydrocephalus, neural tube defect or neurofibromatosis

## Neural tube defects

A tuft of hair over the lower back may herald the presence of a minor defect of the bony spinal processes without any abnormality of nervous tissue, i.e. spina bifida occulta. This is of no consequence and is only rarely associated with problems such as a tethered cord (diastematomyelia), syringomyelia, or a dermoid sinus connecting the skin to the dura. Failure of closure of the neural tube by the fourth week in utero results in *spina bifida*, with exposure of the meninges (meningocoele) and spinal cord (myelomeningocoele) (Fig. 56). The latter is the most serious defect, arising in 0.1% of live births, and may be related to a genetic predisposition, radiation, drugs (e.g. valproic acid) and malnutrition (e.g. folic acid deficiency). Myelomeningocoele is associated with leakage of fetal α-fetoprotein, resulting in a raised level in the mother's bloodstream. The defects can be demonstrated on antenatal ultrasound scanning. Spina bifida is often associated with an abnormality of the posterior brain (Chiari defect), obstructing the flow of cerebrospinal fluid and resulting in hydrocephalus. This is more likely the higher the lesion, with the surprising exception of high thoracic and cervical lesions, which may not be associated with major neurological deficit and hydrocephalus. Exposed, weeping lesions are at great risk of ascending infection. Lumbar lesions account for 75% of cases: affected infants assume a frog position because of flaccid paresis of the lower limbs, and may also have a patulous anus

and incontinence of stool and urine. A patulous anus and perineal anaesthesia are evident with lower sacral lesions.

### Management

Management requires sympathetic counselling and a multidisciplinary team approach. Supportive care alone may be appropriate for those infants with very large lesions, severe neurological deficit and gross hydrocephalus at birth. With exposed myelomeningocoeles surgical closure shortly after birth is essential if infection is to be prevented, and the hydrocephalus generally necessitates a ventriculoperitoneal (V-P) shunt. Closed lesions may be repaired after a few days. Long-term management involves intensive physiotherapy to the lower limbs, attention to bowel habit and the neurogenic bladder, and intermittent catheterisation to avoid urinary retention and urinary tract infection. Orthopaedic review is required, particularly for any associated kyphoscoliosis, dislocated hips and talipes (club feet).

## Hydrocephalus

Obstructive (non-communicating) hydrocephalus results from a blockage to cerebrospinal fluid (CSF) flow. Decreased absorption or increased production of CSF fluid causes non-obstructive (communicating) hydrocephalus. Congenital abnormalities of brain development may affect the flow of CSF, whereas intraventricular haemorrhage is the most common cause for acquired obstruction and diminished CSF absorption (Box 28).

### Signs and symptoms

Hydrocephalus presents with symptoms and signs of raised intracranial pressure. In neonates this manifests as decreased feeding, vomiting, lethargy, irritability, and occasionally convulsions. The fontanelles are wide, tense, convex, and connected together by widely open sutures. Distended veins over the scalp, downward displacement of the orbital globes (sunsetting), cranial nerve palsies (especially of the sixth nerve), long tract signs and papilloedema are late signs. The head circumference should be measured daily and plotted on appropriate centile charts. Accurate serial measurements of the ventricular system are documented on ultrasound, and specific anatomical abnormalities/growths confirmed on CT or MRI scans of the brain. Symptoms and an excessive increase in head size are indications for drainage of the CSF by lumbar or ventricular tapping until a formal shunt is inserted. An

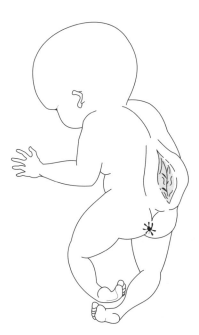

**Fig. 56** Clinical appearance of spina bifida. The figure shows a newborn with 'open' thoracolumbar myelomeningocoele with patulous anus, flaccid lower limbs, bilateral talipes and hydrocephalus.

**Box 28** Congenital abnormalities of brain development that may affect the flow of CSF

|  | Congenital | Acquired |
|---|---|---|
| Obstructive causes | Spina bifida | Intraventricular haemorrhage |
|  | Aqueductal stenosis | Meningitis/encephalitis |
|  | Dandy Walker cyst of fourth ventricle | Obstructing tumour |
|  | Chiari malformation of fourth ventricle |  |
| Non-obstructive causes | Choroid plexus papilloma | Intraventricular haemorrhage |
|  |  | Meningitis |
|  |  | Leukaemic infiltration |

underlying cause for the hydrocephalus, such as a congenital cyst, must be decompressed neurologically, as appropriate.

In older children the triad of lethargy, vomiting and headaches, often with a diurnal variation (usually worse first thing in the morning), and especially if associated with hypertension and bradycardia, is suggestive of raised intracranial pressure. Cranial nerve palsies (especially nerves VI and III) may be false localising signs, whereas long tract signs and papilloedema develop early compared with infants. Dexamethasone and sometimes mannitol diuresis are used to reduce the intracranial pressure in the first instance, and an urgent CT scan will confirm hydrocephalus and may show the primary cause (e.g. a brain tumour). An urgent V–P shunt is required, followed by treatment for the primary lesion (e.g. surgery, radiotherapy). The outcome is largely dependent on the underlying cause. However, children with hydrocephalus have a lower IQ than their peers and an increased risk of neurodevelopmental, visual and learning problems.

## Microcephaly

Microcephaly is defined as a head circumference three standard deviations below the mean for both age and gender. It may be a primary defect or follow an insult that impedes normal brain development (Box 29). A thorough antenatal, perinatal and family history should be obtained. The head circumference should be measured serially, and those of other family members also noted. Many microcephalic children will be developmentally delayed and require appropriate supportive treatment.

## Craniosynostosis

Craniosynostosis occurs about once in every 2.5–4000 births and results from the early fusion of cranial sutures. It can be non-syndromic or associated with syndromes such as Crouzon's, where the cranial sutures fuse early, or Apert and Carpenter syndromes, where

**Box 29** Primary and secondary causes of microcephaly

**Primary**
Familial (recessive or dominant)
Trisomies (18 and 21)
Deletions (e.g. Cri-du-chat, 5p-)
Certain syndromes (e.g. Opitz, de Lange)

**Secondary**
Hypoxic–ischaemic encephalopathy
Cerebral palsy
Congenital infection
Meningitis and encephalitis
Metabolic (e.g. hyperphenylalaninaemia)
Drugs and alcohol

there is early fusion of multiple sutures. There is often a marked cosmetic deformity, brain underdevelopment, hydrocephaly, and syndactyly of the digits. Management should be directed by a multidisciplinary team, including neurological and maxillofacial surgeons.

## Neurocutaneous syndromes

Neurocutaneous syndromes are characterised by neurological disorders together with cutaneous stigmata.

**Neurofibromatosis** (NF) is the most common type, arising in 1 in 4000 of the population. NF-1 is typified by more than five *café-au-lait* pigmented spots (>5 mm diameter), axillary freckling, neurofibromas (soft and small, or large, pigmented plexiform lesions), Lisch spots in the iris and skeletal deformities. Neurological abnormalities include macrocephaly, hydrocephaly, optic gliomas and CNS hamartomas. An increased incidence of malignant lesions occurs in the CNS and elsewhere (e.g. leukaemia, phaeochromocytoma, Wilms' tumour). Bilateral acoustic neuromas are typical of NF-2.

**Tuberous sclerosis** is also an autosomal dominant condition, characterised by hypo- and hyperpigmented skin patches (enhanced under Wood's light), subungual fibromas, facial adenoma sebaceum, and tubers in the retina (phakomata), heart, kidneys and brain. The last often calcify, and many of these patients are mentally handicapped and have troublesome epilepsy.

## 6.4 Handicap

### Learning objectives

You should:

- be able to examine a child with cerebral palsy and estimate the degree of disability

- be familiar with the multidisciplinary approach for children with multiple disabilities

### Cerebral palsy

Cerebral palsy is a disorder of movement that follows a non-progressive insult to the developing brain, including anoxia, infection, haemorrhage, trauma and toxins. Despite the static nature of the insult, clinical signs evolve as the child grows older. Cerebral palsy is commonly associated with disorders of speech, hearing, vision and intellect, and seizures. Classification depends on the distribution and type of motor disorder, which in turn depends on which part of the brain is primarily affected (Table 40). Those with *spastic cerebral palsy* have increased clasp-knife rigidity and decreased movement in the affected limbs (Fig. 57). The upper motor neuron signs (weakness, increased tone, brisk reflexes) are more marked in the upper limb in *spastic hemiplegia* (bilaterally in *double hemiplegia*). Both lower limbs are affected in *spastic diplegia* and all four in *spastic quadriplegia* (Fig. 57), when associated contractures, severe mental retardation and seizures are extremely likely. *Athetoid cerebral palsy* was common following neonatal hyperbilirubinaemia leading to kernicterus. Weakness is associated with marked hypotonia, poor head control and repetitive athetoid movements affecting the limbs and bulbar muscles. Consequently, feeding and speech are often badly affected, and these children are at particular risk of recurrent aspiration pneumonia. Initial investigation should exclude progressive forms of physical and mental handicap and confirm the extent of damage with imaging (CT or MRI) and electrophysiological studies (EEG). Management requires a dedicated multidisciplinary medical and surgical team, with support from educational psychologists and speech, occupational and physiotherapists. Attention to nutrition is important and often requires nasogastric or indwelling gastrostomy (e.g. PEG) tube feeding. Tendon-lengthening procedures to relieve contractures, correction of squints and

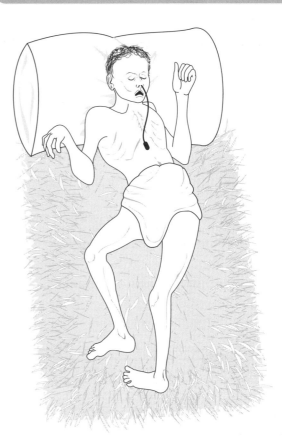

**Fig. 57** Clinical manifestations of cerebral palsy. A school-aged child with severe cerebral palsy showing generalised 'windswept' deformity due to contractures and marked muscle wasting. The child is still in nappies, requires a nasogastric tube for feeding, and is lying on a sheepskin rug to prevent pressure sores.

**Table 40** Types of cerebral palsy

| Cerebral palsy | Motor distribution | Seizures (%) | Mental handicap (%) |
|---|---|---|---|
| Spastic | Diplegia | <10 | <10 |
| | Hemiplegia | 25 | 25 |
| | Quadriplegia | >50 | >50 |
| Athetoid | Extrapyramidal | <20 | <20 |

nystagmus, and hearing aids may improve the quality of life. Baclofen is sometimes useful in cases with severe spasticity.

### Neurodegenerative conditions

Neurodegenerative conditions are rare and result from a number of disorders:

- Inborn errors of metabolism that result in the accumulation of abnormal metabolites in the brain (e.g. lipidoses, leukodystrophies)

**Box 30** Causes of visual impairment

**Orbit**
Cataracts
Amblyopia
Optic atrophy
Retinopathy of prematurity
Retinal degeneration (retinitis pigmentosa)
Retinal detachment/haemorrhage (trauma, non-accidental injury, NAI)
Coloboma

**Central**
Hypoxic–ischaemic encephalopathy (cerebral palsy)
Postinfective (meningitis, encephalitis)
Congenital occipital anomalies (encephalocoele)
Hydrocephaly
Tumours
Demyelinating/neurodegenerative diseases

**Box 31** Causes of hearing impairment

**Peripheral conductive**
Otitis media
Impacted cerumen, foreign body
Perforated tympanic membrane
Disrupted ossicles (trauma)
Bony disruption (craniofacial syndromes)

**Peripheral sensorineural**
Ototoxics (aminoglycosides, irradiation)
Congenital infections
Excessive noise

**Central**
Postinfective (viral, meningitis)
Tumours
Demyelinating diseases
Familial/genetic
Certain syndromes (Pendred, Waardenburg, Alport)
Trisomies

- Abnormal mitochondrial function (e.g. Leigh's encephalopathy)
- Progressive postinfection syndromes (e.g. subacute sclerosing panencephalitis following measles, Creutzfeldt–Jakob Dementia, CJD)
- Toxins (e.g. lead, irradiation).

Patients may be relatively normal at birth but deteriorate over a period of months or years until terminal dementia associated with coma is established.

## Decreased special senses

### Visual impairment

In the UK, severe visual impairment and blindness occurs in 6 of every 10 000 children under the age of 16 years. It occurs commonly in the context of complex non-ophthalmic disorders, and there is an increased rate in low-birthweight children. It should be suspected in any child who does not seem to take an interest in their surroundings, who responds preferentially to sounds or tactile stimuli, and in those with a predisposing abnormality (e.g. cerebral palsy, congenital infection). Every effort should be made to establish a firm diagnosis (Box 30) and instigate the appropriate therapy. Peripatetic teachers and special educational methods are essential if the child is to overcome this severe handicap and achieve their full potential.

### Hearing impairment

The prevalence of confirmed permanent hearing impairment (>40 dB) is around 2 of every 1000 children aged 9 years or older. As with visual impairment, there are often complex problems associated with hearing loss

(Box 31). As auditory input is required before language can develop, hearing loss is often manifest by delayed or unintelligible speech. The distraction test (see viva voce question in Chapter 1) allows a rapid assessment of hearing in young infants who are able to be propped up (>6 months) and still young enough to be taken in by the test (<18 months). Free-field audiometry and auditory evoked responses are required for older children.

## 6.5 Infections

### Learning objectives

You should:

- know the common infections of the central nervous system in children

- be familiar with the signs, symptoms and management of bacterial meningitis

### Meningitis

Meningitis is a rapidly progressive, diffuse infection involving the meninges and CSF. Although potentially fatal, it can result in no neurological sequelae if diagnosed early and treated effectively. The microbiological cause of meningitis varies with age group (Box 32). Before the advent of *Haemophilus influenzae* type b (Hib) vaccine this was the most common infecting organism outside the neonatal period, followed by *Neisseria meningitides* and *Streptococcus pneumoniae*. Patients at particular risk include infants, the immunosuppressed,

**Box 32** Causes of bacterial meningitis

**Neonatal period**
Group B streptococci
Gram-negative bacilli
Staphylococci
*Listeria monocytogenes*
*Haemophilus influenzae*

**Children**
*Neisseria meningitides*
*Streptococcus pneumoniae*
Staphylococci
Gram-negative bacilli if immunosuppressed
*Haemophilus influenzae*

and those with cranial or spinal defects, CSF leak, penetrating trauma and ventricular shunts. Most organisms are acquired by droplet inhalation from close contact with colonised individuals: nasal carriage with *H. influenzae* type b is seen in 5%, whereas *N. meningitides* is present in up to 10% of healthy individuals, especially during the winter months. Most cases are sporadic (e.g. *N. meningitides* group B), although epidemics do occur, especially with *N. meningitides* groups A and C.

Meningitis should always be considered in a child with a fever who has an altered level of consciousness. Although there may be a preceding upper respiratory infection for a few days, the natural history is often rapidly progressive over a few hours. Children may present with fulminating septicaemia, shock and disseminated intravascular coagulation (DIC), especially with meningococcaemia. Indeed, a rapidly evolving purpuric or ecchymotic rash in a toxic child is indicative of meningococcaemia until proved otherwise. Infants are more likely to present with fever, poor feeding, vomiting and drowsiness. Meningism is characterised by irritability, photophobia, neck stiffness, pain on leg extension with the hip flexed (Kernig's sign), and reflex hip flexion when the neck is flexed while supine (Brudzinki's sign). These signs are often absent in infants, who develop signs of raised intracranial pressure with a bulging fontanelle. Focal neurological signs follow vascular occlusion. Convulsions occur in 25% of patients but are less likely with infection with *N. meningitides*. Subdural effusions usually resolve without the need for surgical drainage and, together with resistant organisms or inadequate treatment, may result in a fever persisting beyond 10 days. Hyponatraemia and a hypo-osmolar state occur as a result of inappropriate antidiuretic hormone (ADH) secretion (SIADH).

The diagnosis is confirmed by a lumbar puncture and examination of the CSF, which classically reveals an increase in neutrophils and protein and a decrease in CSF glucose. A Gram stain may help in the initial identification of the causative organism. In those with raised intracranial pressure or severe cardiorespiratory compromise the lumbar puncture is preferably delayed or omitted, particularly if the diagnosis is not in doubt in those with a typical rash and rapidly deteriorating course due to fulminant meningococcaemia. In all cases, several blood cultures should be taken. *N. meningitides* may be cultured from nasopharyngeal swabs, and in those with a purpuric/haemorrhagic rash skin scrapings may provide a useful source of microbiological confirmation, even 2 days after starting antibiotics. The latter should be started empirically, employing third-generation cephalosporins such as cefotaxime or ceftriaxone, and continuing for 10 days. Where antibiotics have already been given, rapid bacterial antigen detection tests can be applied to the CSF to help to identify the organism.

The advent of *H. influenzae* type b (Hib) vaccine has reduced the incidence of this type of meningitis. Vaccines are available against *N. meningitides* groups A and C but not against the more common group B. Nevertheless, a recent significant increase in the incidence of *N. meningitides* type C in the UK has led to the widespread routine introduction of the C vaccine to the general population (see Table 62, p. 212 ). Prophylaxis with rifampicin should be prescribed to all close contacts under the age of 5 years of an index case of *N. meningitides*, and for close contacts below the age of 4 years with *H. influenzae* meningitis. Ciprofloxacin is given to older children and adult contacts of *N. meningitides*. It is not required for contacts of *S. pneumoniae*. Long-term sequelae in survivors include sensorineural deafness (up to 30%), reduced vision, epilepsy, neurodevelopmental delay and mental retardation.

## Viral meningitis

Viral meningitis is usually caused by enteroviruses (80%), arboviruses, herpesviruses and mumps. A non-specific febrile illness generally precedes signs of meningism, and convulsions, focal neurological signs and coma may ensue. The CSF contains an increased number of polymorphs but near-normal levels of protein and glucose. Viruses can sometimes be isolated from the CSF, but confirmation is more likely on sequential serum antibody levels. Aciclovir is effective against herpes; otherwise the treatment is supportive and involves control of complications.

## Encephalitis

Encephalitis, a diffuse infection of the brain parenchyma, is usually seen with viral agents, including

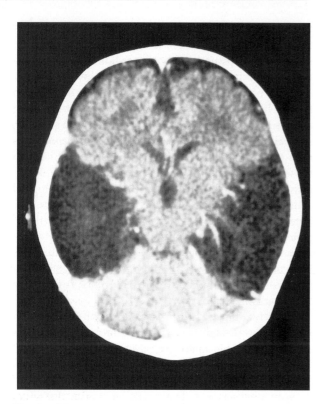

**Fig. 58** CT scan showing bilateral temporal lobe involvement in herpes encephalitis

enteroviruses (80%), arboviruses, herpes (simplex, varicella), measles, mumps, rubella and HIV, and occasionally with toxoplasma, mycobacteria and mycoplasma. The disease is mild and self-limiting (enteroviruses) or severe and rapidly progressive (herpes, mycoplasma). Fever associated with altered consciousness, sometimes seizures, is the hallmark of these conditions. Hallucinations, vomiting, photophobia, neck stiffness and a non-specific erythematous rash develop over a few days and, in the majority, subside as recovery ensues. The CSF shows an increase in white cells but no bacterial organisms. Serological investigation of the CSF and body secretions may confirm the infecting agent. EEG shows a generalised encephalopathic pattern, and CT or MRI confirms changes in the grey–white matter. The last characteristically involves the temporal lobes in herpes simplex encephalitis (Fig. 58). Treatment includes supportive measures to control complications, including raised intracranial pressure and seizures. Specific antimicrobial drugs are indicated with mycoplasma and TB, whereas aciclovir is the drug of choice with herpes infection.

## Brain abscess

Brain abscesses generally occur in early school-aged children and follow penetrating trauma, meningitis,

septic embolisation (e.g. with tetralogy of Fallot), and invasive infection in the scalp, skull, ears and ventricular shunts. They usually involve the frontoparietal lobes, initially presenting with fever, headaches and lethargy, followed by seizures, focal neurological signs and coma. Causative agents include *Staphylococcus aureus*, streptococci, Gram-negative bacilli, anaerobes, and occasionally fungi. If suspected, the diagnosis is confirmed on CT or MRI scanning. A lumbar puncture is avoided because of the significant risk of precipitating cerebellar herniation (coning). Treatment involves combination antibiotics given intravenously in high doses. Surgical aspiration is required with multilocular or fungal abscesses, and in those complicated by gas formation and pressure effects.

## 6.6 Seizures and headaches

### Learning objectives

You should:

- know the features of the common types of childhood seizure

- be able to give advice to the parents of a child with febrile seizures

- know the steps to manage children with epilepsy and status epilepticus

## Epileptic seizures

Seizures occur in 0.5–0.1% of the population and, if febrile seizures are included, affect up to 3–5% of children. They involve episodic involuntary movement and behavioural or sensory activity, often associated with loss of consciousness. Although they are an overt manifestation of abnormal electrical activity in the brain, in the majority of cases investigation will not reveal an underlying cause. Recurrent seizures unrelated to an acute cerebral insult or fever constitute epilepsy. A detailed history is fundamental in making the diagnosis. The clinical examination is usually unremarkable, but must exclude evidence of raised intracranial pressure, hypertension and neurocutaneous stigmata, and evidence of a metabolic or storage disorder. Investigation should focus on excluding an underlying metabolic or CNS abnormality, and should include an electroencephalogram (EEG). The EEG is a recording of the electrical activity of the brain that may provide useful information on the seizure type, its treatment and prognosis.

**Table 41** Types of epileptic seizure

| Partial | Generalised |
|---|---|
| Simple | Absences |
| Complex | Tonic–clonic |
| Secondary generalisation | Tonic |
| | Clonic |
| | Myotonic |
| | Atonic |
| | Infantile spasms |

## Classification of seizures

Epileptic seizures can be divided into partial or generalised types (Table 41).

### Partial seizures

Simple partial seizures (SPS) involve brief tonic or clonic movements of the face and extremities that may follow an aura but are not associated with impaired consciousness.

Complex partial seizures consist of attacks of altered or impaired consciousness associated with strange sensations or complex semi-purposeful movements.

### Generalised seizures

**Absence (generalised) seizures** usually affect girls, who experience a sudden loss of consciousness for less than 30 seconds, often associated with staring and eyelid flickering but no aura or postictal state. Typical absences (petit mal) produce 3 per second spike and generalised discharges on the EEG. Atypical absences (complex) are associated with myoclonic movements of the head and extremities and 2 per second discharges on EEG. An adverse outcome is expected in those with other, tonic–clonic or multiple seizures, a positive family history and low IQ (<90).

**Tonic–clonic (generalised) seizures** are the most common type of convulsion, commencing with an aura and followed by loss of consciousness, tonic contractures and rhythmic clonic movements in the limbs lasting several minutes. Cyanosis, tongue biting and incontinence of urine are common during the fit, which is followed by a postictal phase, generally involving a variable period of sleep.

**Myoclonic epilepsy** includes a heterogeneous group of conditions characterised by sudden loss of muscle tone, which may result in injury. Some forms are associated with a positive family history and a benign course, whereas others are associated with mental retardation and are refractory to treatment.

**Dravet syndrome** is a severe form of myoclonic epilepsy which begins with febrile seizures in early childhood, followed by episodes of repeated short convulsions which are refractory to therapy. Subsequently marked mental retardation is a feature.

**Infantile spasms** (West syndrome) usually commence around 3–6 months of age and involve repetitive, symmetrical contractions of the neck, trunk and limbs. The last are mostly flexor spasms producing the characteristic salaam attacks, but may be interspersed with extensor contractions. Infantile spasms are common just before or after sleep. Up to 20% are idiopathic; the remainder are secondary to hypoxic damage, CNS infection and trauma, neurocutaneous syndromes and storage diseases. Indeed, around 40% of children with infantile spasms have evidence of cerebral palsy and 80% have significant cognitive disability. The EEG is usually chaotic (hypsarrhythmia), and the treatment difficult, especially in non-idiopathic types, when the risk of mental retardation is high. Steroids and, more recently, vigabatrin have been shown to be effective.

**Multiple seizures** are characteristic of the Lennox–Gastaut syndrome. These often include myoclonic seizures associated with tonic activity, atypical absences and infantile spasms. Most children with this syndrome have delayed development, with significant motor and cognitive impairment. The condition is often refractory to therapy and only 10% have a reasonable outcome. Occasionally, recourse to surgical resection is necessary (e.g. callostomy for drop attacks).

## Management of epilepsy

It is important to establish the type of seizure activity through a detailed history and EEG evidence. Any underlying cause and complications must be controlled and any associated problems addressed (e.g. physical or mental handicap etc.). A decision must then be taken as to the need for and type of treatment, if any. An expectant approach can be applied for patients with a single, non-febrile seizure in whom there are no abnormal physical signs and a normal EEG. Having established a diagnosis of epilepsy, a single anticonvulsant is started and the dose built up over a number of weeks until fit control is adequate without drug-related side effects (Table 42). Dose increases should be considered at intervals of at least five times the interseizure intervals (e.g. every 5 weeks in a child who has one seizure per week). Serum anticonvulsant levels should be used only *as a guide* to management, but may be helpful especially with sodium valproate, phenytoin and phenobarbitone (Table 43). Indeed, for most anticonvulsants there is very little correlation with serum levels, efficacy and side effects. The drug of choice is dependent on the seizure type (Table 40). Monotherapy should be tried with a first drug, then a second single drug in appropriate doses for several months. If, despite this approach, the child is still experiencing more than one

**Table 42** Anticonvulsants: indications and side effects

| Anticonvulsant | Seizure type | Side effects |
|---|---|---|
| **First-line** | | |
| Sodium valproate | Tonic–clonic, absences, myoclonic, atonic, partial, Lennox–Gastaut | Tremor, liver dysfunction, thrombocytopenia |
| Carbamazepine | Tonic–clonic, partial, complex | Sedation, ataxia, liver dysfunction, leukopenia |
| Ethosuximide | Absences | Rashes, headaches, behavioural changes, leukopenia |
| Phenobarbitone (in neonates) | Tonic–clonic, partial | Rashes, cardiorespiratory depression, behavioural changes |
| **Second-line** | | |
| Phenytoin | Tonic–clonic, atonic, partial, status epilepticus | Rashes, ataxia, hirsutism, gum hypertrophy, cognitive and liver dysfunction |
| Benzodiazepine | Myoclonic, atonic, status epilepticus, infantile spasms, partial, absences | Sedation, excess salivation, behavioural changes, cognitive and liver dysfunction |
| Lamotrigine | Tonic–clonic, atonic, absences, myoclonic, partial, refractory seizures | Rashes, headache, fever, ataxia, liver dysfunction |
| Vigabatrin | Infantile spasms, behavioural changes, tonic–clonic, refractory, partial | Sedation, increased appetite, visual field restriction |
| **Others** | | |
| Steroids | Infantile spasms, myoclonic, Landau–Kleffner | Weight gain, hypertension, hyperglycaemia |
| Levetiracetam | Tonic–clonic, myoclonic, complex, refractory | Somnolence, ataxia, tremor, behavioural changes |
| Gabapentin | Tonic–clonic, partial, complex | Somnolence, behavioural changes |
| Topiramate | Tonic–clonic, partial, Lennox–Gastaut | Somnolence, anorexia, ataxia, behavioural changes |
| Oxcarbazepine | Partial seizures | Sedation, ataxia, liver dysfunction, leukopenia |
| Tiagabine | Partial seizures | Somnolence, dizziness |
| Visabatrin | West syndrome | Somnolence |
| Paraldehyde | Status epilepticus | Sterile abscesses, anal irritation |
| Thiopentone | Status epilepticus | Cardiorespiratory depression, sedation, arrhythmias, muscle twitching, irritant on extravasation |
| Ketogenic diet | Tonic–clonic, multiple | Difficult to establish and maintain diet |

**Table 43** Common blood tests while on antiepileptic drugs (AEDs)

| Test | Blood count | Liver function | Electrolytes | AED level* |
|---|---|---|---|---|
| Carbamazepine | + | + | + | + |
| Sodium valproate | + | + | | + |
| Phenytoin | + | + | | + |
| Ethosuximide | + | | | + |
| Lamotrigine | | + | | |
| Phenobarbitone | | | | + |

* Serum AED (anti-epileptic drug) levels are only a guide to management.

seizure per month, a second drug is added in combination. Care is required in view of the high incidence of drug interactions between several anticonvulsants (Table 44). After a sufficiently long period of control, usually spanning a few months, the initial drug can be discontinued.

Cessation of medication can be considered after a 1–2-year fit-free period in those without risk factors. Weaning should take place over a minimum of 3 months, and up to 70% of these patients will have no further fits. A good outcome is suggested by a single seizure type of short duration and infrequent occurrence, with clear provoking phenomena (e.g. intercurrent illness) and no neurological impairment in between seizures. Features indicative of a poor outcome include multiple seizure types, refactoriness to anticonvulsants, frequent episodes, prolonged duration, early onset, absence of provoking phenomena and additional neurological impairment.

Surgery is developing as a viable treatment option for intractable epilepsy, particularly in those with a demonstrable clinical, radiological or electroencephalographic focus. Vagal nerve stimulation (VNS) has also been shown to reduce seizures by up to 50% on average, in those with intractable seizure disorders in whom multiple anticonvulsants have previously failed to achieve satisfactory control.

**Table 44** Interactions between antiepileptic drugs

| | Valproate | Carba-mazepine | Phenytoin | Ethosux-imide | Phenobar-bitone | Benzodi-azepines | Topira-mate | Vigabar-trin | Lamot-rigine |
|---|---|---|---|---|---|---|---|---|---|
| Valproate | | ↑ | ↓↑ | ↑* | ↑ | | | | ↑ |
| Carbamazepine | ↓ | | ↓↑ | ↓* | | ↓ | ↓ | | ↓ |
| Phenytoin | ↓ | ↓ | | ↓* | ↑ | ↓ | ↓ | | ↓ |
| Ethosuximide | | | ↑* | | | | | | |
| Phenobarbitone | ↓ | ↓ | ↓ | ↓* | | ↓ | | | ↓ |
| Benzodiazepines | | | | | | | | | |
| Topiramate | | | ↑* | | | | | | |
| Vigabatrin | | | ↓ | | ↓* | | | | |
| Lamotrigine | | ↑* | | | | | | | |

\* Denotes variable effect.
Note that the new antiepileptic levetiracetam is unrelated to and does not interact with the other AEDs.

## Non-epileptic seizures

Non-epileptic seizures include those related to a fever or to a CNS insult such as trauma, metabolic derangement and infections. They do not necessarily lead to lifetime seizure activity. *Febrile convulsions* are the most common seizures in childhood, usually affecting 4% of children aged 6 months to 6 years, often with a positive family history. They comprise symmetrical, generalised tonic–clonic seizures lasting less than 15 minutes, associated with loss of consciousness and no focal neurological signs. The convulsion is generally triggered with spikes of fever and usually responds to cooling and antipyretic measures. Following a febrile convulsion, all children should be examined to exclude a serious underlying infection. If in doubt, a lumbar puncture should be performed. All those with atypical febrile convulsions require investigation with neuroimaging and an EEG. Although there is a slightly increased risk of non-febrile seizure activity later in life in 10% of children, there is no place for routine anticonvulsant therapy in uncomplicated febrile seizures. Adverse factors suggesting continuing seizure activity include complex or atypical initial seizures, a positive family history of epilepsy and preceding neurological abnormality. Treatment involves the administration of rectal diazepam during subsequent convulsions and, where indicated, prophylactic sodium valproate.

## Status epilepticus

Constant seizure activity, or recurrent fits with no resumption of consciousness persisting beyond 30 minutes, constitutes status epilepticus. This is usually seen after prolonged febrile seizures or in patients with preceding neurological or metabolic disease, but also occurs de novo in those without a CNS insult. The excessive convulsive activity causes cerebral hypoglycaemia,

**Table 45** Seizure-like disorders

| Preschool children | School children |
|---|---|
| Breath-holding attacks | Night terrors |
| Paroxysmal vertigo | Syncopal attacks |
| Benign myoclonus | Rage attacks |
| | Narcolepsy |
| | Munchausen syndrome by proxy |

lactic acidosis and hypoxia, and in 5% of patients results in death. This medical emergency requires active resuscitation, protection of the airway, correction of the metabolic derangements and anticonvulsants. Intravenous diazepam is the first drug of choice, and can be repeated and followed by paraldehyde, phenytoin, valproate or phenobarbitone. In refractory cases, general anaesthesia with thiopentone is required.

## Seizure-like disorders

A thorough history is essential to differentiate seizures from the non-convulsive disorders listed in Table 45. In particularly difficult cases a period of in-hospital observation combined with repeated EEGs and, preferably, continuous EEG videotelemetry may be necessary.

## Headaches

### Tension headaches

Tension headaches are extremely common in school-aged children, particularly in sensitive, introverted types. They manifest as continuous pressure-like pain, usually over the forehead or crown, that lasts several minutes or hours. They are generally related to stress and anxiety and are worse towards the end of the day. If prolonged, they may be indicative of serious underlying discord at home or at school, depression, and occasionally child abuse. All children reporting such headaches should have a thorough examination, including fundoscopy and blood pressure recording. Reassurance and simple analgesics are usually sufficient treatment.

## Migraine

A positive family history of migraine is commonly present in children who present with recurrent, severe, throbbing headaches, usually over the eyes, frontal, temporal and occipital areas (often unilaterally). These headaches may be preceded by a visual or sensory aura, are associated with nausea and vomiting, and last several hours or days. Abdominal pain is a frequent accompaniment, especially in younger children. Migraine may be precipitated by stress, chocolate, cheese, nuts and meat extracts; it improves with rest in a quiet, dark room, and sleep. Rarely, migraine may be associated with transient unilateral weakness (*hemiplegic migraine*), a third-nerve palsy (*ophthalmoplegic migraine*), and vertigo with ataxia (*basilar migraine*). Again, a full examination is mandatory and investigation is usually unnecessary. Analgesics and antiemetics are required during the acute attack. For those experiencing more than three attacks a month, treatment may be supplemented with prophylaxis in the form of propranolol.

## Raised intracranial pressure

Raised intracranial pressure results in headaches that have a diurnal variation, usually worse in the early morning. They are usually accompanied by photophobia, progressive lethargy, nausea and vomiting, and improve after vomiting. Bradycardia, hypertension and papilloedema in the presence of these symptoms suggest raised intracranial pressure and are an indication for an urgent brain scan.

## Subarachnoid bleed

A severe, sudden-onset headache associated with an altered level of consciousness and meningism may herald a subarachnoid bleed. The presence of blood and xanthochromia in the CSF necessitates a contrast-enhanced CT scan in order to identify a vascular malformation. An arteriogram or MR angiogram may be necessary, especially when delicate surgery is contemplated.

# 6.7 The spinal cord and peripheral nerves

## Learning objectives

You should:

- be aware of the symptoms of cord compression
- know the congenital causes for a 'floppy' baby

## Cord compression

Spinal cord compression may result from tumours within the spinal canal, vertebral collapse and trauma. It presents with lower limb weakness, gait and sphincter disturbances. Back pain may point toward the site of compression, and sensory loss in the limbs can localise the block at spinal level. Lower motor neuron signs develop at the site of the lesion, whereas upper motor neuron signs are seen in neurons arising below the obstruction.

In children where a cervical fracture is suspected, the neck must be immobilised immediately. Cord compression from whatever cause is a medical emergency. The diagnosis is confirmed on radiology and neuroimaging (where MRI excels), and neurosurgical decompression performed as soon as possible. Radiotherapy and/or chemotherapy may be required with spinal tumours, depending on the histology.

## Neuropathies

Disorders affecting peripheral neurons may have a congenital, degenerative, postinfectious or toxic aetiology (Box 33).

## Spinal muscular atrophy

Congenital spinal muscular atrophy (SMA) describes a group of progressive, degenerative conditions that

---

**Box 33** Causes of peripheral neuronal dysfunctions

| Congenital | Acquired |
|---|---|
| Hereditary | Toxic |
|   Peroneal atrophy |   Heavy metals |
|   Familial dysautonomia |   Organophosphates |
| Degenerative |   Vincristine |
|   Werdnig–Hoffmann |   Uraemia |
|   Kugelberg–Welander | Postinfectious |
| |   Guillain–Barré |
| |   Poliomyelitis |
| |   Diabetes mellitus |

affect the peripheral nerves. Severe forms (e.g. Werdnig–Hoffmann, SMA type I) present in the neonatal period with marked hypotonia, areflexia and fasciculation, and patients die within 2 years from respiratory involvement. Patients with less severe forms (SMA types II/III) may survive into adult life with variable degrees of handicap. The diagnosis is confirmed on muscle and nerve biopsy and, where applicable, by detection of the abnormal mutation in genetic studies.

## Sensorimotor neuropathies

Hereditary sensorimotor neuropathies generally present in late childhood with gait disturbance, foot drop and distal lower limb muscle wasting, producing a champagne-glass appearance. Slow velocities on nerve conduction tests confirm the diagnosis. Management involves supportive orthopaedic splints and avoidance of injury to the limbs.

## Toxic neuropathies

Toxic neuropathies often involve large nerve fibres (e.g. lead poisoning) and may result in ptosis, constipation and loss of reflexes (e.g. vincristine).

## Poliomyelitis

Infection with the poliovirus (poliomyelitis) was a common cause of infective motor neuron disease before vaccination became routine. Up to 95% of infected individuals are asymptomatic or simply develop a mild coryzal illness. A minority develop headache, nausea, vomiting, muscle discomfort and stiffness, which resolves (*non-paralytic poliomyelitis*). Asymmetrical muscle, bladder and bowel weakness can occur in *paralytic poliomyelitis*. Milder disorders with involvement of the anterior horn cells, causing acute flaccid paralysis, weakness and loss of reflexes, can develop after the live attenuated polio vaccine, and after infection with echoviruses and Coxsackie viruses.

## Guillain–Barré syndrome

Guillain–Barré syndrome is a demyelinating disorder that usually follows 10 days or so after a non-specific illness. The presentation of postinfectious neuronitis is similar to that of polio, although the acute febrile manifestations are less prominent, the flaccid paralysis is symmetrical, and sensory involvement can sometimes develop. Weakness progresses slowly from distal to proximal groups, eventually involving bulbar, respiratory and cranial nerves in severe cases. Recovery occurs in reverse pattern and is complete in most patients

within 3 weeks. A few patients develop a chronic, relapsing or unremitting polyneuropathy and are left with permanent weakness. The CSF protein level is typically raised, but glucose and white cells are normal. Nerve conduction velocity is greatly reduced (motor is greater than sensory). All patients require admission in the acute phase until the disease has stopped progressing. A 5-day course of intravenous immunoglobulin is now standard treatment in the first instance, backed up with plasmapheresis in those with severe or rapidly progressive disease. Physiotherapy is required to mobilise weak muscle groups, and artificial ventilation is necessary for those with respiratory embarrassment.

## 6.8 Neuromuscular disorders

### Learning objective

You should:

- be able to perform a relevant clinical examination of a child with Duchenne muscular dystrophy and discuss the management with his parents

### Dystrophies

Muscular dystrophies (MD) are genetically determined, progressive disorders involving muscle fibre degeneration. They run a variable course, so that children with X-linked recessive *Duchenne MD* are generally wheelchair bound by the end of the first decade, and do not survive much beyond three decades. Duchenne MD occurs in 1 in 3600 males and presents with progressive limb weakness and delayed motor milestones. Examination reveals calf pseudohypertrophy, muscle weakness and lumbar lordosis (Fig. 59). Pelvic girdle weakness results in affected boys having to climb up their own limbs in order to stand (Gower sign), and a waddling gait. All patients have a mild degree of intellectual deficit, cardiomyopathy of variable clinical significance and, ultimately, respiratory failure. Investigation reveals a several thousandfold increase in serum creatinine kinase (also raised in most, but not all, female carriers), a myopathic EMG but normal nerve conduction. Muscle biopsy and the identification of abnormal *dystrophin* in muscle or an abnormal dystrophin gene in DNA confirms the diagnosis. Physiotherapy and supportive braces are essential to prolong mobility as long as possible, delaying the onset of scoliosis. Recently steroids have been shown to delay the need for a wheelchair, but their use in this condition remains controversial. Surgery may be required for troublesome contractures. Nutrition should be optimised and chest

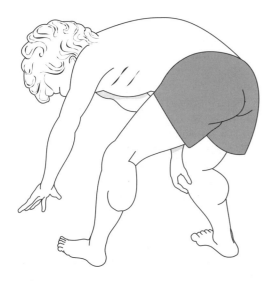

**Fig. 59** Boy with Duchenne muscular dystrophy climbing up himself to stand (Gower manoeuvre) and showing marked pseudohypertrophy of the calves.

infections treated aggressively. A genetically engineered cure is still awaited.

Boys with *Becker MD* have a similar but milder X-linked disorder and remain ambulatory until early adulthood. Nevertheless, few survive beyond their 40s, by which time physical handicap is severe. Other dystrophies are inherited as dominant or recessive traits, and are characterised by weakness in specific muscle distributions, e.g. proximal limbs in *limb girdle dystrophy*, face and distal groups in *myotonic dystrophy*, and face plus shoulder girdle in *facioscapulohumeral dystrophy*.

## Myopathies

Muscle weakness, wasting and myopathic changes observed on electromyography (EMG) may follow congenital disease (mitochondrial myopathy) or be secondary to endocrine disease (hyper- and hypothyroidism, Cushing syndrome, hyperparathyroidism), electrolyte imbalance (hypo- and hyperkalaemia), and inborn errors of lipid and glycogen storage. Drugs, and in particular corticosteroids, may also be associated with myopathic side effects.

## Myasthenia gravis

Myasthenia gravis is seen transiently in neonates born to affected mothers. An immune response against the motor endplate rarely develops in older children, who present with ptosis, facial weakness, difficulty in swallowing and limb weakness. Rapid onset of fatigue is the hallmark of myasthenia. Hence symptoms are worse toward the end of the day, and clinical signs can be enhanced by asking the child to perform repeated exercises. A similar trend is observed on EMG that, like the clinical signs, can be reversed with a cholinesterase inhibitor (e.g. edrophonium). Treatment entails the use of similar, longer-acting drugs such as neostigmine.

# Self-assessment: questions

## Multiple choice questions

1. The following statements describe meningitis:
   a. Meningococci are the most common bacteria to invade the CSF in neonates
   b. *Streptococcus pneumoniae* meningitis is not associated with deafness
   c. Antibiotic prophylaxis is required for all contacts of bacterial meningitis
   d. Viral meningitis is associated with very low glucose levels in the CSF
   e. Viral meningitis usually resolves without long-term complications.

2. The management of cerebral palsy may include:
   a. Tendon release operations
   b. Nasogastric feeding
   c. Attention to pressure areas
   d. Control of seizures
   e. Regular chest physiotherapy.

3. Abnormalities of the cranial nerves result in the following:
   a. Foot drop with a tenth-nerve palsy
   b. Failure of abduction of the eye with a seventh-nerve palsy
   c. 'Down and out' position of the globe with a third-nerve palsy
   d. Total facial palsy with an upper motor neuron defect of the seventh nerve
   e. Deviation of the protruded tongue to the affected side with a twelfth-nerve palsy.

4. The following features are observed in neurocutaneous syndromes:
   a. Strawberry naevi
   b. Recurrent purpuric spots
   c. Plexiform neurofibromas
   d. Retinal phakomata
   e. Port-wine stain.

5. The following are indicative of raised intracranial pressure:
   a. Hypotension
   b. Hypertension
   c. Tachycardia
   d. Unilateral papilloedema
   e. Somnolence.

6. The following drugs and side effects are correctly matched:
   a. Phenytoin and gum hypertrophy
   b. Clonazepam and respiratory depression
   c. Sodium valproate and sterile abscesses
   d. Carbamazepine and liver dysfunction
   e. Ethosuximide and hirsutism.

7. In Guillain–Barré syndrome:
   a. Sensory deficit does not occur
   b. Evidence of recovery within 3 weeks is a good prognostic indicator
   c. Reflexes are lost early but recover rapidly
   d. Respiratory depression is an indication for plasmapheresis
   e. Steroids are the mainstay of treatment.

8. The following are causes of peripheral neuropathy:
   a. Organophosphates
   b. Chemotherapeutic agents
   c. Steroids
   d. Carbamazepine
   e. Mercury poisoning.

9. The following are characteristics of febrile convulsions:
   a. They affect children aged 6 months to 6 years
   b. They are the most common seizure type observed in childhood
   c. They are mainly observed in boys
   d. They last more than 30 minutes
   e. They result in chronic epilepsy in the majority of children.

10. Regarding the intelligence quotient (IQ) in children:
    a. IQ is an extremely precise measurement of intelligence
    b. The IQ score can vary from day to day
    c. The IQ may be low in children with glue ears
    d. An IQ of less than 90 implies severe mental retardation
    e. Children with Down syndrome average an IQ of about 50.

## Case histories

### Case history 1

A 10-year-old boy presents with 'funny turns', whereby he becomes vacant for a few seconds, sometimes associated with flickering of his eyelids. He is bullied at school, where recently his performance has deteriorated.

How would you determine the diagnosis?

### Case history 2

A 10-year-old boy is admitted to A&E at 23.30 h in a semicomatose state. Earlier that same day he had returned from a school outing to a nearby pharmaceutical factory. He had complained of tiredness and a headache, had refused supper and had gone to bed at 19.45 h. His parents heard him moaning in bed at 22.50 h and brought him to hospital, where you confirm his altered conscious level and note a few purpuric spots over the lower limbs and torso.

1. What important features would you check on clinical examination?
2. What is the presumptive diagnosis?
3. How would you confirm the diagnosis?
4. What immediate therapeutic steps would you take in A&E?

Despite the initial management, his conscious level continues to deteriorate such that he is not rousable 1 hour after admission. By this time he is centrally cyanosed, the blood pressure is 65/35 and the rash has spread over most of his body and is partly confluent over the toes. Some bleeding is noted around the IV cannulae insertion sites.

5. What complications have developed?
6. What further investigations are required at this point?
7. What further therapeutic intervention is required at this point?
8. What would you tell the parents at this point?
9. What community-based precautions are required?

Despite incipient gangrene of two toes, the patient's condition stabilises and starts to improve over the next 3 days. Although he is lucid and fully orientated on day 10, he remains slightly irritable, with a fever of around 38°C.

10. What might explain his condition, and how would you investigate the temperature?

### Case history 3

A 7-year-old boy is rushed to A&E by his mother. He had been slightly off colour that same morning, and at midday had cried out and fallen to the floor, where he was found unconscious and shaking all four limbs.

a. What questions directly relating to this episode would you ask at this point?

He was apyrexial but still unresponsive and jerking all four limbs 3 minutes after his arrival in A&E.

b. What preliminary clinical diagnosis would you make at this point?
c. What other history would you seek from the boy's mother?

He is placed in the recovery position and given oxygen by face-mask. However, there is no change in his condition after a further 2 minutes and you decide to intervene.

d. What would you do to abort the event, and how would you implement this in practice?

By 20 minutes he is back to 'normal', albeit slightly drowsy. A detailed examination at this point is entirely normal.

e. What investigations would you organise, indicating the relative timeframe/urgency of each investigation?

These investigations are normal but he has a further two similar episodes over the next 4 months.

f. What medication would you prescribe?

## Short notes

Outline the key points in the management of status epilepticus.

## Viva voce question

A 5-year-old boy is brought to A&E in a coma following a fall on to the head from a height. What would you be concerned about and what steps would you take to confirm this? Outline your initial management.

## OSCE questions

### OSCE 1

Figure 60 was taken from a 6-year-old girl who presented with repeated vomiting.

a. What is the abnormality shown on fundoscopy?
b. What other symptoms may have been present?
c. What other clinical signs may be present?

### OSCE 2

Figure 61 was taken shortly after birth.

a. What is the abnormality?
b. What other clinical signs may be associated with this lesion?

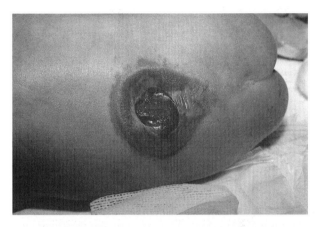

**Fig. 61**

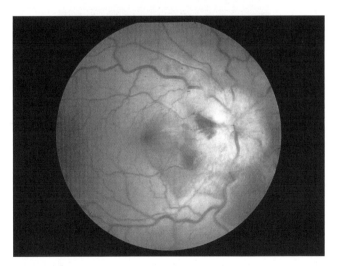

**Fig. 60**

**OSCE 3**

Figure 62 was taken from a 12-year-old girl who suffered with recurrent tonic–clonic and myoclonic seizures.

a.  What is the abnormality?
b.  What is the most likely cause in this child?
c.  Name two other side effects.

**OSCE 4**

An 8-year-old boy had difficulty walking and getting up from a sitting position.

a.  What abnormality is shown on Figure 63?
b.  What is the most likely cause at this age?
c.  What investigations would confirm the diagnosis?

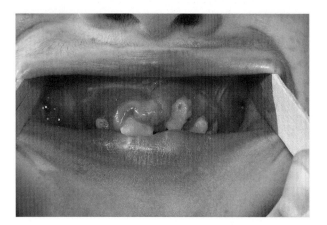

**Fig. 62**

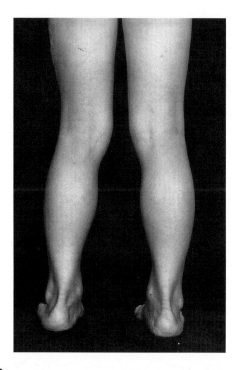

**Fig. 63**

# Self-assessment: answers

## Multiple choice answers

1. a. **False**. Gram-negative bacilli are most common.
   b. **False**. As with other types of bacterial meningitis.
   c. **False**. It is not necessary with *Streptococcus pneumoniae*.
   d. **False**. CSF glucose is normal or slightly reduced.
   e. **True**. Although persistent neurological deficit is not uncommon if an associated encephalitis is also present, especially with herpes simplex and CMV infections.

2. a. **True**. This will help with contractures.
   b. **True**. This maintains enteral feeds when there is bulbar and pseudobulbar involvement, general debility and weakness.
   c. **True**. Pressure sores develop easily at pressure points in relatively immobile patients.
   d. **True**. Seizures are common complications of cerebral palsy.
   e. **True**. Chest infections are common in the immobile patient.

3. a. **False**. A tenth-nerve palsy produces difficulty in swallowing.
   b. **True**. Abduction is primarily limited in the horizontal plane.
   c. **True**. This position is the result of the unopposed, combined action of the fourth (downward) and sixth (lateral) cranial nerves.
   d. **False**. Preservation of the upper division occurs with upper motor neuron defects; total paralysis occurs with lower motor neuron defects.
   e. **True**. It is pushed over by the normal side.

4. a. **False**. Cutaneous manifestations of neurocutaneous syndromes include *café au lait* spots (neurofibromatosis); adenoma sebaceum, shagreen and hypopigmented patches (tuberous sclerosis); and port-wine naevi (Sturge–Weber syndrome).
   b. **False**. See above.
   c. **True**. This is neurofibromatosis type 1 (NF1).
   d. **True**. This occurs in tuberous sclerosis.
   e. **True**. Occurs on the face in Sturge–Weber syndrome.

5. a. **True**. Occurs in end-stage raised intracranial pressure.
   b. **True**. Occurs together with bradycardia.
   c. **False**. Bradycardia is an indication.
   d. **True**. Initially papilloedema may be unilateral.
   e. **True**. This completes the classic triad, with vomiting and headaches.

6. a. **True**. This is a classic side effect of phenytoin.
   b. **True**. As with all benzodiazepines.
   c. **False**. This occurs with paraldehyde.
   d. **True**. Hence the need to perform regular liver function tests in patients taking carbamazepine.
   e. **False**. This occurs with phenytoin.

7. a. **False**. Sensory nerves may be affected.
   b. **True**. This implies a greater chance of total recovery.
   c. **False**. Weakness improves well before the reflexes.
   d. **True**. Plasmapheresis is indicated with rapidly progressive neuropathy, bulbar and respiratory involvement.
   e. **False**. Intravenous immunoglobulin is the mainstay of treatment.

8. a. **True**. These irreversibly inhibit acetylcholinesterases and cause accumulation of acetylcholine at muscarinic and nicotinic synapses.
   b. **True**. Occurs particularly with vincristine.
   c. **False**. Steroids may cause a myopathy.
   d. **False**. Neuropathy is not a recognised complication of carbamazepine.
   e. **True**. As with other heavy metals, e.g. lead.

9. a. **True**. Although febrile convulsions occasionally develop in older children.
   b. **True**. Febrile convulsions affect 3-5% of children.
   c. **False**. They are seen in both sexes.
   d. **False**. They last less than 15 minutes.
   e. **False**. Very few develop epilepsy.

10. a. **False**. It is no more than a good guide.
    b. **True**. IQ assessment depends on a child's wellbeing, mood and cooperation.
    c. **True**. Most IQ tests are language based and rely on hearing.
    d. **False**. Less than 70 is the value used.
    e. **True**.

## Case history answers

### Case history 1

Despite the potential psychosomatic element introduced by the bullying, the history is sufficiently suspicious of seizure activity, particularly of generalised absences. A causal relationship to the bullying should be sought, and a drug and family history obtained. Features such as definite loss of consciousness, incontinence, cyanosis and rhythmic, jerky movements of the limbs, as well as 'runs' of these episodes, several times daily including during sleep, point strongly toward epilepsy. A thorough examination is mandatory to exclude signs of raised intracranial pressure, hypertension, and neurological and metabolic disease. A period of in-hospital observation may be helpful in distinguishing between organic and psychosomatic symptoms. An EEG is required and performed at rest, with photic stimulation and hyperventilation. In addition, in a child with previously undiagnosed seizure activity, neuroimaging (e.g. CT scan) is indicated.

### Case history 2

1. The peripheral and central temperature, pulse rate and volume, blood pressure, state of peripheral perfusion and signs of meningeal irritation, i.e. photophobia, neck stiffness and resistance to extension of the knees while flexing the hips (Kernig's sign). Papilloedema is unlikely at this early stage.
2. Meningococcal septicaemia, probably with meningitis, caused by *Neisseria meningitides* (groups A, B or C).
3. Immediate blood cultures and serum for rapid antigen testing. The latter is not always reliable, especially with *N. meningitides* group B. A sample of CSF would be helpful but is contraindicated in a child with a deteriorating conscious level. Scraping of the purpuric lesions for culture can reveal the organism even up to 48 hours later.
4. One, preferably two, large-bore intravenous cannulae should be inserted and the blood cultures taken from the same access site. Plasma substitute follows immediately (20 mL/kg over 15–20 minutes and repeated as required), as well as intravenous ceftriaxone.
5. Progressive cardiovascular collapse (shock), associated with respiratory failure owing to pulmonary oedema and possibly cerebral oedema, and disseminated intravascular coagulation.

Bleeding into the adrenal glands may account for the deteriorating hypotension (Waterhouse–Friderichsen syndrome). Renal failure is likely to ensue.

6. An urgent blood gas analysis and chest X-ray, electrolyte, urea and creatinine assessment, cross-match and clotting profile, including fibrinogen degradation products, are required.
7. He requires urgent plasma expansion using colloid, fresh frozen plasma and, probably, blood. The introduction of a central line would be extremely important at this stage for the immediate commencement of inotropic support (e.g. dopamine and adrenaline by infusion). In addition, he requires intubation, ventilation, and transfer to the intensive care unit.
8. Explain the nature and severity of their son's condition. You will need to point out the possibility that he may not survive the acute episode and that, if he does, he may be left with residual sequelae, including neurological handicap. You will also need to introduce the need for antibiotic prophylaxis for all close contacts.
9. Hence the local public health authority must be notified. A thorough investigation into close 'contacts' is indicated. These include all individuals within the same household and friends with whom he may have had close (almost touching) contact for several hours within the preceding 24 hours, including contacts during the school trip. These should be given chemoprophylaxis with rifampicin (children) or ciprofloxacin (adults). There is no indication for mass 'blind' prophylaxis – indeed, this will encourage the emergence of resistant strains.
10. Provided there is no other obvious focus of infection, the fever may be caused by persistent low-grade infection in the CSF, a cerebral abscess or a subdural collection. It may be related to the antibiotic (or other medication). A full septic screen, including blood cultures and CT brain scan, possibly followed by a lumbar puncture, is necessary.

### Case history 3

a. Incontinence of urine
   Incontinence of faeces
   Frothing at mouth
   Cyanosis
   Any injuries; tongue biting, bang to head
   Symmetry/type of jerking/abnormal movements
   Duration of episode

b. Grand mal seizure/generalised convulsion *(but not febrile convulsion)*

c. History of headaches
   Recent illness with temperature
   Family history of fits/related problems
   Past history – similar episodes
   Birth history/risk factors
   Possibility of ingestion/drugs in household

d. Administer diazepam (5 mg), preferably per rectum or IV
   Repeat at least once, if necessary

e. Urgent/immediate: serum electrolytes ($Na^+$, $K^+$, $Ca^{2+}$, $Mg^{2+}$, urea); glucose; toxicology screen
   Note: lumbar puncture is not indicated.
   Within few days/weeks: CT (or MRI) brain scan.
   Within few days or weeks: EEG.

f. Sodium valproate or carbamazepine.
   Note: phenytoin, ethosuximide, vigabatrim, lamotrigine, thiopentone, benzodiazepine and steroids are not usually first-line drugs.

## Short notes answer

The management of status epilepticus involves: (i) control of the fits, and (ii) determining and treating any underlying cause, as follows:

a. Place child in left lateral position.
b. Administer oxygen by face-mask with oral airway in situ.
c. Cool child (undress, give rectal paracetamol).
d. Give diazepam per rectum while obtaining intravenous access.
e. Blood sent for glucose, electrolytes, calcium, blood gas and culture.
f. Correct hypoxia, acidosis, hypoglycaemia, metabolic derangements.
g. Repeat IV diazepam, followed by paraldehyde if fits not controlled.
h. Continuous IV phenytoin or IV valproate and benzodiazepine are third-line agents.
i. Thiopentone with full ventilatory support in refractory cases.
j. Transfer to intensive care unit with continuous ECG and EEG monitoring in refractory cases.

Investigation is aimed at excluding infection (septicaemia, meningitis, encephalitis), intracranial pathology (e.g. space-occupying lesion, intractable epileptic focus) and metabolic and neurodegenerative disease. Subsequent treatment will depend on the specific cause.

## Viva voce answer

Given that the child is in coma, it is reasonable to assume that he has sustained a significant injury to the brain and/or neck. These could include depressed or multiple skull fractures, major intracranial contusion(s) and haemorrhage(s), as well as fracture(s) of the cervical vertebrae with spinal compression. The neck must be immobilised immediately with an appropriate collar prior to a detailed examination to assess for signs of shock, raised intracranial pressure, focal neurological signs and injuries elsewhere (e.g. limb fractures, pneumothorax, acute abdomen etc.). If shocked, the child must be resuscitated. Intravenous access is obtained and fluids commenced: initially at 50% of maintenance in view of the risk of raised intracranial pressure and incipient brain oedema. Inotropic support may be required if he is hypotensive. Comprehensive X-rays of the skull and cervical spine, together with a brain CT scan, are mandatory and must be reviewed with the neurosurgical team. In addition, a cervical MRI scan may be required. Further management will depend on the result of these investigations, and may involve neurosurgery for intracranial haematoma and treatment of cerebral oedema with hyperventilation and fluid restriction.

## OSCE answers

### OSCE 1
a. Papilloedema, blurred disc edges, obscured and congested vessels
b. Headaches, drowsiness, blurred vision, weakness
c. Long tract signs, cerebellar signs, hypertension with bradycardia.

### OSCE 2
a. 'Open' spina bifida/myelomeningocoele/neural tube defect
b. Hydrocephalus, flaccid paralysis of lower limbs, urinary and bowel retention/dysfunction.

### OSCE 3
a. Gum or gingival hyperplasia
b. Anticonvulsant therapy, probably phenytoin
c. Hirsutism, liver dysfunction, rashes.

### OSCE 4
a. Bilateral pseudohypertrophy of calves
b. Duchenne muscular dystrophy
c. Raised CPK level, positive dystrophin gene.

# 7 The urinary system

**7.1** Introduction      145

**7.2** Symptoms and examination      145

**7.3** Congenital abnormalities      146

**7.4** Infections      146

**7.5** Proteinuria      149

**7.6** Haematuria      151

**7.7** Renal failure and dysfunction      153

Self-assessment: questions      156

Self-assessment: answers      159

## Overview

Structural abnormalities of the renal tract are common in children and often identified on antenatal screening. Other diseases of the urinary system are often either asymptomatic or have non-specific symptoms. Urinary tract infections, vesicoureteric reflux (VUR) and urinary obstructions have the potential to damage the growing kidney, therefore it is important to diagnose these conditions early. Unlike in adults, nephrotic syndrome is steroid sensitive and only rarely progresses to chronic renal disease. Thus an understanding of the investigation of a child with proteinuria and haematuria is essential. Finally, although few children develop end-stage renal failure, those that do contribute a significant workload on paediatric services and students should be familiar with the basic symptoms and signs suggestive of renal failure, and have a working overview of its management.

## 7.1 Introduction

Because of its non-specific symptoms and a paucity of signs, pathology in the urinary system in childhood is often 'forgotten'. However, in many cases the routine measurement of blood pressure and a simple urinalysis can alert one to the possibility of renal disease. Infection is the most common problem involving the urinary tract in childhood. When associated with congenital anomalies and reflux, this may result in significant morbidity. A clear understanding of its aetiology, clinical manifestations, investigation and treatment is required in order to prevent long-term complications, including renal failure.

Proteinuria and haematuria are manifestations of the renal tract as well as systemic diseases, and are easily confirmed on simple urinalysis. Both require further investigation of renal function. Although rare in childhood, renal failure results in acute and chronic complications that necessitate prompt intervention if morbidity and mortality are to be avoided. Children with end-stage renal failure require renal-replacement therapy and, ultimately, a percentage will go on to renal transplantation. The undergraduate should be familiar with the indications but not necessarily the details of these treatment modalities.

## 7.2 Symptoms and examination

### Learning objective

You should:

* know the symptoms and signs of renal diseases in childhood

### Symptoms of urinary tract disease

Symptoms specific to the urinary tract are generally absent in young children and a high level of suspicion is required. A *fever* without an obvious focus should raise the possibility of urinary tract infection (UTI). In neonates, prolonged jaundice, vomiting and weight loss are subtle pointers toward a UTI, and the urine and renal tracts should be investigated. Older children may complain of pain or a burning sensation on micturition (*dysuria*) and loin and/or abdominal pain. *Frequency* and an alteration in urinary habit, particularly with regression to incontinence, are relatively common presenting complaints. An alteration in *urinary consistency* and/or *colour* is rarely volunteered and should be asked for specifically. Offensive-smelling cloudy urine is suggestive of urinary infection, frothy urine of proteinuria, and 'smoky' urine of haematuria. Marked lethargy with a waxy pallor and, at times, itching may suggest uraemia in children with renal failure.

## Signs of urinary tract disease

Clinical signs may be conspicuous by their absence. Many *dysmorphic syndromes* are associated with renal anomalies. Some congenital anomalies are specifically indicative of renal disease, e.g. preauricular pits, two instead of three vessels in the umbilical cord, perineal and genital anomalies. *Anaemia* is a common association in children with renal failure and should be looked for. All those with suspected renal disease should have their *blood pressure* measured and *urinalysis* performed. Large kidneys and *renal masses* in the loin can be ballotted using both hands. A *distended bladder* is confirmed by finding a firm, rounded mass that rises out of the pelvis and is dull to percussion.

## 7.3 Congenital abnormalities

### Learning objective

You should:

* know the common renal anomalies of childhood and be able to discuss the diagnosis and management of an infant with vesicoureteric reflux

### Renal agenesis

Bilateral renal agenesis results in complete renal failure antenatally, culminating in oligohydramnios followed by stillbirth. Affected infants have the *Potter facies*, with a broad, flat nose, widely spaced eyes, epicanthic folds and low-set ears. Severe renal dysplasia and obstructive uropathy may produce a similar appearance. Unilateral agenesis may be suspected with the presence of a single umbilical artery and is compatible with a normal existence, provided there are no other major anomalies of the genitourinary, skeletal, cardiac and gastrointestinal systems.

### Maldevelopment

Incomplete upward migration of the embryonic kidney results in an *ectopic* kidney, usually sited in the pelvis. Fusion of the lower poles of each kidney produces a *horseshoe* kidney, whereas underdevelopment of the number of nephrons constitutes *renal hypoplasia*. The latter carries a risk of hypertension in early childhood and, if bilateral, renal failure later in life. Renal *dysplasia*

describes structurally abnormal nephrons and renal parenchyma, and may present with renal masses, hypertension and renal failure.

## Polycystic kidney disease

### Autosomal dominant polycystic kidney disease

Autosomal dominant polycystic kidney disease is associated with large cystic lesions in the kidneys and liver that increase in size over several decades. Children are generally asymptomatic, although enlarged kidneys may be palpable. Hypertension and renal failure may ensue in adulthood. Subarachnoid haemorrhage may result from associated cerebral aneurysms.

### Autosomal recessive polycystic kidney disease

Autosomal recessive polycystic kidney disease may present in the neonatal period through to the teenage years, often with bilateral flank masses. The earlier-presenting types are associated with pulmonary hypoplasia and early death. Surviving patients develop multiple cysts of the collecting ducts, progressive renal fibrosis, tubular atrophy and inexorable renal failure. The diagnosis is confirmed on renal ultrasound scanning, intravenous pyelography and renal biopsy.

## Hydronephrosis and hydroureters

These are discussed in Chapter 12.

## Vesicoureteric reflux

Vesicoureteric reflux (VUR) is a common problem in childhood caused by lower ureteric sphincter incompetence, sometimes as a result of malinsertion of the ureter into the bladder. It is commonly associated with ureterocoeles and, if severe, results in varying degrees of hydroureter and hydronephrosis. Reflux is graded according to the level to which urine flows retrogradely on voiding (Fig. 64). When associated with recurrent urinary infections, reflux carries a high risk of renal scarring and, eventually, renal failure (*reflux nephropathy*).

## 7.4 Infections

### Learning objective

You should:

* know the diagnosis and management of a toddler with an urinary tract infection

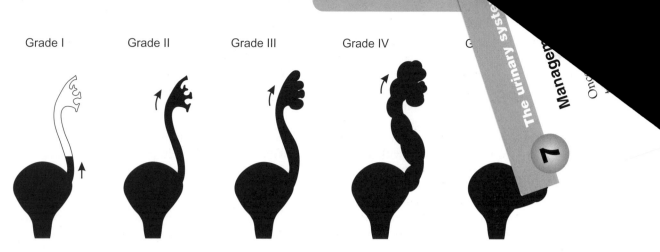

Grade I   Grade II   Grade III   Grade IV   G

**Fig. 64** Grading of vesicoureteric reflux.

---

**Box 34** Predisposing factors for urinary tract infection

**Renal**
Congenital anomalies
Vesicoureteric reflux
Urinary obstruction
Urinary stasis
Urinary calculi
Bladder dysfunction

**Non-renal**
Chronic constipation
Sexual abuse
Immunosuppression
Diabetes mellitus

---

**Box 35** Causes of urinary tract infection

**Gram-negative bacteria**
*Escherichia coli* (85%)
*Klebsiella* spp.
*Proteus* spp.
*Pseudomonas* spp.

**Gram-positive bacteria**
*Streptococcus faecalis*
*Staphylococcus saprophyticus*

**Viruses:** several

**Fungi**
*Candida* spp.

---

**Box 36** Common symptoms of urinary tract infections

| | |
|---|---|
| Neonates: | Sepsis; poor feeding; failure to thrive; irritability |
| Toddlers: | Vomiting; chronic diarrhoea; failure to thrive; fever |
| Older child: | Dysuria; abdominal pain
May be asymptomatic |

---

## Pathophysiology of urinary tract infection

Urinary tract infection (UTI) is the most common bacterial infection in childhood, affecting up to 1% of boys and 2% of girls. As many as 25% of those with recurrent UTIs develop renal scarring, especially if VUR is also present. Children with congenital abnormalities of the renal tracts, reflux, urinary stasis and repeated catheterisation are at a considerably increased risk of UTI. The risk of renal scarring is particularly great in infancy and can, with time, result in hypertension and chronic renal failure. UTI is usually caused by Gram-negative organisms that gain entry via the bloodstream or by retrograde passage from the external genitalia and perineum.

## Diagnosis of UTI

The clinical symptoms suggestive of a UTI are listed in Box 36. It is essential to obtain a clean specimen of urine *prior to commencing antibiotics*. A bag specimen is suitable for infants after appropriate cleansing of the perineum, whereas a 'clean catch' midstream specimen is possible in older children. A suprapubic aspirate should be performed whenever there is a delay in sampling and other methods have failed. Catheter specimens are generally reserved for those with neurogenic bladders. Simple urinalysis may confirm the presence of increased white cells, with or without red cells and protein. In addition, every urine sample should be sent to the laboratory for culture and sensitivity. Dipslide cultures are extremely useful when immediate microbiological services may not be available. The presence of $>10^5$ colony-forming units in a voided specimen constitutes significant bacteriuria, whereas any growth in a suprapubic sample is significant. In an ill-looking, poorly perfused child a UTI is usually accompanied by a raised white cell count and positive blood cultures.

## ...ent of UTI

...e infection is confirmed, a 7-day course of oral ...imethoprim, first-generation cephalosporin, amoxycillin or nitrofurantoin will treat common organisms, including *Escherichia coli*. A subsequent urine sample should be assessed to ensure eradication of the infection. Infants should be treated aggressively with intravenous antibiotics (e.g. cefotaxime and gentamicin). Following a first infection, infants and those under the age of 4 years should be started on prophylactic trimethoprim as a single night-time dose. This will prevent recurrences until renal tract investigations can be organised, as shown in Figure 65. Ultrasound, in order to exclude congenital anomalies, dilatation resulting from obstruction and calculi, should be carried out in all patients. A plain abdominal X-ray is useful to exclude spinal abnormalities and detect small calculi. Renal scarring is best evaluated by means of a renal isotope DMSA scan (technetium-labelled 2,3-dimercaptosuccinic acid), 6 weeks after the UTI, especially in preschool and school-aged children at risk (Fig. 66a). Isotope renography using DTPA scan (technetium-labelled diethylenetriamine penta-acetic acid), or MAG3 is useful in demonstrating differential renal function, excretion

and obstruction (Fig. 66b). A micturating cystogram (MCUG) is necessary to assess ureteric reflux and bladder emptying. It should be performed once the UTI has cleared in all children aged 4 years or under, and in those with renal scarring, a positive family history of reflux nephropathy or other renal anomaly. Serum electrolytes, urea, creatinine and glomerular filtration rate (GFR) are indicated in patients with evidence of renal damage where renal dysfunction is a possibility. An intravenous urography (IVU) assessment is carried out if there is no reflux.

The indications for antibiotic prophylaxis are shown in Table 46. For those whose imaging is normal, follow-up should include urine cultures if symptoms recur. Children in whom VUR is present should continue on prophylactic antibiotics and have their urine checked routinely every 3 months. Prophylaxis should continue for the first 4 years, provided renal scarring on DMSA scanning remains absent. For those with renal scars but no VUR, biannual DMSA scans are required. Recurrent breakthrough infections, the persistence of reflux on repeat MCUG, the development of scars on DMSA, deteriorating renal function and underlying renal tract anomalies are indications for surgery. All patients with scars should have annual blood pressure measurements,

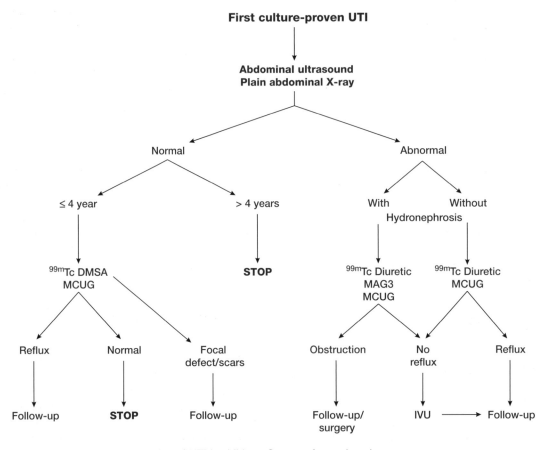

**Fig. 65** Protocol for investigation of UTI in children. See text for explanation.

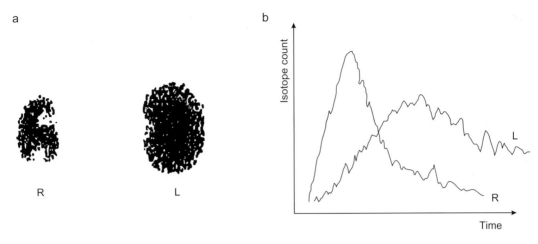

**Fig. 66** Renal scans. (a) DMSA scan showing an atrophied right kidney with filling defects representing renal scars. (b) A DTPA excretion curve shows a normal pattern in the right, with reduced and delayed excretion in the obstructed left kidney.

| **Table 46** Indications for antibiotic prophylaxis |
| --- |
| First UTI prior to results of ultrasound/DMSA MCUG |
| Recurrent UTIs |
| Reflux |
| Renal tract anomalies |
| Renal scars |
| Compromised renal function |

together with urinalysis for proteinuria. The potential risk of a deterioration in renal function during pregnancy must be explained.

## Renal abscess

Pyelonephritis with abscess formation is a rare complication of UTI. The toxic, febrile patient presents with bacteriuria, pyuria and haematuria. A painful loin mass is confirmed on ultrasound scanning (and, if necessary, by CT scan). The urine may be sterile in children previously treated with antibiotics. The pus must be drained by means of a nephrostomy tube under direct imaging or surgery, and antibiotics given intravenously for at least 10 days.

## 7.5 Proteinuria

### Learning objective

You should:

- be able to make a diagnosis of nephrotic syndrome in a child and discuss the management

## Estimation of proteinuria

Protein loss in the urine amounting to not more than 150 mg in 24 hours lies within normal limits and comprises mainly albumin and Tamm–Horsfall mucoprotein. Dipsticks are highly sensitive for albuminuria but less so for other proteins, and may result in many false-positive results. If suspected, proteinuria is best quantified in a 24-hour urine collection, but a good estimate is obtained by calculating the urine protein:creatinine ratio (normal <0.5 and <0.2 in infants and older children, respectively). Proteinuria in excess of 1000 mg in 24 hours is almost always pathological, especially when associated with oedema.

## Benign proteinuria

*Transient* proteinuria <1 g in 24 hours (<2+ on dipstick) may arise during exercise and intercurrent febrile illnesses. Increased urinary protein loss on standing (*orthostatic* proteinuria) can be shown to resolve on comparing daytime samples with night-time urine voided in the supine position. Children with postural proteinuria require long-term monitoring of blood pressure, renal function and protein loss.

## Pathological proteinuria

Damage to the proximal renal tubules by congenital or acquired disease can result in *tubular proteinuria*, which does not usually exceed 1 g in 24 hours (Box 37). It is generally associated with obvious features of the underlying disease process and other features of tubular dysfunction. In contrast, *glomerular proteinuria* is far more common and may be present in asymptomatic patients. The amount of protein loss varies enormously,

**Box 37** Non-benign causes of proteinuria

| Acquired | Congenital |
|---|---|
| **Glomerular** | |
| Nephrotic syndrome | Nephrotic syndrome |
| Glomerulonephritis | |
| Toxins (heavy metals) | |
| Drugs (captopril, phenytoin) | |
| **Tubular** | |
| Tubular necrosis | Tubular acidosis |
| Interstitial nephritis | Cystinosis |
| Toxins (heavy metals) | Wilson disease |
| Drugs (antibiotics) | Galactosaemia |

**Box 38** Nephrotic syndrome (minimal change disease)

**Symptoms and signs**

| Oedema | Periorbital |
|---|---|
| | Pedal |
| | Ascites |
| | Pleural effusion |
| Diminished urine output | |

**Diagnosis**

| Urinary protein | >2 g/24 h |
|---|---|
| | Early morning urine protein/ creatinine ratio 200 mg/dL |
| Serum albumin | <25 g/dL |

**Complications**

| Peritonitis | *Streptococcus pneumoniae*; Gram-negative organisms |
|---|---|
| Viral infections | Chickenpox, measles (result of steroid therapy) |
| Arterial and venous thrombosis | |

**Treatment**
Restricted-salt diet
Moderate fluid restriction
Prednisolone 60 mg/m$^2$/day for 28 days, followed by 40 mg/m$^2$ every alternate day for 28 days

and may include albumin and low-molecular-weight proteins (selective) or albumin plus large proteins (non-selective).

## Nephrotic syndrome

Nephrotic syndrome is typified by proteinuria, hypoproteinaemia, oedema and hyperlipidaemia. It is *idiopathic* in 90% of patients and histopathology will show minimal change disease (85%), focal sclerosis (10%) or mesangial proliferation (5%). The remaining 10% are secondary to glomerulonephritis, malignant tumours (e.g. lymphoma), drugs and toxins. Autosomal recessive *congenital nephrotic syndrome* (Finnish type) is extremely rare and associated with a poor outcome, with the majority developing end-stage renal failure requiring renal replacement therapy and, ultimately, transplantation. In all cases, increased glomerular permeability results in protein loss (especially albumin) and oedema develops as the serum albumin falls. Hyperlipidaemia is caused by decreased lipid catabolism and increased lipoprotein production in the liver. Patients are at an increased risk of infection, partly through loss of complement and protein-bound immunoglobulins. Peritonitis caused by *Streptococcus pneumoniae* is common. This may be masked by the effect of steroid therapy and may not present with overt signs; a high index of suspicion must be maintained. An increased thrombotic tendency arises because of elevated coagulation factors and reduced fibrinolysis. It is exacerbated by the low plasma oncotic pressure, which results in loss of intravascular fluid to the interstitial space and a subsequent decrease in circulatory volume (Box 38).

Idiopathic nephrotic syndrome due to *minimal change disease* is characterised by normal appearances on light microscopy but fusion of epithelial cell foot processes on electron microscopy. The majority (95%) are responsive to steroids and the prognosis is excellent. Steroid resist-

ance is seen in up to 50% of those with mesangial proliferation and 80% with focal sclerosis, where progressive disease leading to end-stage renal failure is likely. Minimal change disease usually affects boys (more than girls) aged between 2 and 6 years. Ascites and diminished urine output follow. A few patients with minimal change disease are hypertensive, and occasionally there is microscopic haematuria. Renal biopsy is only indicated in those with atypical features and a failure to respond to steroids. Any suspicion of infection must be treated with systemic Gram-positive and Gram-negative antibiotic cover. Diuretics must be used with caution as there is intravascular volume depletion. Severe oedema requires careful fluid restriction and the combination of frusemide (furosemide) and metolazone, with monitoring of serum electrolytes as there is underlying hypovolaemia despite the obvious oedema. Infusions of 25% albumin are likely to produce only transient improvement.

In those who have had no relapses steroids can be tailed off rapidly, although corticosteroids must be provided during subsequent illness or surgery in the following 12 months. Persistence of proteinuria after 4 weeks of steroid therapy constitutes *steroid resistance* and is an indication for renal biopsy. Relapses involve recurrence of proteinuria with oedema and are initially treated with steroids in a similar fashion. Cyclophosphamide is also useful in steroid-resistant and frequently relapsing disease, and is usually given for 12 weeks, during which time weekly estimates of the white cell count are mandatory. Although many patients will suffer multiple relapses, the nephrotic syndrome generally burns out during the teenage years. A significant risk of end-stage renal failure is present with steroid-resistant disease secondary to focal and segmental glomerulosclerosis.

## 7.6 Haematuria

### Learning objective

You should:

- know the common causes of haematuria in a child and know how a diagnosis is established

Microscopic haematuria describes more than five red cells per high-power field in urine and may be present in up to 1% of asymptomatic schoolchildren. Blood in the urine may originate as a result of diseases primarily affecting the kidneys and lower urinary tract, as well as coagulopathies, drugs and exercise (Boxes 39 and 40).

---

**Box 39** Renal causes of haematuria

**Glomerular**
Glomerulonephritis
Recurrent haematuria
Haemolytic uraemic syndrome (HUS)
Henoch–Schönlein purpura
Systemic lupus erythematosus (SLE)

**Non-glomerular**
Polycystic disease
Congenital anomalies
Infection
Trauma
Tumours
Calculi

---

**Box 40** Non-renal causes of haematuria

**Haematological**
Coagulopathies
Thrombocytopenia
Renal vein thrombosis
Sickle cell disease

**Non-haematological**
Exercise
Drugs

---

## Glomerular causes of haematuria

### Glomerulonephritis

Glomerular damage that follows various immunological or toxic insults may result in glomerular bleeding together with loss of protein. In addition, some types of glomerulonephritis can be associated with acute renal failure, whereas others progress to chronic disease with end-stage renal failure.

#### Poststreptococcal glomerulonephritis

The incidence of poststreptococcal glomerulonephritis is declining and it is now a less common cause of haematuria than IgA nephropathy (see below). It affects young children over 3 years of age, who present with low-grade fever, lethargy and 'smoky' or red urine, sometimes accompanied by oedema and hypertension. The acute nephritis develops 1–2 weeks after a preceding upper respiratory tract or skin infection caused by group A β-haemolytic streptococci. Urinalysis confirms haematuria, often in the form of casts, as well as proteinuria and increased urinary white cells. Characteristically, investigation reveals a mild anaemia, leukocytosis, decreased C3 levels, haemolytic streptococci on throat swab culture, and positive antistreptococcal antibodies (e.g. ASOT or DNAase B antigen). Renal biopsy would confirm an increase in glomerular size, mesangial and inflammatory cell proliferation with few, if any, crescents. However, biopsy is only necessary in children with 'non-classic' features, such as acute renal failure, nephrotic syndrome, normal C3 levels, no evidence of streptococcal infection and persistence of symptoms beyond 2–3 months. Up to 95% of patients make a full recovery. Treatment is essentially supportive. Complications such as renal failure and hypertension must be controlled. Although penicillin is given for 10 days to clear residual streptococci, it has no effect on the nephritic process.

#### Other infection-related glomerulonephritis

Glomerulonephritis caused by damage resulting from the deposition of immune complexes in the glomeruli may be associated with chronic infection, including hepatitis B and C, malaria, syphilis, candidiasis, subacute endocarditis and chronically infected ventriculoperitoneal shunts. Patients develop a nephrotic or nephritic syndrome, often with low C3 levels, which resolves on treatment of the infection.

#### Membranoproliferative glomerulonephritis

Membranoproliferative glomerulonephritis is the most common cause of *chronic* glomerulonephritis. It affects children over the age of 10 years, who present with gross or microscopic haematuria, proteinuria, hypertension and a moderate decrease in C3 levels and renal function. These symptoms persist beyond 2 months, at which point a biopsy will show an increase in mesangial cells with deposition of C3 rather than immunoglobulin in the subendothelial region, and crescent formation. The outcome is poor, the severity increasing with increasing number of crescents. Some response may follow renal supportive measures and prednisolone, but the majority develop end-stage renal failure.

## Rapidly progressive glomerulonephritis

Although crescents are a feature of several types of glomerulonephritis, they are typical of idiopathic, rapidly progressive crescentic nephritis. Patients present with nephrotic or nephritic features and renal dysfunction, which progresses within a few weeks to end-stage renal failure. Only a small minority respond to immunosuppression with steroids, azathioprine, cyclophosphamide and plasmapheresis.

## SLE-related glomerulonephritis

SLE-related glomerulonephritis is one of the most serious complications of this condition. All adolescent girls with SLE and haematuria or proteinuria, with or without renal dysfunction, should undergo renal biopsy. This reveals varying degrees of mesangial and subendothelial deposits, and focal or segmental cellular proliferation with crescent formation and necrosis. Thickening of the capillary wall produces the *wire loop appearance*. Aggressive immunosuppression with multiple agents is usually required to keep the disease under control.

## Goodpasture disease

Goodpasture disease involves antibodies against lung and glomerular basement membrane (GBM), resulting in pulmonary haemorrhage and a glomerulonephritis similar to rapidly progressive disease with crescents. Patients present with haemoptysis, haematuria, proteinuria and renal failure. Few respond to immunosuppression and plasmapheresis, and the mortality from pulmonary haemorrhage is high.

## Recurrent haematuria

Some conditions are characterised by recurrent haematuria, which may be gross or microscopic. The latter may follow a brief latent period of 1–3 days after a nonspecific viral illness, and recurs with subsequent infections. Mild proteinuria is common, but complications such as hypertension, oedema and renal failure are

unusual. Blood tests and renal imaging are normal. The diagnosis is confirmed on renal biopsy. A normal biopsy characterises *idiopathic haematuria*, which carries a good prognosis. Predominant IgA mesangial deposits are seen in *IgA (Berger) nephropathy*, 30% of cases of which develop complications and require immunosuppressant therapy. *Alport syndrome* is an X-linked dominant nephritis associated with sensorineural deafness that presents with haematuria and mild proteinuria. Biopsy shows splitting of the GBM, sometimes with sclerosis and fibrosis; if these are present, renal failure in the second to third decade can be expected.

## Henoch–Schönlein purpura

Henoch–Schönlein purpura is discussed in Chapter 11.

## Haemolytic uraemic syndrome

Haemolytic uraemic syndrome (HUS) is the commonest cause of acute renal failure in preschool children. Most cases follow a few days after gastrointestinal (sometimes upper respiratory) infections, often with verotoxin-producing *E. coli*. (0157:H7) or, rarely, other bacterial or viral agents. Thickening of the glomerular capillaries and fibrin deposition may result in glomerular sclerosis and cortical necrosis. Damage to red cells as they pass through the abnormal renal vasculature results in microangiopathic haemolytic anaemia. Similarly, platelet damage and consumption in intrarenal clot formation result in thrombocytopenia. Patients present with oliguria together with severe lethargy and marked pallor, sometimes with petechiae. Investigation will show an anaemia, thrombocytopenia, and often an elevated white cell count. Blood film analysis shows fragmented cells (Fig. 67) and the Coombs' test is negative. Full-blown disseminated intravascular coagulopathy is unusual. Microscopic haematuria and proteinuria is coupled with raised serum urea and creatinine levels. Ultrasound of the kidneys is helpful in excluding renal vein thrombosis, and renal biopsy is not required. Management entails aggressive treatment of renal failure with dialysis, control of complications such as hypertension and hyperkalaemia, and careful anticoagulation with heparin. The majority of patients make a full recovery but require long-term follow-up of their blood pressure and renal function.

## Tubular causes of haematuria

Haematuria is a feature of urinary infections and tumours, when it is usually microscopic. Macroscopic haematuria may result from congenital anomalies that

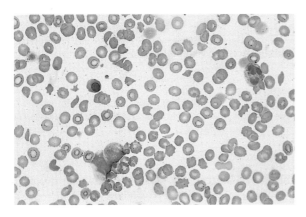

**Fig. 67** Blood film in haemolytic uraemic syndrome, showing anaemia with fragmented red blood cells (microangiopathic haemolytic anaemia) and an absence of platelets, resulting in thrombocytopenia.

Box 41 Causes of acute renal failure

| Prerenal disease | Renal disease | Postrenal disease |
|---|---|---|
| Hypotension | Glomerulonephritis | Obstructive |
| Hypovolaemia | Acute tubular | uropathy |
| Anoxia | necrosis | Posterior urethral |
| Sepsis | Haemolytic | valves |
| Poor cardiac | uraemic | Reflux |
| output | syndrome | nephropathy |
| | Renal vein | Calculi, blood |
| | thrombosis | clot |
| | Drugs, toxins, uric | |
| | acid | |
| | Congenital | |
| | anomalies | |

bleed, e.g. haemangiomas, cysts and polycystic disease. In the majority of school-aged children gross haematuria is secondary to the formation of a renal haematoma after blunt trauma (e.g. caused by falling astride bicycle handlebars). Urinary calculi themselves may lead to epithelial trauma and subsequent bleeding (see Chapter 12).

## Non-renal causes of haematuria

Any severe coagulopathy can present with haematuria. Indeed, microscopic haematuria is frequent in patients with thrombocytopenia (e.g. with idiopathic thrombocytopenic purpura (ITP), or those receiving myelosuppressive chemotherapy) and in those taking anticoagulants. Other drugs that may cause renal damage or cystitis may also precipitate haematuria (e.g. antibiotics, cytotoxics). Sickling within the kidneys can result in haematuria in children with both sickle cell disease and sickle trait. *Renal vein thrombosis* is a complication seen in critically ill neonates and presents with renal mass(es) and haematuria. Some individuals develop haematuria after strenuous exercise, which resolves with a few days of rest. In all cases, tests of renal function and urinary tract imaging are normal.

## 7.7 Renal failure and dysfunction

### Learning objective

You should:

- know the causes of renal failure in childhood and the associated complications

Neonates have a diminished glomerular filtration rate and ability to excrete ions such as hydrogen, potassium, sodium and phosphate, and can only concentrate urine to a maximum of 700 mmol/L. Older children can concentrate urine beyond 1000 mmol/L. Urine output below 1.0 and 0.5 mL/kg/h for newborns and older children, respectively, constitutes *oliguria* and is indicative of renal failure. *Anuria* is the total absence of urine output.

## Acute renal failure

Most children who present in renal failure have a decreased renal perfusion pressure from prerenal causes. The majority have hypotension associated with dehydration, hypoxia, sepsis and diminished cardiac output (congenital heart disease or postcardiac surgery). Renal and postrenal causes of renal failure are listed in Box 41.

Patients with acute renal failure present with lethargy, pallor, vomiting and decreased urine output. Examination reveals anaemia, hypertension and fluid overload. The last manifests as dependent oedema, heart failure, pulmonary oedema, behavioural changes and even coma. Other signs related to the primary cause may be evident (e.g. diarrhoea, rashes etc.). Investigative findings may vary widely depending on the cause, although anaemia, hyponatraemia, hyperkalaemia, hyperphosphataemia with hypocalcaemia, acidosis, uraemia and a raised serum creatinine are usual. With renal causes of renal failure urine quality is poor, with low osmolality (<400 mmol/L) and high sodium ions (>30 mmol/L). Urgent abdominal X-rays and ultrasound scans are required to exclude an obstructive cause.

A stringent *fluid balance* must be maintained in all cases of diminished renal function. Prerenal failure caused by hypovolaemia usually responds to careful fluid replacement using isotonic saline or colloid solutions (10–20 mL/kg over 0.5–1 h). In underfilled oliguric (not anuric) patients a bolus dose of 20 mL/kg colloid followed by a potent diuretic may encourage urine output. Frusemide (furosemide) may be repeated twice in increasing doses (2 and 10 mg/kg), whereas mannitol (up to 1 g/kg) should only be administered once. Dopamine at 5 µg/kg/min may improve renal perfusion and urine output. If there is no response, this implies incipient or established renal failure. In this situation, in order to maintain an accurate fluid balance, patients should be catheterised, weighed twice daily and, if possible, measurement of the central venous pressure established. Continuous ECG monitoring is mandatory.

**Fluid restriction** should be limited to insensible losses (approximately 400 mL/m$^2$ daily), plus the daily urine output (if any) and any other losses (e.g. from gastrointestinal tract). Regular monitoring of serum electrolytes is paramount, and fluid should be given as glucose solutions with the appropriate addition of electrolytes.

**Hyperkalaemia** is the most serious complication, resulting in arrhythmias and death if uncontrolled. No potassium-containing solutions should be given in any guise. A serum potassium ion level >6 mmol/L without ECG changes should be treated with a potassium chelating resin (orally or per rectum). Levels >7 mmol/L with peaked T waves or other ECG changes require urgent treatment with slow intravenous 10% calcium gluconate (0.5 mL/kg over 10 minutes) to counteract cardiac irritability. The elevated potassium can be lowered using 8.4% sodium bicarbonate (1 mL/kg over 30 minutes), β-agonists (e.g. salbutamol) and a dextrose–insulin infusion. A poor response to these measures necessitates urgent dialysis.

**Hyponatraemia** usually responds to fluid restriction and extra NaCl given when the plasma sodium ion level is <120 mmol/L.

**Acidosis** with a pH <7.1 or a bicarbonate level <8 mmol/L is managed by partial correction to maintain the pH above 7.2. Sodium bicarbonate is given intravenously in the acute setting and by the oral route as the situation stabilises.

**Hypocalcaemia–hyperphosphataemia** is controlled by phosphate-binding oral calcium carbonate.

**Hypertension** that is moderate is treated with salt and fluid restriction, frusemide and propranolol. Severe hypertension may respond to labetalol infusion (or sodium nitroprusside).

**Anaemia** is corrected only in severe cases and by using small amounts of packed cells.

**Renal dialysis.** Failure to control the above complications, fluid overload, congestive heart failure and hypertensive seizures are indications for renal dialysis

**Table 47** Indications for acute renal dialysis

| Complications | Manifestations |
|---|---|
| Electrolyte disturbance | Hyperkalaemia, hyperphosphataemia, acidosis |
| Fluid overload | Heart failure, pulmonary oedema |
| Hypertension | Uncontrolled, accelerated, with seizures |

(Table 47). This can be performed by continuous or intermittent flushing of diasylate fluid across the peritoneum (peritoneal dialysis), or extracorporeal haemofiltration (haemodialysis).

## End-stage renal failure

Persistence of renal failure, often as a result of the causes listed in Box 41, results in *chronic renal failure* that, in due course, culminates in end-stage renal failure. Chronic renal failure is exacerbated by a high-protein diet, hypertension, persistent proteinuria and recurrent urinary infections. Management entails optimising nutritional intake utilising carbohydrate and fats, controlling electrolyte levels (especially potassium, hydrogen and phosphate ions), and the provision of iron, folic acid and trace elements. Inadequate growth can be enhanced using growth hormone and chronic anaemia by means of erythropoietin. Acidosis is corrected with bicarbonate to maintain levels above 20 mmol/L. Renal osteodystrophy is manifest by hyperphosphataemia, hypocalcaemia, raised alkaline phosphatase and parathyroid hormone, with ricket-like changes on X-ray examination. Treatment involves a low-phosphate diet, antacids such as calcium carbonate to bind phosphate in the gut, and vitamin D supplements. Hypertension and urinary infections must be treated aggressively. Renal replacement therapy via dialysis is instituted once the glomerular filtration rate falls below 20% of normal, usually with a serum creatinine level around 900 µmol/L.

## Renal transplantation

Ultimately, all children on long-term renal-replacement therapy will require a renal transplant. In the meantime, most patients are stabilised on *continuous ambulatory peritoneal dialysis* (CAPD) involving three to six daily exchanges via an abdominally sited Tenckhoff catheter. A minority require haemodialysis through a prosthetic arteriovenous fistula. Catheter/fistula failure and infection is an ever-present risk for these patients. Kidney transplantation is effected using a donor with matching human leukocyte antigens (HLA). These are encoded on the major histocompatibility complex (MHC) on chromosome 6. The best fit is likely with an identical twin and, to a lesser extent, another living family member. Alternatively, a matched cadaveric donor organ is used. Up to 80% of living related and 65% of cadaveric grafts function adequately after 3 years. Despite the problems associated with immunosuppressive therapy (steroids, ciclosporin A and tacrolimus), the improvement in quality of life of successful transplant recipients is tremendous. Transplant failure is primarily through rejection (50%), recurrence of primary renal disease (33%) and thrombotic phenomena (15%).

## Renal dysfunction

### Proximal renal tubular acidosis

In proximal renal tubular acidosis (RTA) bicarbonate is insufficiently reabsorbed in the proximal tubules, and the excess load spilling into the distal tubules cannot be totally reclaimed and is lost as sodium bicarbonate in the urine. Compensatory mechanisms, including the absorption of sodium (and chloride) in exchange for potassium ions, result in hypokalaemia and hyperchloraemia. Loss of bicarbonate results in acidosis. Proximal RTA may be an isolated defect. However, in the *Fanconi syndrome* it is associated with generalised tubular dysfunction, resulting in RTA with glycosuria, phosphaturia and aminoaciduria. Rickets is an added complication of this type of RTA.

### Distal renal tubular acidosis

Defective hydrogen ion secretion in the distal tubules results in distal RTA, whereby the urine cannot be acidified below a pH of 5.8, even in the presence of marked systemic acidosis. Associated loss of sodium bicarbonate results in hypokalaemia and hyperchloraemia. Distal RTA, unlike proximal RTA, is also associated with hypercalciuria, leading to the formation of renal calculi and nephrocalcinosis.

The diagnosis is suspected when, in the presence of systemic acidosis with a serum bicarbonate level of less than 16 mmol/L, the urine pH remains above 5.5 or 5.8 for proximal and distal RTA, respectively. Treatment entails alkalinisation of the plasma with sodium bicarbonate (or citrate) and potassium supplementation.

### Renal osteodystrophy

Loss of nephrons, as well as significant glomerular and tubular dysfunction, can result in renal osteodystrophy (renal rickets). Insufficient production of vitamin D at the renal level, together with secondary hyperparathyroidism, results in malabsorption of calcium and phosphate from the gut. A compensatory increase in parathyroid hormone (PTH) ensures normocalcaemia but low or normal phosphate levels, owing to increased excretion of phosphate in the urine. This leads to bone resorption, resulting in osteopenia, increased bone turnover, and replacement with disorganised lamellae, producing characteristic ricket-like changes seen on X-ray. Renal osteodystrophy contributes toward growth failure in children with chronic renal failure and is treated with calcium and vitamin D supplements, together with phosphate-lowering binding agents.

### Renal diabetes insipidus

Failure to reabsorb water at the renal level despite the presence of antidiuretic hormone (ADH) constitutes nephrogenic diabetes insipidus. This may be an X-linked dominant condition where boys, and to a lesser extent girls, present with marked polydipsia and polyuria, sometimes with hypernatraemic dehydration. Hypernatraemia with serum hyperosmolality >295 mmol/L in the presence of a dilute urine is suggestive of this diagnosis. Failure to concentrate the urine after intramuscular ADH and during a carefully monitored water deprivation test provides confirmatory evidence. Treatment includes regular fluid intake and, paradoxically, diuretics (e.g. chlorothiazide).

# Self-assessment: questions

## Multiple choice questions

1. The following statements describe urinary tract infection:
   a. It is the most common bacterial infection in childhood
   b. It is more common in those with ectopic ureters
   c. It carries a high risk of end-stage renal failure
   d. It is usually caused by *Proteus* species
   e. In school-aged children it is best treated with intravenous antibiotics.

2. Asymptomatic bacteriuria:
   a. Is more common in girls
   b. Is always associated with significant urinary tract infection
   c. May be associated with vesicoureteric reflux (VUR)
   d. Is not associated with renal scarring
   e. Should be treated with antibiotics.

3. The following features are observed in the nephrotic syndrome:
   a. Hypoalbuminuria
   b. Hyperlipidaemia
   c. Hypocalcaemia
   d. Increased intravascular volume
   e. Minimal change disease in the majority of idiopathic cases.

4. The following are associated with a good prognosis for renal function:
   a. Nephrotic syndrome caused by glomerulosclerosis
   b. Nephrotic syndrome with minimal change disease
   c. Rapidly progressive glomerulonephritis
   d. SLE-related glomerulonephritis
   e. Poststreptococcal glomerulonephritis.

5. The following are causes of haematuria in childhood:
   a. Urinary calculi
   b. Wilms' tumour
   c. Haemolytic uraemic syndrome (HUS)
   d. Hyperbilirubinaemia
   e. Rifampicin therapy.

6. The following are associated with acute renal failure:
   a. Hypertension
   b. Hypovolaemia
   c. Hypervolaemia
   d. Hypokalaemia
   e. Hypophosphataemia.

7. The following statements describe the treatment of acute renal failure:
   a. Sodium supplements are an important addition to the diet
   b. Hyperkalaemia can be reduced using calcium gluconate
   c. Diuretics should not be used in oliguric patients
   d. Accelerated hypertension may be treated using labetalol
   e. Dialysis may be required for excessive fluid overload.

8. The following are complications of chronic renal failure:
   a. Osteomalacia
   b. Hypertension
   c. Hypokalaemia
   d. Uraemia
   e. Anaemia.

9. The treatment of chronic renal failure includes:
   a. A high-protein diet
   b. A low threshold for blood transfusion
   c. Potassium supplementation
   d. Growth hormone
   e. Phosphate-binding agents.

10. In renal-replacement therapy and transplantation:
    a. Most children are stabilised on haemodialysis not peritoneal dialysis
    b. Recurrent peritonitis is a serious complication with dialysis therapy
    c. Erythropoietin is only given after and not before transplantation
    d. Ciclosporin A therapy is commonly associated with hirsutism
    e. Cadaveric kidneys have an improved prognosis compared to live-related kidneys.

## Case history

As a senior house officer in A&E you see a 4-year-old girl who presents with a 2-day history of lower abdominal pain, fever and vomiting. Despite being undernourished for her age, clinically she appears well and there are no localising signs of infection, although you cannot be sure that the left eardrum is not a bit congested. A full blood count shows a haemoglobin of 8 g/dL, a white cell count of $6 \times 10^9$ cells/L and a normal differential and a platelet count of $190 \times 10^9$ cells/L. A urine dipstick shows 2+ protein and 2+ blood. You send off a midstream urine (MSU) sample for culture, prescribe paracetamol and amoxycillin, and ask the patient to come back the next day. The next day, you find that she has now stopped vomiting and her fever is lower. The urine culture has been reported to show more than $10^5$ colonies and the haematologist informs you that she has a normochromic normocytic anaemia.

1. What is the most probable diagnosis?
2. Why do you think she is anaemic?
3. Is your choice of antibiotic appropriate?
4. What advice would you give the parents regarding the immediate management?
5. Which part of the renal tract is most likely infected, and why?

6. How long should the therapy continue for?
7. Name at least four other initial investigations that are needed, and give the rationale for them.
8. Based on the results of these investigations, what advice would you need to give to the parents on the long-term prognosis?
9. Name three causes of haematuria other than the one illustrated here.
10. Name three possible complications of urinary tract infections.

## Short notes

1. Outline the main problems and key points in the management of chronic renal failure.
2. Tabulate the tests that may be performed during the course of investigation of gross haematuria, indicating the reason for each test in a second column.
3. A 5-year-old girl presents with a 2-week history of polyuria, and examination confirms mild hypertension together with facial, sacral and ankle oedema.

a. What is the most likely diagnosis?
b. How would you confirm the clinical diagnosis?
c. What is the most likely cause?
d. What complications may this child develop?
e. What treatment is indicated?

## OSCE questions

### OSCE 1
Examine Figure 68.

a. What is shown on the figure?
b. Name TWO symptoms possibly associated with this lesion.
c. What is it commonly associated with?
d. Name TWO complications.

### OSCE 2
Examine Figure 69.

a. What is shown on this figure?
b. Name TWO causes associated with this appearance.

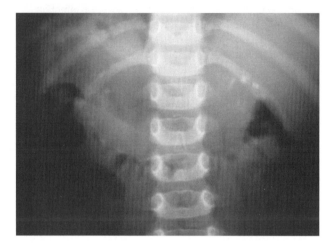

**Fig. 69**

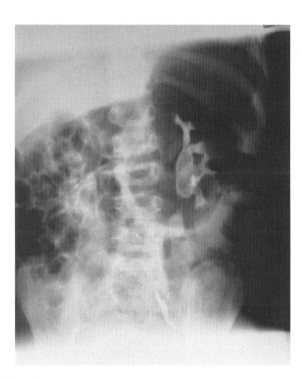

**Fig. 68**

# Self-assessment: answers

## Multiple choice answers

1. a. **True**. It affects up to 1% of boys, 2% of girls.
   b. **True**. Ectopic ureters generally insert lower down the urinary tract (e.g. urethra or vagina), thereby allowing increased access to ascending organisms.
   c. **False**. There is a low risk at all ages, although the risk is greater in those under 3 years, especially if vesicoureteric reflux is also present.
   d. **False**. *E. coli* infection occurs in over 80%. *Proteus* sp. are associated with staghorn calculi, which are rare in childhood.
   e. **False**. Intravenous antibiotics are used in neonates.

2. a. **True**. It occurs in 1% of girls and 0.03% of boys.
   b. **False**. Hence the dilemma of how to manage patients with asymptomatic bacteriuria.
   c. **True**. VUR occurs in 25%.
   d. **False**. Scarring occurs in 15%.
   e. **False**. Only treated with antibiotics if symptoms develop.

3. a. **False**. Hyperalbuminuria occurs with hypoalbuminaemia.
   b. **True**.
   c. **True**. This is secondary to hypoalbuminaemia.
   d. **False**. Decreased plasma oncotic pressure results in interstitial leakage, with decreased intravascular volume.
   e. **True**. The most common cause of nephrotic syndrome in childhood.

4. a. **False**. There is a high risk of end-stage renal failure.
   b. **True**. The majority of children with minimal change disease make a full recovery.
   c. **False**. It is associated with numerous glomerular crescents and renal failure.
   d. **False**. SLE-related disease often results in end-stage renal failure.
   e. **True**. Poststreptococcal glomerulonephritis is usually a transient disease.

5. a. **True**. Calculi may traumatise the urinary endothelium.
   b. **True**. Usually microscopic haematuria occurs.
   c. **True**. Usually associated with microscopic haematuria and proteinuria.

d. **False**. Bilirubinuria occurs, but no blood.
e. **False**. Pink discoloration of urine occurs, but no blood.

6. a. **True**. This is a major debilitating complication.
   b. **True**. It results in prerenal failure (e.g. following dehydration).
   c. **True**. Fluid overload occurs secondary to poor urine output.
   d. **False**. Hyperkalaemia is associated with acute renal failure.
   e. **False**. Hyperphosphataemia is associated with acute renal failure.

7. a. **False**. Sodium ion intake must be severely restricted.
   b. **False**. Calcium acts as a cardioprotective agent; it does not lower the potassium ion level.
   c. **False**. They may be very useful in establishing urine output, especially when given after a volume load.
   d. **True**. It provides both $\alpha$ and $\beta$ blockade.
   e. **True**. Dialysis is appropriate with fluid overload, congestive heart failure, hypertension, acidosis, hyperkalaemia and central nervous system complications (e.g. seizures).

8. a. **True**. This is a feature of renal osteodystrophy.
   b. **True**. Hypertension is common in all types of renal failure.
   c. **False**. Hyperkalaemia can occur in chronic disease.
   d. **True**. This is a hallmark of renal failure.
   e. **True**. Due to diminished erythropoietin production.

9. a. **False**. A low-protein diet is used to reduce nitrogen load.
   b. **False**. Blood transfusion is avoided unless absolutely necessary.
   c. **False**. Potassium must be excluded.
   d. **True**. It is used to enhance growth potential.
   e. **True**. These are used to lower phosphate in renal osteodystrophy.

10. a. **False**. Most children cope well with peritoneal dialysis.
    b. **True**. It occurs with peritoneal dialysis.
    c. **False**. It is used both before and after transplantation.

d. **True**. This is a common, cosmetically unwelcome side effect.

e. **False**. The reverse is true.

## Case history answers

1. The most likely diagnosis is a urinary tract infection. An acceptable alternative is cystitis.

2. Any child with an infection may have suppression of normal erythropoiesis. However, as this child has failed to thrive, a more chronic cause must be ruled out. Chronic renal insufficiency or failure could be a cause. Previous urinary tract infections may have been asymptomatic and resulted in reflux nephropathy and damage to the kidneys.

3. An antibiotic with action against Gram-negative bacilli is appropriate as they are the most common pathogens. Commonly co-trimoxazole, trimethoprim, nitrofurantoin or amoxycillin are used. The final choice should depend on the reported sensitivity of the organism. In this child there appears to have been a therapeutic response, and it is best to wait for the final culture and sensitivity report.

4. Urinary tract infections are common in childhood and are seen more often in girls. It is usually an ascending infection and responds quickly to a course of antibiotics. The course must be completed even though the symptoms may subside quickly; she can be managed as an outpatient and need not be hospitalised. Fever can be controlled with paracetamol and the child should be given small amounts of fluid frequently to ensure that she remains well hydrated. She will need to be followed up once she recovers, and a repeat urine culture must be performed a week after stopping therapy to ensure that the urine remains sterile.

5. The bladder is the commonest site of infection. In this child there is associated microscopic haematuria and lower abdominal pain, again a common presenting feature of cystitis. The absence of toxic signs and symptoms, colic and tenderness in the renal area argues against pyelonephritis.

6. The acute episode must be treated for 7–10 days. Thereafter, the child should be started on prophylactic antibiotics pending results of further investigations to rule out any underlying cause.

7. Four other investigations would be: serum creatinine to establish renal function; a plain abdominal X-ray to look for calculi and vertebral anomalies such as spina bifida; ultrasonography of the renal tract to rule out abnormalities of the renal tract, and a $^{99m}$Tc-labelled DMSA scan to assess renal function.

8. The prognosis is based on the presence or absence of any underlying abnormality. Simple urinary tract infections with normal imaging may recur, and if so acute exacerbations will need to be treated with a course of antibiotics. Cultures should be obtained at regular intervals and the child kept on a low single daily dose of either trimethoprim or nitrofurantoin for at least a year. The problem will resolve with age, usually without any chronic sequelae. In those with renal scarring (shown by DMSA scan) or dilated renal tracts (ultrasound) further investigations, including a MAG3 scan (to look for obstructive uropathy) and micturating cystourethrogram (for reflux), need to be performed. In some of these children, surgical reconstruction of the collecting tract may be required to prevent further damage to the kidney. In the majority with focal or reflux abnormalities, conservative management with long-term antibiotic prophylaxis is usually successful.

9. Causes can be divided into:

   - Glomerular: IgA nephropathy, poststreptococcal glomerulonephritis, Henoch–Schönlein purpura
   - Urinary calculi
   - Systemic: sickle cell disease, idiopathic thrombocytopenic purpura
   - Drugs: cyclophosphamide.

10. Complications include pyelonephritis, renal scarring, hydronephrosis, perinephric abscess, chronic renal failure, anaemia and failure to thrive.

## Short notes answers

1. The main complications associated with chronic renal failure include:

   - Electrolyte imbalance: hyperkalaemia, hyponatraemia, hypocalcaemia, hyperphosphataemia
   - Metabolic problems: acidosis with low bicarbonate, low pH, hyperuraemia
   - Fluid imbalance: overload
   - Anaemia: chronic disease, folate and iron deficiency, reduced erythropoietin
   - Nutritional problems: catabolic state, rickets (renal osteodystrophy), growth failure
   - Hypertension.

   The management is aimed at preventing further deterioration in renal function and controlling existing complications, initially by non-invasive means and, later, by renal-replacement therapy (dialysis) prior to transplantation. A low-protein diet and aggressive treatment of UTIs and hypertension reduce the risk of exacerbating renal dysfunction. Electrolyte problems are controlled via a low-salt, low-potassium and low-phosphate diet and the use of phosphate-binding agents with vitamin D supplements. Bicarbonate supplements are required to maintain a serum bicarbonate level above 20 mmol/L. Anaemia is prevented with folic acid and iron, together with regular erythropoietin in those receiving renal-replacement therapy. Growth is enhanced by optimising nutritional intake, mainly via a diet rich in carbohydrate and fat, if necessary via nasogastric tube feeding. Growth and an anabolic state may be augmented by the use of growth hormone. Failure of non-invasive therapeutic measures and inexorable progression of the underlying renal disease necessitates the introduction of regular dialysis, with a view to transplantation in the long term.

Tests performed during investigation of gross haematuria are given in Table 48.

3. a. Nephrotic syndrome
   b. Urine for proteinuria, albuminuria
      Serum protein/albumin
      Abnormal triglycerides.
   c. Minimal change nephrotic syndrome
   d. Hypertension/hypotension
      Severe oedema
      Ascites
      Pulmonary oedema/CCF
      Increased risk of infection
      Hypercoagulopathy
      Persistent proteinuria
      Renal failure.
   e. High-dose steroids (e.g. prednisolone 60 mg/m$^2$/day for 4 weeks, followed by 40 mg/m$^2$ given on alternate days for another 4 weeks)
      Treat any complications.

**Table 48** Tests performed in gross haematuria

| Test performed | Reason for test |
| --- | --- |
| **Blood tests** | |
| Blood count* | Anaemia, thrombocytopenia |
| Blood film, sickle screen | Abnormal red cells/haemoglobin |
| Clotting profile* | Clotting disorder |
| Electrolytes, urea, creatinine* | Renal dysfunction with glomerulonephritis, haemolytic uraemic syndrome |
| Calcium, uric acid, amino acids | Causes of urinary calculi |
| Antistreptolysin O titre (ASOT)/DNAase B | Poststreptococcal glomerulonephritis |
| C3 level* | Glomerulonephritis |
| Immunoglobulin levels | Glomerulonephritis |
| Antibody levels | For example antinuclear antibody (ANA) associated with systemic lupus erythematosus (SLE) nephritis |
| **Urine tests** | |
| Urinalysis* | Amount of haematuria, also proteinuria |
| Urine culture* | To exclude UTI |
| Calcium and creatinine in 24-hour sample* | Hypercalciuria, renal concentrating ability |
| **Microbiology** | |
| Throat/skin cultures | Poststreptococcal glomerulonephritis |
| Mantoux, urine for acid-fast bacilli (AFB) | Tuberculosis |
| **Imaging** | |
| Plain abdominal X-ray* | Renal calculi, mass in flank |
| Renal tract ultrasound* | Renal anomaly, malformation, tumour, renal vein thrombosis, haematoma |
| CT/MRI scan | Tumour, invasion of inferior vena cava |
| **Invasive tests** | |
| Cystoscopy | Renal calculi, bladder/urethral anomalies, tumours |
| Renal biopsy | Glomerulonephritis, SLE |

* These tests are carried out on all patients.

## OSCE answers

### OSCE 1

a. A large staghorn calculus
b. Abdominal/flank pain
   Haematuria
   Recurrent UTIs
c. *Proteus* infection in urine
d. Recurrent UTIs
   Stranguria.

### OSCE 2

a. Bilateral 'freckled' renal calcification or nephrocalcinosis
b. Distal renal tubular acidosis
   Idiopathic hypercalciuria
   Idiopathic hypercalcaemia
   Hyperparathyroidism
   Excess vitamin D
   Steroids and frusemide
   Hyperuricosuria and oxaluria.

# 8 The endocrine system

**8.1** Introduction     163

**8.2** Disorders of sexual differentiation     163

**8.3** Disorders of stature     165

**8.4** Disorders of puberty     169

**8.5** Disorders of the thyroid gland     171

**8.6** Disorders of the adrenal gland     173

**8.7** Disorders of calcium homeostasis     175

**8.8** Disorders of glucose homeostasis     177

**8.9** Disorders of antidiuretic hormone secretion     179

Self-assessment: questions     182

Self-assessment: answers     186

## Overview

This chapter outlines the basic physiology of the various endocrine glands, normal processes of growth and pubertal development, and the symptoms and signs associated with various endocrinopathies. The undergraduate would be expected to have a good understanding of the more common problems associated with the endocrine system, such as short stature, hypothyroidism, problems associated with puberty and diabetes mellitus. The more common endocrinological tests that are required to confirm a diagnosis, and their interpretation, are presented, together with a basic outline of the treatment of the common endocrinopathies.

## 8.1 Introduction

The endocrine system includes the pituitary, thyroid, adrenals, parathyroids, pancreas and gonads. These glands control the processes of growth and development in childhood and adolescence, and are vital for the maintenance of normal homeostasis in the body and the wellbeing of the individual.

## 8.2 Disorders of sexual differentiation

### Learning objective

You should:

- know the causes of ambiguous genitalia in the newborn

One in 4500 newborn babies has *ambiguous genitalia* (Fig. 70). Uncertainty about the gender of a newborn baby is extremely distressing for the parents, and it is important to reassure them as soon as possible that the baby is either male or female, and not 'in between'. Nevertheless, the registration of birth should be delayed until gender is established. To understand how to approach this problem, one needs to understand the development of the genitalia.

### Development of the genitalia

The undifferentiated gonad develops into a male testis around the sixth week of gestation, under the influence of the sex-determining region on the Y chromosome (SRY). Testicular Leydig cells secrete testosterone in response to placental human chorionic gonadotrophin (hCG) and fetal luteinising hormone (LH), which in turn stimulates wolffian ducts to develop. These form the epididymis, vas deferens and seminal vesicles. The external penis and scrotum develop as a result of the action of dihydrotestosterone that is formed from testosterone by the enzyme $5\alpha$-reductase. Testicular Sertoli cells produce müllerian inhibiting hormone (MIH), which inhibits the development of female internal structures from the müllerian ducts.

In the female ovary, primordial follicles develop and reach a peak at 20–25 weeks of gestation under the influence of fetal follicle-stimulating hormone (FSH). Wolffian ducts disappear and müllerian ducts develop into fallopian tubes, the middle into the uterus and the upper third of the vagina. The clitoris is formed from the genital tubercle, the labia majora from the labio-scrotal folds, and the labia minora from the urethral

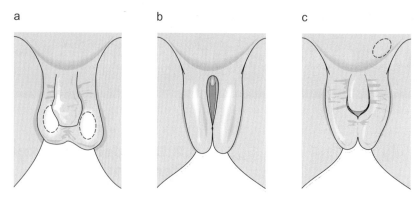

**Fig. 70** External genitalia in (a) the normal male, (b) the normal female and (c) ambiguous genitalia, showing clitoromegaly (or underdeveloped penis), fused labia minora (or marked hypospadias), fused and rugose labia majora (or bifid scrotum). A partially descended gonad (if present) is usually a testis, implying XY karyotype.

folds. The urogenital sinus forms the lower two-thirds of the vagina.

The hormones that control the development of the genitalia are all derived from cholesterol. In general, ambiguity results due to a defect in the metabolic pathways that convert cholesterol into mineralocorticoids, glucocorticoids or sex hormones.

## Clinical features and assessment

Attention should be paid to the details of drugs taken during pregnancy, a family history of primary amenorrhoea or infertility, late puberty and unexplained neonatal deaths. An urgent karyotype analysis is required.

### Ambiguous genitalia with no palpable gonads

The commonest cause is a virilised female with congenital adrenal hyperplasia (CAH, or female pseudohermaphroditism). This is due to a deficiency in the enzyme 21-hydroxylase, and may also result in salt loss. The salt loss can lead to dehydration and shock. Rarely other enzyme deficiencies may cause a similar picture. The diagnosis is confirmed by measuring urine and serum levels of cortisol precursors. Male pseudohermaphroditism with intra-abdominal testes and true pseudohermaphroditism is rare (Box 42).

### Ambiguous genitalia with one gonad palpable

This is usually due to mixed gonadal dysgenesis (with an XO/XY karyotype). Pelvic ultrasound, genitogram, hCG test and laparoscopy with genital biopsy may be required.

---

**Box 42** Causes of female virilisation

**Excess fetal androgens**
Congenital adrenal hyperplasia: usually due to 21-hydroxylase deficiency
Testis or ovotestis present: from partial gonadal dysgenesis

**Male pseudohermaphroditism**
Excess maternal androgens crossing placenta
Drugs: anabolic steroids, danazol, testosterone, progestagens
Maternal disease: ovarian or adrenal tumours

---

**Box 43** Causes of incomplete masculinisation

**Inadequate androgens**
Gonadal dysgenesis: caused by the SRY gene mutation
LH deficiency
Leydig cell agenesis or hypoplasia
Errors of testosterone synthesis: defect in adrenals, testes or both

**Impaired response to testosterone**
Impaired conversion of testosterone to dihydrotestosterone: 5α-reductase deficiency
Androgen insensitivity: androgen receptor/postreceptor defect

---

### Both gonads palpable

The commonest cause is an incompletely virilised male or male pseudohermaphroditism. These are due to impaired Leydig cell activity, impaired androgen metabolism, receptor defects or abnormal secretion of MIH (Box 43).

Management is designed to achieve unambiguous and functionally normal external genitalia and reproductive capacity. The penile size and its ability to respond to testosterone are vital considerations. The karyotype may therefore be less relevant in the management. Treatment may be medical (e.g. glucocorticoid and mineralocorticoid therapy in CAH, androgens in errors of testosterone biosynthesis), or surgical (e.g. clitoral reduction, separation of labia and vaginoplasty). In males with hypospadias, reconstructive surgery is indicated to ensure that the patient can urinate standing up before going to school. Gonadectomy is indicated with dysgenetic or non-functional gonads, especially in those with Y-bearing cell lines, because of an increased risk of malignant change in later life. Pubertal induction and maintenance by means of sex hormone replacement therapy may be required.

## 8.3 Disorders of stature

### Learning objectives

You should:

- be able to plot a child's height and weight on a centile chart
- know the causes of short stature
- know the causes of tall stature

### Physiology

Growth is greatest in terms of height velocity in the second trimester of pregnancy, when the crown–heel length increases at a rate of 52 cm/year. Influences on fetal growth include ethnic origin, maternal height, mid-pregnancy weight, nutrition, smoking and alcohol intake, fetal sex, the presence of congenital abnormalities and growth factors. Postnatal growth is best described by the infancy–childhood–pubertal model (Fig. 71). The figure shows the height and velocity curves of a normal child, highlighting the three phases of growth in childhood and adolescence:

1. There is a rapidly decelerating growth phase in infancy, dependent on nutrition.
2. The steady, slowly decelerating growth phase in childhood is dependent on growth hormone (GH); growth rate may be enhanced by a mid-childhood growth spurt.
3. The rapidly accelerating and decelerating pubertal growth spurt is dependent upon the normal secretion of GH and sex steroids. This growth spurt occurs with breast development in girls (breast stage 2–3) and a testicular volume of 10–12 mL in boys, as measured by a Prader orchidometer.

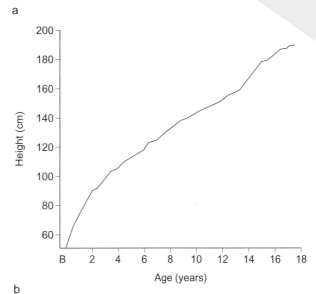

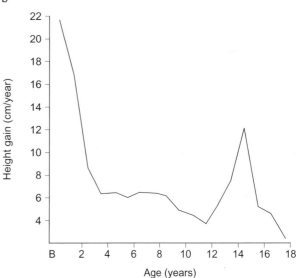

**Fig. 71** The infancy–childhood–pubertal model of growth. (a) The height-distance chart and (b) the height velocity chart of a normal child.

### Assessment of growth

The assessment of growth is vital and involves several parameters.

**Linear height** should be measured using a stadiometer and plotted on a distance chart. The parents' heights should also be plotted and the mid-parental centile calculated (add 12.5 cm to the mother's height for a boy; subtract 12.5 cm from the father's height for a girl). The distance chart simply compares the child's height to that of other children of the same age, and a child may lie below the third centile and still be normal.

**Height velocity** is calculated by measuring the height at 4-monthly intervals and dividing the incre-

...s by the time interval in years. A ...rmal if the height velocity lies close ... on a height-velocity chart.

...esses skeletal maturity and is delayed ...al growth delay, hypothyroidism and ...ess. It is advanced in precocious

**Pub...staging** employs standard references for the development of breast, pubic hair, testicular and penile size.

## Short stature

Short stature is defined as a height below the third percentile for chronological age. Short stature may be disproportionate (e.g. achondroplasia) or proportional, depending on the upper : lower body segment ratios. The management of short stature is shown in Figure 72 and Table 49.

### Achondroplasia

Children with achondroplasia, a common, autosomal dominant form of short-limbed dwarfism, may not have a positive family history as there is a high rate of spontaneous mutations. Patients have frontal bossing, hydrocephalus, a low nasal bridge, lumbar lordosis, and the three middle fingers are trident-shaped. The use of growth hormone in this condition is still controversial.

### Low-birthweight infants

Low birthweight may be caused by problems during pregnancy, such as hypertension and intrauterine infection. Children with the Russell–Silver syndrome have a low birthweight, feeding difficulties in the first year of life, small triangular facies, clinodactyly and body asymmetry, especially pronounced in the face. Their growth velocity is generally normal; if so, no further investigation or treatment is indicated.

### Turner syndrome

Girls with Turner syndrome have characteristic features (see Section 9.3) including short stature and gonadal failure (Fig. 73). Although 20% of girls with Turner

**Table 49** Investigations for short stature according to age

| Age group | Investigations | Treatment |
|-----------|----------------|-----------|
| Infancy | Nutritional Karyotype Skeletal survey | Dietary management |
| Childhood | Growth hormone provocation test Thyroid function Adrenal function | Hormone replacement |
| Puberty | Hypothalamopituitary –gonadal function | Sex steroid treatment |

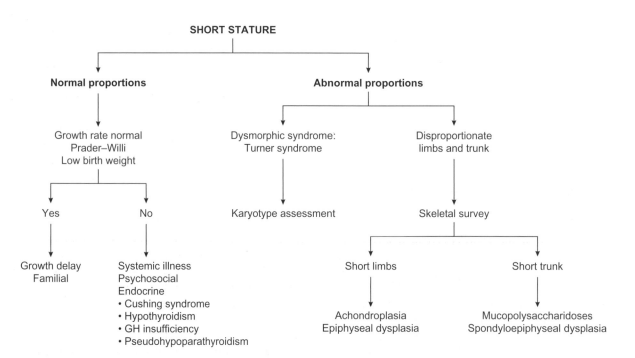

**Fig. 72** Algorithm for the management of short stature.

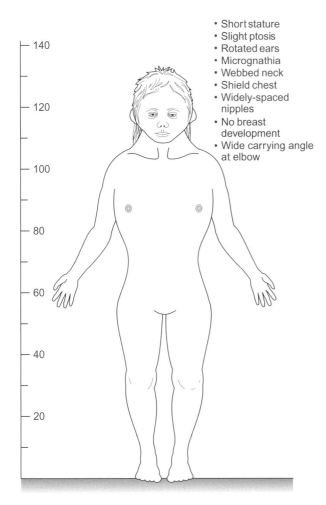

- Short stature
- Slight ptosis
- Rotated ears
- Micrognathia
- Webbed neck
- Shield chest
- Widely-spaced nipples
- No breast development
- Wide carrying angle at elbow

**Fig. 73** 12-year-old girl with Turner syndrome.

syndrome will start puberty spontaneously, most will require oestrogen at some stage. GH can be used to maximise their height potential. Psychological counselling is important, and the use of donor eggs to achieve pregnancy may be appropriate in later life.

## Systemic causes of short stature

Short stature secondary to systemic disease is often characterised by a delayed bone age and may occur in severe Crohn's, coeliac, renal and cardiovascular diseases, cystic fibrosis, asthma, rickets and metabolic disorders. The potential for catch-up growth is present if the underlying systemic disorder is treated successfully.

## Psychosocial emotional deprivation

Infants suffering from severe neglect or non-accidental injury may develop endocrine abnormalities, such as short stature and delayed skeletal and sexual maturation. The biochemical picture may indicate GH deficiency. Following prolonged admission to hospital an

---

> **Box 44** Causes of growth hormone deficiency
>
> **Congenital**
> GH gene deletion
> Developmental abnormalities: pituitary aplasia, pituitary hypoplasia, midline brain defects
>
> **Acquired**
> Hypothalamopituitary tumours: craniopharyngioma, Langerhans' cell histiocytosis
> Secondary to cranial irradiation
> Secondary to head injury
> Secondary to infection

improvement in height ensues, together with an increase in spontaneous and stimulated GH secretion. Treatment may involve placing the child in foster care on either a temporary or a permanent basis.

## Endocrine causes of short stature

The important hormones concerned with growth are thyroxine (T$_4$), GH and sex steroids. Deficiency of any of these may result in short stature. Other endocrine disorders leading to short stature (e.g. Cushing syndrome) are discussed in the appropriate sections.

## Growth hormone deficiency

Deficiency of GH may be isolated or may occur with other pituitary hormone deficiencies (Box 44). GH has a pulsatile pattern of secretion from the anterior pituitary gland that is controlled by growth hormone-releasing hormone (GHRH) and somatostatin, which are themselves secreted by the hypothalamus. GH secretion is stimulated by sleep, exercise, hypoglycaemia, physical and emotional stress, and a high protein intake. It is inhibited by psychogenic stress, malnutrition and CNS trauma. GH has indirect actions on the musculoskeletal system mediated via insulin-like growth factor-1 (IGF-1), leading to protein synthesis and cell proliferation. GH also has direct anti-insulin effects, resulting in lipolysis and breakdown of carbohydrate.

### Clinical features
GH deficiency is typified by a height equal to or less than three standard deviations (SD) from the mean (Fig. 74), a slow height velocity and delayed bone age. Normal body proportions are associated with crowded midface structures, a high-pitched voice and increased skinfold thickness.

### Diagnosis
GH secretion can be assessed in several ways. GH profiles over 24-hour periods are mainly used as a research

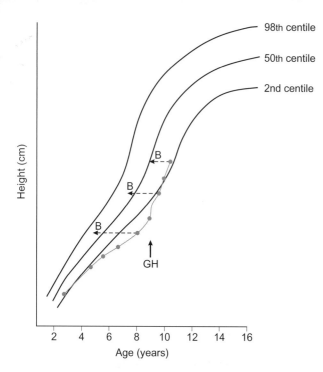

**Fig. 74** Linear growth before and after treatment with GH in a patient with GH deficiency. After starting therapy, the height approaches and then crosses the second percentile. The delay in bone age (B) is reduced and bone age becomes more appropriate for the chronological age.

tool. Provocative tests induce GH secretion by means of a suitable stimulus, such as sleep, exercise, insulin, arginine, L-dopa, glucagon, clonidine, propranolol and GHRH. The insulin-induced hypoglycaemia test is the most reliable, but should only be performed in a tertiary centre *under strict medical supervision*. Glucagon is safer and more widely used. Normally a peak GH of >10 µg/L is achieved, although the absolute value depends on the assay used.

**Treatment**
The response to daily subcutaneous injections of recombinant human GH (hGH) is usually excellent, with an initial catch-up phase followed by a normal height velocity.

## Constitutional delay of growth and puberty

Constitutional delay is more common in boys than girls and is often associated with a positive family history. It is the commonest cause of short stature, characterised by a delay in growth, puberty and bone age. The growth rate is normal, given the stage in puberty. The final height prognosis is good, and treatment is unnecessary unless short stature leads to psychosocial distress. In

severe cases a short course of anabolic steroids (e.g. oxandrolone) or slow-release testosterone (sustanon) may accelerate the pubertal growth spurt. The condition is difficult to differentiate from hypogonadotrophic hypogonadism.

## Tall stature

Tall stature is defined as a height above the 97th percentile for chronological age. Tall children with normal body proportions and a normal appearance are unlikely to have any underlying pathological cause for tall stature. A height prediction can be made using the bone age and the height velocity. An algorithm for the assessment of children with tall stature is shown in Figure 75.

## Tall stature in children with normal proportions

### Tall stature associated with a normal height velocity
If a tall child has a normal appearance and normal growth velocity, constitutional tall stature is the most likely diagnosis. Obese children are often taller than average for their age, and if bone maturity is advanced puberty may also occur earlier. Tall stature may represent a considerable disadvantage, especially in girls, and if necessary limitation of growth can be achieved using sex steroids.

### Tall stature associated with increased growth velocity
Tall children with increased growth velocity and signs of puberty should be investigated for CAH and precocious puberty. In precocious puberty, accelerated linear growth and bone maturation result in tall stature at presentation, but the final height is likely to be compromised because of early fusion of the epiphyses. If there are no signs of puberty, the following conditions should be considered:

**Growth hormone excess.** Excess GH secretion in childhood or adolescence causes gigantism. GH levels are elevated but the bone age is not advanced. The pituitary fossa may be enlarged because of a GH-secreting tumour. Patients present with rapid linear growth, overgrowth of soft tissues, and hyperglycaemia. Treatment entails dopamine agonists (e.g. bromocriptine) to reduce the excess GH secretion and the removal of an adenoma by trans-sphenoidal surgery and/or radiotherapy.

**Thyrotoxicosis.** An increase in growth rate and advanced bone age are seen in thyrotoxicosis. In addi-

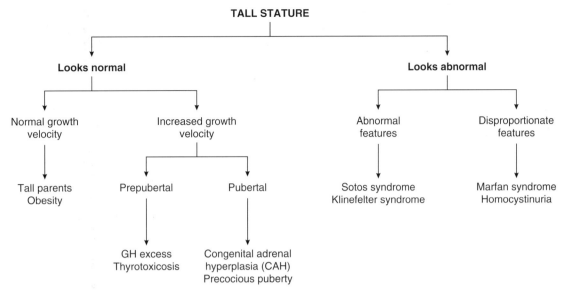

**Fig. 75** Algorithm for the management of tall stature.

tion, free thyroxine levels are high and thyroid-stimulating hormone (TSH) levels low.

## Tall stature in children with abnormal appearance

### Sotos syndrome
Sotos syndrome is characterised by tall stature, a large elongated head, prominent forehead, large ears, elongated jaw, coarse facial features and subnormal intelligence.

### Marfan syndrome
Patients with Marfan syndrome, an autosomal dominant condition, are tall with long limbs, narrow hands and slender fingers. Their arm span is greater than their height. Hyperextensible joints, kyphoscoliosis, ribcage deformities, upward lenticular dislocation, mitral and aortic valve lesions and aortic aneurysms are other features of this condition.

### Homocystinuria
Homocystinuria is an autosomal recessive condition with features caused by the absence of cystathionine synthetase. Phenotypic features are similar to those of Marfan syndrome, except for downward dislocation of the lens. Mental retardation and venous and arterial thrombotic disease are also common.

### Klinefelter syndrome
Klinefelter syndrome results from an XXY karyotype and manifests in tall stature, eunuchoid features, gynaecomastia, seminiferous tubule dysgenesis and testicular atrophy.

## 8.4 Disorders of puberty

### Learning objectives

You should:

- know the causes of delayed puberty
- know the causes of precocious puberty

## Normal puberty

Puberty is the period during which sexual maturation occurs and reproductive capacity is attained. It is characterised by the adolescent growth spurt, the appearance of secondary sexual characteristics and profound psychological changes.

In girls, puberty is heralded by an increase in height velocity followed by breast and then pubic hair development, and finally menarche. Peak height velocity coincides with stage 3 breast development and menarche with stage 4, so that about 5–8 cm of growth follow the first menstrual period. In boys, testicular enlargement is followed by penile growth, the growth of pubic hair and an increase in height velocity.

Profound changes in hormone levels occur with puberty. Pulsatile gonadotrophin (FSH and LH) secretion stimulates the release of testosterone and oestradiol to adult concentrations. In addition, in girls, gonadotrophin secretion is cyclical, resulting in increases in oestrogens in mid-cycle. Initially, the ovary does not secrete sufficient oestrogen to induce the LH surge required for ovulation, and during the first 2 years post menarche 50–90% of cycles are anovulatory, decreasing to <20% after 5 years. The initial appearance of multi-cystic ovaries is replaced by one with a dominant follicle. During this time, the uterus develops an adult configuration, with endometrium formation leading to menarche when the endometrium is 7–8 mm thick. At around 8 years of age, the adrenal gland matures and secretes adrenal androgens, leading to the development of pubic and axillary hair.

## Delayed puberty

Delayed puberty may be a manifestation of severe systemic illness, central nervous system disease and gonadal disease (Box 45).

### Constitutional delay of growth and puberty

This is described earlier in the chapter.

### Hypogonadotrophic hypogonadism

Children with hypogonadotrophic hypogonadism fail to achieve puberty without assistance. It may follow congenital or acquired malformations of the hypothalamo-pituitary area (Box 46).

Micropenis and small or cryptorchid testes are seen in boys, and in girls the reproductive organs are pre-pubertal in size. There is no FSH and LH response to luteinising hormone releasing hormone (LHRH).

**Treatment** includes pulsatile gonadotrophin-releasing hormone (GnRH) and testosterone or oestrogen replacement.

### Prader–Willi syndrome

Prader–Willi syndrome results from a deletion in the paternally derived chromosome 15. Poor activity in utero is followed by hypotonia, obesity owing to an insatiable appetite, mental retardation and hypogonadotrophic hypogonadism. Patients have a characteristic facies with almond-shaped eyes and often die prematurely from a Pickwickian syndrome with hypoventilation.

### Anorexia nervosa

Anorexia nervosa usually arises in females and results in marked weight loss and secondary amenorrhoea. Gonadotrophin secretion is reduced in these girls.

## Precocious puberty

Though initially associated with tall stature, precocious puberty leads to early fusion of the epiphyses and a short final height. The increased production of sex steroids results in early physical maturation and menstruation in mentally immature young children, and behavioural problems are common. Precocious puberty may be gonadotrophin dependent (central) or gonadotrophin independent (Box 47).

### Gonadotrophin-dependent precocious puberty

Gonadotrophin-dependent precocious puberty is characterised by the normal pubertal sequence: breast devel-

---

**Box 45** Causes of delayed puberty

**Central disorders**
Constitutional delay
Congenital abnormalities
Gonadotrophin deficiency
Panhypopituitarism
Severe systemic disease

**Gonadal disorders**
Turner syndrome
Noonan syndrome
Gonadal dysgenesis
Trauma and neoplasia

---

**Box 46** Causes of hypogonadotrophic hypogonadism

| **Congenital** | **Acquired** |
|---|---|
| Malformations of hypothalamic area | Neoplasia |
| Intrauterine infections | Encephalitis, meningitis |
| Perinatal hypoxia | Trauma |
| Kallman syndrome | |

---

**Box 47** Causes of precocious puberty

**Gonadotrophin-dependent causes**
Idiopathic: common in girls, rare in boys
CNS disorders: space-occupying lesions (benign or malignant), congenital CNS anomalies, post infection or trauma, hCG-producing neoplasms

**Gonadotrophin-independent causes**
Exogenous sex steroids: tumours of the adrenal, ovary and testis, congenital adrenal hyperplasia
McCune–Albright syndrome

opment followed by pubic and axillary hair growth and menarche in girls; testicular development followed by penile enlargement, then pubic and axillary hair development in boys. The condition is more common in girls and is often idiopathic. In boys, it often results from an intracranial lesion. Patients have a pubertal LH and FSH response after an LHRH test, and girls may have multicystic ovaries as a result of pulsatile gonadotrophin secretion. The bone age is usually advanced.

## McCune–Albright syndrome

McCune–Albright syndrome is associated with gonadotrophin-independent precocious puberty, large unilateral irregular *café-au-lait* spots and polyostotic fibrous dysplasia. Excessive oestrogen in girls or excess testosterone in boys is seen, together with no LH or FSH response to LHRH.

## Premature thelarche

Isolated breast development (thelarche) is usually a benign isolated finding in girls with a normal growth rate, appropriate skeletal maturity for chronological age and normal final height. Pelvic ultrasound is indicated to exclude an ovarian cyst.

## Premature pubarche

Isolated pubic hair development may arise because of excess androgens (adrenarche), CAH, an adrenal neoplasm and Cushing syndrome.

## Treatment of precocious puberty

LHRH analogues are only effective in centrally mediated, gonadotrophin-dependent precocious puberty. Cyproterone acetate can be effective in gonadotrophin-independent precocious puberty but can cause adrenal insufficiency.

# Polycystic ovary syndrome

Polycystic ovary syndrome (PCOS) may be idiopathic or follow central precocious puberty or CAH. These girls are tall, obese and hirsute, with acne, large ovaries, amenorrhoea, dysfunctional menstrual bleeding and infertility. Biochemical findings include hyperinsulinism, raised adrenal and ovarian androgens, testosterone, LH : FSH ratio, and lowered sex hormone-binding globulin.

**Treatment** is complicated, involving multiple hormone manipulation.

# 8.5 Disorders of the thyroid gland

## Learning objectives

You should:

- know the clinical features of congenital hypothyroidism and be able to discuss the diagnosis and management

- know the causes, symptoms and signs of hyperthyroidism in a child and be able to discuss the diagnosis and management

## Physiology

The thyroid gland forms in the third week of gestation. Thyroid follicular cells synthesise, iodinate and store thyroglobulin, and release the thyroid hormones thyroxine ($T_4$) and triiodothyronine ($T_3$) after organification of the trapped iodide. The gland stores thyroglobulin, $T_3$ and $T_4$, and is responsible for deiodination and recycling of the iodide.

TRH secreted by the hypothalamus leads to TSH secretion by the anterior pituitary, which in turn stimulates the release of $T_4$ from the thyroid gland. Circulating $T_4$ levels are high in the neonate and when the thyroid gland is hyperactive in response to TSH, and decrease during childhood and when the gland is underactive. TSH is inhibited by somatostatin, dopamine and $T_3$, thereby completing the negative feedback loop. The thyroid gland is the sole source of $T_4$, which is bound in plasma by thyroxine-binding globulin (TBG). It is monodeiodinated in peripheral tissues to form $T_3$, the more potent hormone, which is bound by both albumin and TBG. $T_3$ binds to tissue receptors and stimulates mitochondrial activity, catecholamine release, lipid and amino acid turnover, and growth factor production and action.

In the fetus, the pituitary–thyroid axis is independent of the mother's axis, as the placenta is impermeable to TSH, but allows small amounts of $T_3$ and $T_4$ to cross. TSH levels may be elevated in normal neonates and declines to normal levels within the first few days after birth.

## Hypothyroidism

### Congenital hypothyroidism

Congenital hypothyroidism occurs in 1 in 4000 live births and follows maldescent or dysgenesis of the gland, or dyshormonogenesis. Most affected neonates are initially

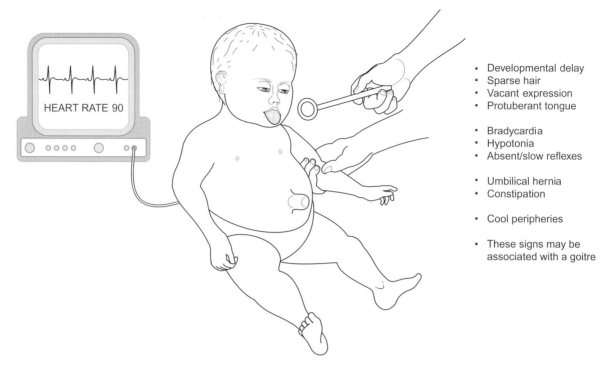

**Fig. 76** Clinical features of hypothyroidism.

- Developmental delay
- Sparse hair
- Vacant expression
- Protuberant tongue

- Bradycardia
- Hypotonia
- Absent/slow reflexes

- Umbilical hernia
- Constipation

- Cool peripheries

- These signs may be associated with a goitre

HEART RATE 90

asymptomatic, the majority being detected on routine biochemical screening. If untreated, clinical features will eventually include coarse facies, large tongue, hoarse cry, hypotonia, lethargy, umbilical hernia, constipation, prolonged jaundice, feeding and respiratory problems (Fig. 76). Routine screening involves the measurement of TSH from blood collected on a Guthrie card between 5 and 7 days of age. If the initial TSH is elevated, free $T_4$ and TSH levels are measured. If free $T_4$ is low and TSH high, a radionuclide thyroid scan is performed to distinguish between thyroid dysgenesis, ectopic thyroid and dyshormonogenesis. Deafness may be associated with dyshormonogenesis and congenital hypothyroidism (Pendred syndrome), and so audiological assessment is also required.

**Treatment**. $T_4$ replacement is necessary for life, with regular monitoring of thyroid function, growth and skeletal maturation. Worsening neurodevelopmental delay is related to lower initial $T_4$ levels and increasing delay in starting hormone replacement, especially if left until after 4–6 weeks.

### Secondary hypothyroidism

Hypothyroidism secondary to TRH or TSH deficiency is rare and usually associated with deficiency of other pituitary hormones and midline defects, e.g. cleft palate.

### Acquired hypothyroidism

The most common cause of acquired hypothyroidism worldwide is iodine deficiency. Autoimmune disease (Hashimoto disease) is the usual cause in childhood and adolescence, whereas local or total body irradiation is the usual cause in those treated for malignant disease. Disease secondary to TSH or TRH deficiency is rare. Poor height velocity, with consequent short stature, is associated with delayed skeletal age, gain in weight and subcutaneous fat, intolerance of cold, constipation and mental slowing. Puberty is usually delayed. Examination may reveal a goitre, coarse facies, bradycardia, a protuberant abdomen and slow relaxation of tendon reflexes. Signs of associated autoimmune disease may also be present, e.g. chronic mucocutaneous candidiasis, hypoparathyroidism, Addison disease, vitiligo, chronic active hepatitis, pernicious anaemia, myasthenia gravis and diabetes mellitus.

**Treatment**. Therapy with $T_4$ is indicated, initially in low dose to avoid dramatic behavioural changes. Cortisol deficiency must also be excluded, as the commencement of $T_4$ may precipitate an Addisonian crisis if untreated hypoadrenalism exists. Regular monitoring of growth and thyroid function is essential.

# Hyperthyroidism

Hyperthyroidism is usually caused by autoimmune disease involving a multinodular goitre. The term Graves' disease is used when eye signs are present. Excess TSH production from the pituitary or $T_4$ from a single thyroid nodule is less common.

Thyrotoxicosis is seven times more common in girls than boys, and generally occurs in the peripubertal period. A family history of other autoimmune disease is common. Patients may present with behavioural problems, including hyperactivity, agitation, weight loss, tall stature, excessive sweating, intolerance of heat and palpitations. A goitre, occasionally with a bruit, tachycardia, tremor, lid lag, exophthalmos and ophthalmoplegia may be found on examination.

Levels of $T_4$ and free $T_3$ are raised, but TSH is suppressed (often undetectable).

**Treatment**. Propranolol controls the acute symptoms and carbimazole or propylthiouracil suppresses the overactive gland. If medical treatment fails or side effects are unacceptable, thyroidectomy or radioactive iodine may be considered.

## 8.6 Disorders of the adrenal gland

### Learning objectives

You should:

- know the aetiology, clinical manifestations and management of Addison's disease

- know the aetiology, clinical manifestations and management of Cushing's syndrome

- know the aetiology and clinical manifestations of congenital adrenal hyperplasia

The adrenal cortex occupies 80% of the gland at term and becomes active during the second trimester. The zona glomerulosa in the outer cortex produces aldosterone under the control of the renin–angiotensin system. Aldosterone modulates sodium and potassium exchange, mainly in the renal distal tubule. The middle zona fasciculata comprises 75% of the adrenal cortex and secretes cortisol under the control of hypothalamic corticotrophin–releasing hormone (CRH), and especially pituitary ACTH. From 6 months of age, cortisol and ACTH levels vary in a circadian rhythm, with higher levels in the morning than at night. The urinary steroid profile provides a useful assessment of the secretion of abnormal steroid metabolites.

The innermost zona reticularis matures in midchildhood to release adrenal androgens, predominantly dehydroepiandrosterone sulphate (DHEAS).

## Adrenal steroid deficiency

Adrenal insufficiency may involve all three zones or affect the production of mineralocorticosteroids or glucocorticoids alone (Box 48). It may result from primary failure of the gland or be secondary to ACTH deficiency.

### Primary adrenal insufficiency (Addison disease)

Adrenal haemorrhage is the most common cause of adrenal insufficiency in the newborn, whereas autoimmune adrenalitis is most common in the older child. Hypoglycaemia, salt and fluid loss and conjugated hyperbilirubinaemia predominate in infants, whereas anorexia, vomiting, fatigue, weight loss, hypotension and hyperpigmentation are seen in childhood. A family history of autoimmune disorders may be present.

**Investigations** show hyponatraemia with hyperkalaemia, raised ACTH, low cortisol throughout a 24-

---

**Box 48** Causes of adrenal insufficiency

| | Primary adrenal insufficiency | Secondary adrenal insufficiency |
|---|---|---|
| All zones | Autoimmune adrenalitis<br>Adrenal haemorrhage<br>Infections (including DIC)<br>Iatrogenic, chemical or surgical<br>Multiple endocrinopathy | Pituitary hormone deficiencies<br>Isolated ACTH deficiency<br>Hypothalamopituitary tumours<br>Glucocorticoid therapy<br>Cranial radiotherapy<br>Surgery |
| Zona glomerulosa<br>Zona fasciculata | Hypoaldosteronism<br>Isolated glucocorticoid deficiency<br>Congenital adrenal hyperplasia | |

hour period, raised plasma renin with low aldosterone levels, and hypoglycaemia. There is failure of the adrenals to respond to exogenous ACTH (synacthen) by increasing cortisol levels. Positive antibodies to the adrenal glands are found in autoimmune adrenalitis. A CT scan of the adrenals may reveal large adrenal glands in CAH.

## Secondary adrenal insufficiency

Secondary adrenal insufficiency should be excluded in those with hypopituitarism. GH, LH and FSH insufficiency are more common than isolated ACTH deficiency. However, ACTH deficiency combined with other pituitary hormone deficiencies is a late feature of hypopituitarism, especially when secondary to cranial irradiation. In congenital hypopituitarism there may be associated midline defects, e.g. agenesis of the corpus callosum, cleft lip and palate.

**Investigations** reveal low cortisol and ACTH levels over a 24-hour period. MRI of the hypothalamopituitary area is essential to exclude local tumours, e.g. craniopharyngioma.

## Treatment of adrenal insufficiency

In an Addisonian crisis resuscitative measures are required to replete the plasma volume. Intravenous hydrocortisone should be administered, to be replaced later by oral hydrocortisone. Mineralocorticoid deficiency, indicated by increased renin levels, requires mineralocorticoid replacement in the form of oral 9α-fludrocortisone. Regular assessment of growth, ACTH, cortisol and plasma renin profiles is mandatory in all those on adrenal replacement treatment.

## Adrenal steroid excess

### Cushing syndrome

Cushing syndrome describes the clinical features of adrenal steroid excess. This is usually iatrogenic due to exogenous steroids, but may follow excess corticosteroids from pituitary tumours (Cushing disease) and, less commonly, adrenal and other neoplasms (Box 49).

A moon-like plethoric facies with acne, interscapular fat pad (buffalo hump), truncal obesity, striae, hirsutism, growth arrest, easy bruising, hypertension, proximal myopathy, cataracts, hypogonadism and glucose intolerance characterises this syndrome (Fig. 77). Loss of the normal diurnal variation in plasma cortisol, with an elevated midnight level, is associated with elevated 24-hour urinary cortisol. There is failure of suppression of cortisol secretion by exogenous low-dose

---

**Box 49** Causes of adrenal steroid excess

**Primary adrenal disorders**
*Glucocorticoids*
Nodular adrenal hyperplasia
Adrenal neoplasm

*Mineralocorticoids*
CAH (11β, 17α-hydroxylase)
Neoplasm (Conn syndrome)
Dexamethasone-suppressible hyperaldosteronism

*Androgens*
CAH (11β, 21-hydroxylase)
Adrenal neoplasm
Premature adrenarche

**Secondary adrenal disorders**
CRH- and ACTH-secreting tumours
Renin-secreting tumours

**Iatrogenic**
Excess steroids

---

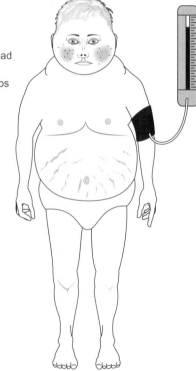

- Moon face
- Facial acne
- Facial plethora
- Interscapular fat pad
- Truncal obesity
- Relatively thin limbs
- Hypertension
- Abdominal striae
- Glycosuria

**Fig. 77** Manifestations of Cushing syndrome.

---

dexamethasone in all cases, although levels may suppress with high-dose dexamethasone in pituitary-dependent Cushing disease but not in adrenal-dependent Cushing syndrome. ACTH levels are raised in Cushing disease but suppressed in Cushing syndrome. CT or MRI scanning of the pituitary and adrenal glands is required to exclude hormone-secreting adenomas or carcinomas.

**Management**. Surgery is required, via an abdominal approach (adrenal tumours) or trans-sphenoidal resection (pituitary tumours).

## Adrenal tumours

Patients with adrenal tumours develop Cushing syndrome and virilising features, e.g. accelerated growth velocity, advanced bone age, pubic hair, acne, hirsutism and phallic enlargement.

**Investigation** confirms elevated adrenal androgens and urinary steroids.

**Management**. Surgical resection is followed by regular monitoring of the growth rate and 24-hour urinary steroid profile.

## Congenital adrenal hyperplasia

CAH describes a group of autosomal recessive conditions where an enzyme block in cortisol synthesis results in excessive CRH–ACTH drive to the adrenal gland, promoting adrenal hyperplasia. The incidence of CAH is 1 in 4000. The mutation can be identified in many patients, allowing for antenatal diagnosis. The enzyme defect prevents the production of particular adrenal steroids, with the accumulation of others higher up the biochemical pathway. Clinical features depend upon which steroids are deficient and which are present in excess.

The commonest defect is 21-hydroxylase deficiency. Female patients have virilised genitalia, whereas males may have a large penis with a pigmented scrotum. In later childhood, males may develop precocious puberty with excessive growth and bone maturation, and virilisation occurs in females. Salt-losing crises occur in early life in two-thirds of patients. Low levels of cortisol and elevated ACTH are associated with hyponatraemia, hyperkalaemia and excess urinary sodium in salt losers. Identification of urinary steroid metabolites will delineate the enzymic block, e.g. elevated 17-hydroxyprogesterone with 21-hydroxylase deficiency. A karyotype and pelvic ultrasound scan are essential to ascertain the gender and internal genitalia in those who present with ambiguous genitalia (see Fig. 70).

**Management**. Treatment entails hydrocortisone and mineralocorticoid replacement. Follow-up includes measurement of the growth rate and estimation of plasma renin activity. The prognosis for fertility is guarded, and girls may develop polycystic ovarian disease. If well controlled, the prognosis for final height is good.

# 8.7 Disorders of calcium homeostasis

## Learning objectives

You should:

- know the aetiology and clinical features of hypo- and hypercalcaemia

- understand the aetiology, clinical presentation, diagnosis and management of rickets in children

## Physiology

Three hormones, vitamin D, parathyroid hormone (parathormone, PTH) and calcitonin, are vital in the maintenance of normal calcium homeostasis. Vitamin D is synthesised in the skin and converted to 25-hydroxyvitamin D in the liver and to 1,25-dihydroxyvitamin D in the kidney. The latter induces the synthesis of mRNA and, in turn, protein messengers that stimulate the transport of calcium and phosphate across the intestine into the blood and assist PTH-stimulated osteoclastic bone resorption. 1,25-Dihydroxyvitamin D has an inhibitory feedback effect on 1α-hydroxylation and PTH secretion.

The secretion of PTH by four parathyroid glands is regulated by plasma calcium concentration. Secretion is maximal with a calcium concentration of 2 mmol/L, but is not totally suppressed even with very high calcium levels. PTH promotes calcium reabsorption in the distal renal tubules and inhibits phosphate and bicarbonate reabsorption in the proximal tubule. It also stimulates 1α-hydroxylation of 25-hydroxyvitamin D and induces osteoclasts to resorb calcium from bone.

In response to a fall in calcium concentration, PTH release leads to reduced renal calcium excretion and, in conjunction with 1,25-dihydroxyvitamin D, to mobilisation of calcium from bone. In addition, enteral calcium and phosphate absorption is promoted. The phosphate concentration remains stable because of the phosphaturic effect of PTH. With hypercalcaemia PTH secretion is inhibited, leading to increased calcium excretion, decreased bone resorption and suppression of calcium binding in the gut. Phosphate loss increases vitamin D synthesis independently of PTH, whereas phosphate retention inhibits it. The primary role of calcitonin, produced by thyroid C cells, is the inhibition of bone resorption by PTH and vitamin D.

## Hypocalcaemia

### Neonatal hypocalcaemia

Hypocalcaemia is a common, usually transient problem in the first few days of life. Hypocalcaemia between 4 and 28 days can be caused by transient or congenital hypoparathyroidism, a high phosphate intake, hypomagnesaemia, calcium malabsorption or maternal vitamin D deficiency. Neonates present with irritability, jitteriness and apnoea.

**Treatment**. Initial correction using intravenous calcium gluconate is followed by maintenance oral calcium lactate.

### The older child with hypocalcaemia

Intractable seizures, paraesthesiae, muscle cramps, weakness and laryngospasm, together with carpopedal spasm and positive Chvostek and Trousseau signs, may all be manifestations of hypocalcaemia. Chronic hypocalcaemia leads to mental retardation, cataracts and dental enamel hypoplasia. Clinical features of rickets may be present (see below).

The plasma phosphate concentration may provide the clue to the underlying diagnosis. If it is high with a low PTH, the cause of the hypocalcaemia is likely to be hypoparathyroidism. Low plasma phosphate suggests hypophosphataemic rickets, whereas a normal phosphate concentration indicates calciopenic rickets.

### Rickets

Rickets follows calcium, phosphate and vitamin D deficiency (Box 50). In the first year of life the child presents with craniotabes, widened cranial sutures, frontal bossing, swollen epiphyses (especially wrists), bulging costochondral joints (rachitic rosary) and a Harrison's sulcus. Later, patients present with growth failure, genu varum and valgum, bone pain, proximal myopathy and/or retarded motor development. The clinical features can be attributed to hypocalcaemia, secondary hyperparathyroidism and hypophosphataemia, resulting in defective bone mineralisation with excessive bone resorption.

**Investigation**. Low calcium and phosphate levels are observed with an elevated alkaline phosphatase. The 1,25-dihydroxyvitamin D level may also be low and serum PTH high. Radiological features include expansion of the growth plate, with fraying, cupping and widening of metaphyses, pseudofractures, and signs of secondary hyperparathyroidism, e.g. subperiosteal erosions (see Fig. 5). Other abnormalities may be found, depending upon the underlying cause, e.g. acidosis, aminoaciduria, chronic renal failure.

**Treatment**. Calcium, phosphate and vitamin D supplements help correct the bony abnormalities. Treatment of end-organ (receptor) resistance to vitamin D can be very difficult, requiring large doses of calcium. Hypophosphataemic rickets is treated with very high doses of oral phosphate, and compliance may be a major problem.

### Hypoparathyroidism

Hypoparathyroidism may result from agenesis or hypoplasia of the parathyroid glands, and presents with hypocalcaemia in the neonatal period. This abnormality may be a feature of DiGeorge syndrome, when it is associated with thymic abnormalities, T-cell defects, and cardiac and facial abnormalities. In older children, hypoparathyroidism usually results from an autoimmune process and may be part of the polyglandular autoimmune syndrome, with chronic mucocutaneous candidiasis, Addison's disease, thyroid disease and malabsorption. Hypoparathyroidism may follow inadvertent removal of the parathyroids during thyroidectomy. End-organ receptor resistance to PTH causes *pseudohypoparathyroidism*, with short stature, round facies, mental retardation, ectopic calcification, and short fourth and fifth metacarpals and metatarsals.

**Diagnosis**. A high plasma phosphate, low plasma calcium and low PTH level are diagnostic of hypoparathyroidism. In pseudohypoparathyroidism the PTH level is elevated. Treatment entails calcium and vitamin D supplements to achieve normocalcaemia.

## Hypercalcaemia

Hypercalcaemia occurs with vitamin D intoxication and hyperparathyroidism. The latter is an uncommon condition caused by a primary parathyroid adenoma, sometimes as part of the multiple endocrine neoplasia

---

**Box 50** Causes of rickets

| Calcium deficiency | Vitamin D deficiency | Phosphate deficiency |
|---|---|---|
| Dietary malabsorption | Dietary malabsorption | Decreased intake |
| | Lack of sunlight | Renal tubular acidosis |
| | Hepatic disease | Renal tubular loss |
| | Anticonvulsants | Fanconi syndrome |
| | Renal disease | X-linked hypophosphataemia |
| | 1α-Hydroxylase deficiency | Nephrotoxic agents |
| | Vitamin D receptor defect | |

syndromes (MEN). Infantile hypercalcaemia may be an isolated abnormality that runs a benign and self-limiting course, or is a feature of Williams syndrome, associated with supravalvular aortic stenosis, peripheral pulmonary artery stenosis, mental retardation and dysmorphic features (elfin-like facies).

Anorexia, nausea, vomiting, constipation and polyuria are symptoms of hypercalcaemia. Urinary stones develop if hypercalciuria is present. With all causes of hypercalcaemia except hyperparathyroidism the PTH level is suppressed. In hyperparathyroidism the elevated plasma calcium level is associated with hypophosphataemia and inappropriately elevated PTH.

**Management**. In infantile hypercalcaemia, adequate hydration and a low-calcium diet should be maintained. If calcium levels remain high, then glucocorticoids should be commenced. In the emergency setting with very high calcium levels, a calcitonin infusion can be effective. Surgery remains the definitive treatment for primary hyperparathyroidism.

## 8.8 Disorders of glucose homeostasis

### Learning objectives

You should:

- know the presenting features and management of a child with insulin-dependent diabetes mellitus

- know the signs, symptoms and management of a child with diabetic ketoacidosis

- appreciate the causes and management of hypoglycaemia in childhood

### Physiology

The blood glucose reflects the balance between glucose intake, its mobilisation from glycogen stores in the liver (gluconeogenesis), its formation from protein (glyconeogenesis) and fat (lipolysis), and the consumption of glucose by body tissues. Glucose mobilisation is controlled by hormones, including cortisol, GH, glucagon and catecholamines, whereas its utilisation is controlled by insulin. In the fed state, an increase in blood glucose and amino acid levels leads to the secretion of insulin from β cells in the islets of Langerhans in the pancreas. Insulin inhibits gluconeogenesis and glycogenolysis and stimulates the deposition of glucose as glycogen in the liver, uptake of glucose and amino acids by muscle, and by adipocytes to form triglycerides. In the fasting state, blood glucose levels fall and insulin secretion is switched off. Counterregulatory hormones such as GH, cortisol and catecholamines inhibit glucose uptake and stimulate glycogenolysis, gluconeogenesis, the release of amino acids by muscle, and lipolysis and the release of free fatty acids from adipose tissue. Subsequent β-oxidation of free fatty acids results in the production of ketone bodies, an alternative fuel for the brain.

## Type 1 diabetes mellitus (TIDM)

Type 1 diabetics are insulin deficient and cannot utilise carbohydrate as fuel. Blood glucose levels are elevated, and the ability of the proximal renal tubules to reabsorb the glucose is exceeded; glycosuria followed by an osmotic diuresis results. The incidence of TIDM varies markedly from 5.3 to 35.3 new cases/100 000 in different countries, with 16.5/100 000 in the UK.

Genetically susceptible individuals with the HLA antigens B8, B15, DR3 and DR4 develop islet cell antibodies that destroy the β cells of the pancreas. The autoimmune process is probably triggered by environmental factors, including viruses such as Coxsackie. Diabetes mellitus may be a feature of other conditions, e.g. cystic fibrosis and chronic pancreatitis. Type 2 diabetes mellitus occurs in obesity, Prader–Willi syndrome, acanthosis nigricans and polycystic ovarian disease.

### Clinical features

TIDM usually presents insidiously at any age, with glycosuria, polyuria, dehydration, thirst and polydipsia. Inefficient energy utilisation results in weight loss despite polyphagia, and lassitude. *Diabetic ketoacidosis* is the mode of presentation in 25–60% (mean 45%) of diabetics. Clinical signs include those of severe dehydration, sometimes coma, with dry mucous membranes, decreased skin turgor, muscle and subcutaneous tissue wasting, odour of ketones on the breath, and Kussmaul (deep sighing) respiration.

Initially, shortly after diagnosis some endogenous insulin secretion is still present and the requirement for exogenous insulin is low. This 'honeymoon phase' is characterised by improved insulin sensitivity but is invariably followed by further destruction of islet cells and an increase in the insulin requirement.

### Investigation

The presence of hyperglycaemia, glycosuria and ketoacidosis confirms the diagnosis. Other useful investigations include blood gas analysis, urea and electrolytes, and a glycosylated haemoglobin level.

## Diabetic ketoacidosis (DKA)

Ketoacidosis affects up to 10% of known diabetics per annum, particularly teenage diabetics and those with poor glycaemic control, a past history or a family history of DKA. Seventy-five per cent of DKA episodes are associated with errors in insulin dosage, and 25% are a result of insufficient insulin administration during intercurrent infections. DKA is a medical emergency that must be managed in a controlled fashion if severe complications are to be avoided. The clinical signs (see above) are associated with hyperglycaemia (>11 mmol/L), metabolic acidosis (pH <7.3 with bicarbonate <15 mmol/L) and ketosis in blood or urine. The steps taken to manage this emergency situation are outlined in Box 51. About 5% of those with DKA may have significant cerebral oedema. The clinical risk features are given in Box 52. As up to 25% of those with cerebral oedema may suffer severe brain injury, these children are often best managed in an intensive care unit.

---

**Box 51** Management of diabetic ketoacidosis

**Assess and correct dehydration**
Slow rehydration *over 48 hours* (dehydration to a maximum of 10% plus maintenance fluids)
Use normal isotonic 0.9% saline until blood glucose is <15 mmol/L, then mixed 5% dextrose/0.45% saline infusion can be introduced. Avoid hypotonic solutions
Careful monitoring of urine output
*Fluid boluses are restricted to those in shock*

**Reduce hyperglycaemia**
Gradual reduction of hyperglycaemia and ketone production
Insulin infusion. Rapid-acting soluble insulin at 0.1 units/kg/h, aiming for a reduction of 2.5–3 mmol/h of glucose

**Replacement of electrolyte losses**
Potassium deficit is generally in the region of 3–6 mmol/kg and supplements should be started immediately unless the patient is anuric
Regular monitoring of electrolytes and pH

**Acidosis**
Adequate hydration and glycaemic control as above are usually sufficient
Bicarbonate supplementation may be considered with profound shock and a pH <6.9

**Prevent cerebral oedema**
Careful monitoring of the cerebral state
Prompt measures to prevent and counteract cerebral oedema

---

## Long-term management of TIDM

Time should be spent discussing the condition, its treatment and possible complications with the entire family prior to discharge. During the inpatient stay an adequate insulin regimen tailored to the individual patient must be devised, ensuring that the control of blood glucose in hospital is not 'perfect', thereby allowing for the inevitable increase in physical activity once discharged. An approximate insulin requirement of 0.5–1.0 unit/kg is usually needed, administered in a twice or three times daily dose, with one-third given as soluble, rapid acting insulin and two-thirds as a long-acting preparation. A balanced, complex carbohydrate-rich low-fat diet is recommended. Careful manipulation of the diet and insulin regimen allows for strenuous exercise, provided exercise-associated hypoglycaemia is avoided. Family education, with emphasis on self blood-glucose monitoring and testing for urinary ketones, particularly during intercurrent illnesses, is essential. The 'sick day' rule should be emphasised, whereby during periods of ill health patients and their carers are encouraged to monitor blood glucose levels at least every 4 hours, and every urine sample for ketones. Patients should be referred to a diabetic health visitor and reviewed regularly in the diabetic clinic, where measurement of glycosylated haemoglobin at 3-monthly intervals gives a good index of glycaemic control.

### Complications
*Acute*

- Cerebral oedema is usually the result of over-rapid correction of hyperglycaemia during ketoacidosis.
- Hypoglycaemia follows insulin overdosage or inadequate carbohydrate intake
- Patients with TIDM, especially if poorly controlled, have an increased susceptibility to infection.

---

**Box 52** Risk factors for cerebral oedema in DKA

New onset of TIDM
Younger diabetics (especially <2 years of age)*
Prolonged duration of DKA symptoms
Altered level of consciousness*
Hyponatraemia at presentation
Elevated urea
Marked dehydration (>10%) ± shock*
Marked acidosis (especially <7.1)* with low $CO_2$
Use of bicarbonate

* These factors in particular should indicate transfer to intensive care.

**Box 53** Chronic complications of poor glycaemic control

Impaired growth
Limited joint mobility
Early cataract formation
Hypertension
Hyperlipidaemia
Nephropathy
Retinopathy
Neuropathy

**Box 54** Causes of hypoglycaemia

| **Inadequate glucose production** | **Excessive glucose utilisation (hyperinsulinism)** |
|---|---|
| Inadequate glycogen stores | Infant of diabetic mother |
| Glycogen storage disease | Beckwith–Wiedemann syndrome |
| Galactosaemia, fructose intolerance | Nesidioblastosis |
| Fat oxidation defects | Insulinoma |
| GH, ACTH, glucocorticoid deficiency | Excessive insulin administration |
| Liver disease | Oral hypoglycaemic agents |
| Alcohol, salicylate poisoning | |

*Chronic* Good diabetic control in childhood reduces the risk of microangiopathic complications in adulthood. Chronic complications are rare in children (Box 53).

### Changes in insulin requirements

During puberty insulin requirements increase, probably because of the increased secretion of growth and sex hormones. The requirements decrease after puberty, and in adulthood they are lower than in adolescence. Any intercurrent illness may disrupt diabetic control by increasing insulin requirements as a result of the increased secretion of catecholamines. Control is also impaired as a result of the dawn and Somogyi phenomena. Nocturnal increase in GH secretion increases circulating glucose concentrations in the early hours of the morning, without preceding hypoglycaemia, and results in the *dawn phenomenon*. The *Somogyi effect* is defined as posthypoglycaemic hyperglycaemia and is thought to be caused by the increase in counterregulatory hormones during hypoglycaemia, which leads to insulin resistance.

## Hypoglycaemia

Hypoglycaemia is usually defined as a blood glucose level of less than 2.6 mmol/L. Its causes are listed in Box 54.

### Clinical features

Hypoglycaemia in the neonatal period presents with feeding problems, irritability, jitteriness, apnoea, hypotonia, convulsions and coma. Older children develop lassitude, headaches, abdominal pain, hunger, irritability, pallor, sweating, confusion, behavioural abnormalities, convulsions and coma.

### Investigations

The normal infusion rate of glucose required to maintain euglycaemia is 5–8 mg/kg/min in neonates and infants. A blood sample taken during hypoglycaemia should be analysed for glucose, insulin, cortisol, growth hormone, lactate, free fatty acids, ketones and C-peptide. A urine sample taken simultaneously should be analysed for organic acids.

Hypoglycaemia associated with low ketone and free fatty acid levels is typical of hyperinsulinaemic states. In factitious hyperinsulinism insulin levels are elevated but C-peptide levels are low. In endogenous hyperinsulinism insulin and C-peptide are both elevated.

### Treatment

Hypoglycaemia is a medical emergency and must be treated promptly with the administration of glucose (given intravenously in the unconscious patient) after taking the appropriate blood and urine samples. Intravenous glucose should not exceed 10–20%, as higher concentrations can cause cerebral oedema. Glucagon can be used as an emergency short-term measure but can lead to hyperinsulinism, with subsequent rebound hypoglycaemia.

## 8.9 Disorders of antidiuretic hormone secretion

### Learning objectives

You should:

- know the causes of polyuria

- know the causes of the syndrome of inappropriate ADH secretion

## Physiology

Water balance is maintained by the action of the hypothalamic thirst centre: osmoreceptors and neurons secrete antidiuretic hormone (ADH or vasopressin), which limits urinary output. ADH is synthesised in the supraoptic nuclei and migrates to the posterior pituitary for storage and release. Its release into the circulation is inhibited at a plasma osmolality of approximately 275 mmol/L, thereby allowing maximal urinary dilution. Conversely, an osmolality of 295 mmol/L stimulates sufficient ADH release to permit maximal urinary concentration.

## Diabetes insipidus

Without normal ADH activity, water is lost through the renal tubules; if the thirst mechanism is intact this will lead to polydipsia. Hence, thirst, polydipsia and polyuria are the cardinal features of diabetes insipidus (DI). This may result from central ADH deficiency (central DI) or renal causes (nephrogenic DI).

### Cranial diabetes insipidus

Cranial DI is caused by ADH deficiency and may follow congenital abnormalities of the hypothalamopituitary axis (e.g. septo-optic dysplasia), surgical or accidental trauma, inflammation (e.g. post meningitis, autoimmune disease), and local infiltrative or invasive lesions (e.g. histiocytosis, sarcoid, craniopharyngioma, optic nerve glioma). Genetic causes of cranial DI include autosomal dominant and X-linked hereditary conditions, and the DIDMOAD syndrome (DI, diabetes mellitus, optic atrophy and deafness).

## Nephrogenic diabetes insipidus

Nephrogenic DI is an X-linked disease resulting in resistance of the renal tubules to ADH. It may also be associated with sickle cell disease and renal abnormalities, e.g. hypokalaemia, hypercalcaemia, polycystic kidneys and chronic renal failure.

## Clinical features

Loss of more than 80% of ADH secretory capacity is required before symptoms of thirst, polydipsia and polyuria develop. If fluids are restricted, severe dehydration with hypernatraemia ensues. In children with associated ACTH deficiency DI will only become evident once glucocorticoid treatment is started, as the ability to excrete a water load is dependent on adequate glucocorticoid secretion.

## Investigations

If hypernatraemia with a high plasma osmolality is present simultaneously with a low urine osmolality a water deprivation test is not necessary. Indeed, this test can be extremely dangerous, and should only be performed under careful supervision. However, in children with compulsive water drinking the kidneys may develop a chronic inability to concentrate urine, and a water deprivation test may be the only method of differentiating this condition from DI. A dose of DDAVP (D-amino-D-arginine vasopressin) will restore the concentrating ability of the kidneys in cranial DI, thereby distinguishing this from nephrogenic DI.

## Treatment

DDAVP given orally or intranasally is used to treat cranial DI. The dose is titrated against symptoms, urine output and biochemical results. Access to water should not be restricted in those with normal thirst sensation. In patients who lack thirst sensation, a strict regimen of fluid intake and DDAVP replacement should be instigated, with careful monitoring of the sodium level, paired plasma and urine osmolalities.

In nephrogenic DI, treatment consists of free access to fluids and therapy with indomethacin or, paradoxically, diuretics such as hydrochlorothiazide and amiloride.

## Syndrome of inappropriate ADH secretion

The syndrome of inappropriate ADH secretion (SIADH) arises with abnormalities of the respiratory and nervous systems, malignancy and drugs (Box 55).

---

**Box 55** Causes of SIADH

**Nervous system abnormalities**
Tumours
Haemorrhage
Trauma
Infection, e.g. meningitis, encephalitis
Guillain–Barré syndrome
Ventriculoatrial shunt blockage

**Respiratory disease**
Pneumonia
Tuberculosis
Hyaline membrane disease

**Malignancies**
Thymoma
Lymphoma

**Drugs**
Narcotics and analgesics
Cytotoxics

---

**Clinical features** of SIADH include headaches, apathy, nausea, vomiting, abnormal neurological signs and impaired consciousness, occasionally convulsions and coma.

**Investigations** reveal hypo-osmolality, hyponatraemia, inappropriately high urinary osmolality, and sodium loss with inappropriately elevated ADH levels.

**Treatment** entails restriction of fluid intake and replacement of sodium losses. In severe cases ADH secretion may be inhibited using demeclocycline.

# Self-assessment: questions

## Multiple choice questions

1. Development of a normal male phenotype is dependent on:
   a. The SRY region of the Y chromosome
   b. Gonadotrophin secretion by the anterior pituitary gland
   c. Normal secretion of adrenal androgens
   d. Normal testicular function
   e. Normal prolactin secretion.

2. The following should be performed in a child with ambiguous genitalia:
   a. Abdominal ultrasound scan
   b. Karyotype analysis
   c. Urinary steroid profile
   d. hCG test
   e. Thyroid function.

3. The following are causes of short stature:
   a. Constitutional delay of growth and puberty
   b. Thyrotoxicosis
   c. Cushing syndrome
   d. Rickets
   e. Soto syndrome.

4. The following are manifestations of Turner syndrome:
   a. Delayed puberty
   b. Webbing of the neck
   c. Abdominal striae
   d. Renal abnormalities
   e. Lenticular dislocation.

5. In normal puberty:
   a. Breast development is the first stage in girls
   b. Pubic hair development heralds the onset of puberty in boys
   c. The growth spurt is only dependent on the normal secretion of growth hormone
   d. Menarche is an early event in girls
   e. Pulsatile gonadotrophin secretion is mandatory for normal puberty.

6. The following are causes of delayed puberty:
   a. Anorexia nervosa
   b. Cranial irradiation
   c. Poorly controlled type 1 diabetes mellitus
   d. Neurofibromatosis
   e. Marfan syndrome.

7. Congenital hypothyroidism:
   a. Caused by dyshormonogenesis is an autosomal recessive condition
   b. Can be associated with development delay
   c. Is detected in the UK by screening for free thyroxine levels
   d. Is usually the result of an autoimmune process
   e. Resulting from secondary causes can be missed on screening.

8. Thyrotoxicosis:
   a. Frequently presents with difficulties in behaviour and schooling
   b. Is associated with delayed relaxation of reflexes
   c. Is invariably associated with exophthalmos
   d. May be associated with vitiligo
   e. May be associated with an absent TSH response to TRH.

9. The following are features of Addison disease:
   a. Hypotension
   b. Retinal haemorrhages
   c. Virilisation
   d. Hyponatraemia
   e. Hyperpigmentation.

10. In Cushing syndrome, the following may be helpful in the diagnosis:
    a. Plasma renin activity
    b. Loss of diurnal variation in cortisol secretion
    c. Synacthen test
    d. Urinary free cortisol
    e. Dexamethasone suppression test.

11. The following are clinical features of rickets:
    a. Proximal myopathy
    b. Bone pain
    c. Ectopic calcification
    d. Genu varum
    e. Craniotabes.

12. The following may be associated with infantile hypercalcaemia:
    a. Mental retardation
    b. Elfin facies
    c. Supravalvular aortic stenosis
    d. Ectopic calcification
    e. Chronic diarrhoea.

13. The following can be used in the treatment of hypercalcaemia in children:
    a. High-dose phosphate
    b. Increased fluid intake
    c. EDTA
    d. Calcitonin
    e. Glucocorticoids.

14. With regard to cranial diabetes insipidus:
    a. It can present with convulsions
    b. Neuroradiological imaging is vital in all cases
    c. A water deprivation test is essential for diagnosis
    d. Water restriction is the treatment of choice
    e. It is a feature of Langerhans' cell histiocytosis.

15. Causes of nephrogenic diabetes insipidus include:
    a. An X-linked recessive condition
    b. Meningitis
    c. Heavy metal poisoning
    d. Hypokalaemia
    e. Intracranial neoplasia.

## Case histories

### Case history 1

A 6-month-old girl presents with bilateral inguinal swellings. A karyotype is performed and shows 46XY.

How would you manage this child?

### Case history 2

A prepubertal 8-year-old boy presents with tall stature and headaches. The bone age is 6 years and growth velocity 12 cm/year, equivalent to the 97th centile on the height velocity chart.

How would you investigate this child?

### Case history 3

A 4-year-old boy presents with tall stature. Examination reveals bilateral papilloedema and penile and testicular enlargement. The bone age is 10 years, and the growth velocity lies on the 97th centile.

Give two further essential investigations and the most likely diagnosis.

### Case history 4

A 6-year-old girl presents with short stature and isolated breast development. Examination confirms a height well below the third centile, weight on the 25th centile and breast stage 3 with no pubic or axillary hair development. Bone age was delayed at 2 years of age. Follow-up revealed a height velocity that lay on the third centile.

What is the most likely diagnosis?

### Case history 5

A 2-year-old girl presents with tall stature and a rapid rate of growth. Examination reveals marked clitoromegaly, and the bone age is advanced, at 7 years.

Name two diagnostic investigations and give the most likely diagnosis.

### Case history 6

A 9-year-old boy presents with a history of recurrent croup, epilepsy, alopecia and mental retardation. His corrected plasma calcium level was 1.3 mmol/L (normal 2.25–2.6 mmol/L), phosphate 2.4 mmol/L (normal 1.4–1.8 mmol/L) and magnesium 0.5 mmol/L (normal 0.8–1.4 mmol/L).

Name one further diagnostic investigation and the most likely diagnosis.

## Short notes

Write short notes on the following:

1. The management of short stature.
2. The immediate management of diabetic ketoacidosis in a comatose 10-year-old child.
3. The symptoms and signs of hypothyroidism in a 3-year-old girl.

## OSCE questions

### OSCE 1
1. Describe the appearance shown in Figure 78.
2. What is essential to complete the relevant clinical examination?
3. Name ONE diagnosis that may present in this way.

a

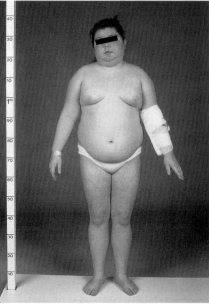

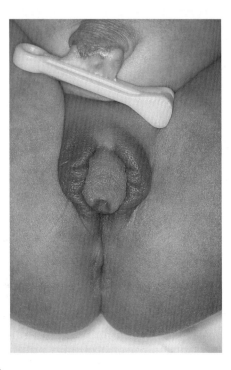

**Fig. 78**

b

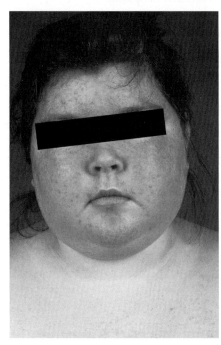

### OSCE 2
Figure 79a and b shows a 14-year-old girl.
1. List TWO abnormalities that appear on the photographs.
2. What is the diagnosis?
3. List THREE other abnormalities associated with this condition.

**Fig. 79**

# Data questions

**Question 1:** A 10-year-old boy was the shortest in his class and suffered with constipation over the past few years. He was obese, with a daytime pulse of 65 bpm. Treatment was started at the age of 10 years (Fig. 80).

1. On which centile does the height measurement lie at 10 years of age (point B)?
2. Describe the growth pattern between points A and B (i.e. between 7 and 10 years of age).
3. What is the most likely cause for the growth pattern seen between points A and B?
4. What treatment was started at 10 years of age?

**Question 2:** This investigation was taken from a short 11-year-old girl (Fig. 81).

1. What is this investigation?
2. What does it show?
3. List five clinical features associated with this condition.

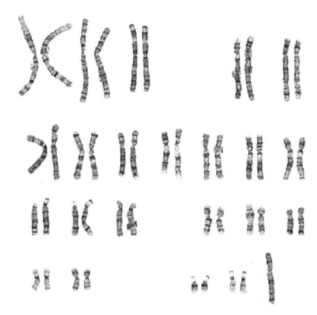

**Fig. 81**

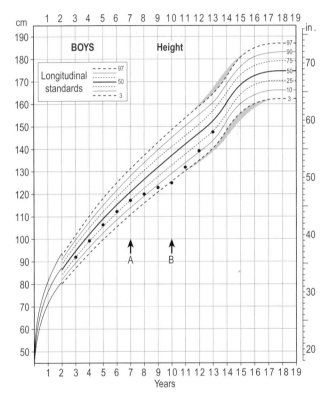

**Fig. 80**

# Self-assessment: answers

## Multiple choice answers

1. a. **True**. This regulates testicular development.
   b. **True**. Vital for the stimulation of the testis.
   c. **False**. They have no role in the development of the male phenotype.
   d. **True**. Testosterone is produced by the testis.
   e. **False**. It has no role in the development of the male phenotype.

2. a. **True**. This will enable assessment of adrenal size/masses, internal genitalia and gonads.
   b. **True**. This is essential.
   c. **True**. In order to diagnose congenital adrenal hyperplasia.
   d. **True**. This assesses functioning testicular tissue, if testes are present.
   e. **False**. Thyroid disease is not associated with ambiguous genitalia.

3. a. **True**. Although these children have a late growth spurt.
   b. **False**. This causes tall stature.
   c. **True**. Excess steroids result in impaired growth, the height often falling below the third percentile.
   d. **True**. Poor skeletal maturation and stunting.
   e. **False**. This is linked with tall stature.

4. a. **True**. Atretic ovaries occur, with failure of sexual maturation.
   b. **True**. This is a typical feature of Turner syndrome.
   c. **False**. This is a feature of obesity and Cushing syndrome.
   d. **True**. Abnormalities include horseshoe kidneys.
   e. **False**. This is a feature of Marfan syndrome or homocystinuria.

5. a. **True**. It is followed by pubic hair, female habitus and finally menses.
   b. **False**. Puberty in the male is heralded by testicular enlargement.
   c. **False**. It also requires sex steroids.
   d. **False**. This is a late event in girls.
   e. **True**. This is the driving force behind pubertal development.

6. a. **True**. Undernutrition results in generalised growth and pubertal delay, including amenorrhoea.
   b. **True**. This results in inhibition of pituitary gonadotrophins.
   c. **True**. Metabolic derangement will impair normal developmental processes.
   d. **False**. This usually leads to precocious puberty.
   e. **False**. It is usually associated with normal pubertal timing.

7. a. **True**. As with most hereditary enzyme deficiencies.
   b. **True**. This is a characteristic feature.
   c. **False**. Screening is based on a raised TSH level.
   d. **False**. It is caused by thyroid agenesis or dyshormonogenesis.
   e. **True**. Congenital hypothyroidism secondary to pituitary failure is associated with a low TSH, which may be missed on many screening programmes that are initially designed to identify *high* TSH levels (and only then go on to check the free thyroxine levels).

8. a. **True**. Aggressive, unruly behaviour and poor concentration with poor school performance can be the presenting picture.
   b. **False**. This is a feature of hypothyroidism.
   c. **False**. Exophthalmos is a feature of Graves' disease but is not *invariably* associated with thyrotoxicosis.
   d. **True**. This is an unusual association.
   e. **True**. Suppression of the hypothalamopituitary axis by excess circulating thyroxine occurs.

9. a. **True**. Collapse with hypotension is typical of Addison's disease.
   b. **False**. These are a feature of hypertension and are therefore seen in Cushing syndrome.
   c. **False**. Virilisation is caused by excessive adrenal androgen secretion.
   d. **True**. In the absence of mineralocorticoids there is a subsequent loss of sodium in the urine.
   e. **True**. This is a consequence of lack of cortisol and excess corticotrophin.

10. a. **False**. Plasma renin activity is of little use in diagnosing Cushing syndrome.

b. **True**. Flattening or loss of the diurnal rhythm in cortisol is a major indicator toward the diagnosis of Cushing syndrome.

c. **False**. The synacthen test is diagnostic in Addison's disease.

d. **True**. This would be elevated in Cushing syndrome.

e. **True**. This test is useful to determine whether the excess corticosteroid secretion can be suppressed (i.e. cases that are ACTH dependent) or not (e.g. ACTH-independent steroid secretion by tumours).

11. a. **True**. It may prevent or delay walking in severely affected patients.
    b. **True**. Pain usually occurs in the long bones.
    c. **False**. Ectopic calcification is a feature of pseudohypoparathyroidism.
    d. **True**. The distal limb is bowed inward below the knee.
    e. **True**. Softening of the skull is a feature seen in young infants.

12. a. **True**. This is part of Williams syndrome.
    b. **True**. Williams syndrome.
    c. **True**. Williams syndrome.
    d. **False**.
    e. **False**.

13. a. **False**. High-dose phosphate is toxic and contraindicated.
    b. **True**. This will help to enhance urinary clearance.
    c. **False**. EDTA is toxic and contraindicated.
    d. **True**. Calcitonin lowers serum calcium levels.
    e. **True**. Steroids also lower serum calcium.

14. a. **True**. Convulsions are caused by dehydration and electrolyte disturbance.
    b. **True**. Imaging is necessary to exclude hypothalamopituitary tumours.
    c. **False**. This test can be very dangerous and is not essential for diagnosis; paired plasma:urine osmolalities may be sufficient.
    d. **False**. This can lead to devastating consequences and death in cranial DI.
    e. **True**. Together with multiple bony osteolytic lesions.

15. a. **True**. This is the usual mode of inheritance.
    b. **False**. This causes cranial DI.
    c. **True**. This is a rare renal complication of poisoning with toxic heavy metals.
    d. **True**.
    e. **False**. This causes cranial DI.

# Case history answers

## Case history 1

The diagnosis in this child is that of complete androgen insensitivity. The bilateral inguinal swellings contain testes. Management is as follows.

**History**. Family history of infertility in phenotypic female members. The condition is X-linked recessive.

**Investigations**. hCG test to assess gonadal function and exclude Leydig cell hypoplasia, in which there is no response to hCG.

**Treatment**. Sex of rearing should be female, and the gonads removed because of the risk of malignant change in the late teenage years.

## Case history 2

In a tall, prepubertal child with a rapid growth rate the differential diagnosis lies between pituitary gigantism and thyrotoxicosis. A GH profile may reveal high basal GH and increased secretion after provocation. The normal secretory pattern of GH peaks and troughs (when GH secretion may be undetectable) is absent. An MRI scan may show a pituitary adenoma. In thyrotoxicosis there are high free $T_4$ and $T_3$ levels, with undetectable TSH and a flat TSH response to TRH.

## Case history 3

Precocious puberty in boys is never idiopathic. In this instance, the presence of papilloedema suggests an underlying brain tumour. The investigations indicated are an LHRH test, which will show an elevation of LH and FSH in response to LHRH, and a CT or MRI scan of the brain.

## Case history 4

Early breast development in a child with short stature, a delayed bone age and a poor height velocity is caused by primary hypothyroidism. All other causes of breast development are associated with a normal or rapid growth rate. The breast development is caused by elevated FSH concentrations, which are increased probably because of an excessive TRH drive.

## Case history 5

Virilisation with tall stature and an advanced bone age in a girl is suggestive of excessive secretion of adrenal androgens as a result of congenital adrenal hyperplasia or a virilising adrenal tumour. The diagnostic investigations include a plasma 17-

hydroxyprogesterone level, a urinary steroid profile and a CT/MRI scan of the adrenal glands.

## Case history 6

The hypocalcaemia, hypomagnesaemia and hyperphosphataemia are indicative of hypoparathyroidism; a serum parathyroid hormone level is therefore the diagnostic investigation of choice.

## Short notes answers

1. The management can be divided into several areas:

   **History**. The following should be assessed: symptoms of raised intracranial pressure, systemic illness, birthweight, feeding difficulties in infancy, family history of short stature, thyroid disease.

   **Examination**. Important points are dysmorphic features, features of Russell–Silver syndrome, signs of systemic illness, wasting, abdominal distension, raised intracranial pressure, hypothyroidism or Cushing syndrome.

   **Auxology**. Compare the child's height with target mid-parental centile; calculate height velocity.

   **Investigations**. Exclude systemic illness, investigate for endocrine causes of short stature, e.g. insulin tolerance test, insulin-like growth factor-1 (IGF-1), IGF-1-binding protein 3.

   **Treatment**. Treat according to diagnosis.

2. Management includes:

   **History**. Take details of weight loss, anorexia, polyuria, polydipsia, fatigue, family history of insulin-dependent diabetes mellitus and other autoimmune conditions.

   **Examination**. Look for dehydration, Kussmaul respiration, altered level of consciousness, ketone odour on breath, signs of precipitating infection.

   **Investigations**. Measure blood glucose, analyse urine for glycosuria and ketonuria, measure arterial blood gas, urea and electrolytes, glycosylated haemoglobin, take blood cultures, and cultures of midstream urine (MSU).

   **Treatment**. Rehydrate slowly over 48 hours, using normal saline initially and sliding scale insulin infusion to reduce the blood glucose slowly. Substitute fluid with dextrose/saline when blood glucose is <15 mmol/L; replace potassium. Carefully monitor electrolytes, pH and blood glucose at regular intervals over the first 24 hours; use antibiotics if sepsis suspected.

3. Symptoms:   tiredness
               constipation
               feel cold
               slowing down at school/daily
                 activities
               weight gain
               neck swelling/goitre.

   Signs:      cold peripheries
               waxy complexion
               thin hair
               obesity
               bradycardia
               slow/slow recovery reflexes
               constipation
               goitre
               hoarse/gruff voice
               pretibial myxoedema.

## OSCE answers

### OSCE 1
1. Ambiguous genitalia or clitoromegaly + bifid scrotum + hypospadias
2. Feel for gonad; check BP; feel abdomen for mass, check salt/sodium output in urine
3. Congenital adrenal hyperplasia; hermaphrodite; pseudohermaphrodite

*Other reasonable but less precise answers:*

1. Hypospadias, clitoromegaly, bifid scrotum alone
2. Other congenital anomalies

### OSCE 2
1. Cushingoid facies (moon face); facial plethora; acne; hirsutism; enhanced interscapular fat pad (buffalo hump), central obesity
2. Cushing syndrome
3. Pituitary adenoma/Cushing's disease; adrenal adenoma; exogenous steroids

## Data answers

### Question 1:
1. *Third centile*
2. *Height or growth deceleration*
3. *Hypothyroidism (acquired)*
4. *Thyroxine replacement*

### Question 2:
1. Karyotype
2. 45 XO or Turner syndrome
3. Webbed neck, wide carrying angle, shield chest, underdeveloped breasts, streak ovaries, amenorrhoea, coarctation of the aorta, abnormal dermatoglyphics, cervical and lower limb oedema in the neonatal period, hypoplastic nails.

*No score for short stature (information provided)*

# 9 Hereditary and metabolic diseases

**9.1** Introduction     189

**9.2** Mendelian patterns of inheritance     190

**9.3** Chromosomal disorders     192

**9.4** Inborn errors of metabolism     194

**9.5** Immunodeficiency disorders     198

**9.6** Diagnosis of genetic disorders and counselling     199

Self-assessment: questions     201

Self-assessment: answers     203

## Overview

The sequencing of the human genome has led to rapid advances in our understanding of the genetic basis of human disease. The underlying genetic causes for many syndromes are now being established, and an in-depth analysis of the genes involved is providing an explanation for the diverse features and presentation of disease. This chapter reviews the basis of inheritance of disease and the approach to diagnosis, including molecular techniques and laboratory tools that have been developed to diagnose genetic disorders. You will need to recognise the clinical features of the common chromosomal disorders and know how to examine for dysmorphic features. You will also need to understand the basis of inheritance and the principles of genetic counselling. Finally, a brief overview of the more common inherited metabolic and immunodeficiency disorders of childhood is presented.

## 9.1 Introduction

### Learning objective

You should:

* understand how malformations occur

## Molecular basis of genetic disorders

Each human cell contains two copies of the entire human genetic programme or *genome*. This is packaged into 46 chromosomes (23 pairs), amounting to approximately 3 billion base pairs (bp) of DNA. *Genes*, the functional units of the DNA, comprise approximately 10% of the human genome, and there are approximately 30 000 of them encoded for by human DNA. Their size varies from several hundred to more than 2 million base pairs. In any one cell, subsets of these genes are actually active and genes will be expressed at varying levels from cell to cell. Genes *transcribe* messenger RNA (mRNA). To do this, the double-stranded DNA separates and a complementary strand is synthesised. The cellular machinery takes out (splices out) the non-coding sequences or *introns*, and the sequences that are retained represent the coding sequences or *exons*. The mRNA is transported to the ribosomal cytoplasm, where it is *translated* into protein. Proteins can then be further modified. Some functional proteins are the products of more than one gene, and these genes do not necessarily lie on the same chromosome. For example, the various components of the human heavy-chain immunoglobulin protein are all located on the long arm of chromosome 14. However, haemoglobin is composed of α chains coded for by genes on chromosome 16 and β chains coded for by a gene on chromosome 11. Whereas the majority of genes are present in the nucleus, the mitochondrion has its own genome and genes. Peculiarly, the sperm does not carry mitochondria into the oocyte, and so all mitochondrial DNA is of maternal origin.

## Genetic variation

### Mutations

Human genetics deals with variations between humans. A change in the linear sequence of bases along the DNA is a *mutation*. Mutations can affect the functioning of a gene or may have no apparent impact on the organism. The latter are called *polymorphisms*, and will include changes in the intronic sequences. The effect of mutation varies with the number of base pairs affected and with the role of the genes involved.

**Mutations in the coding sequence.** These may result in a change in a single amino acid (*missense mutation*) or may truncate a protein (*nonsense mutation*). They may also destroy stop or start codons. Small deletions (or insertions) can cause a *frameshift* affecting all subsequent translation.

**Mutations in introns**. These may destroy or create splicing sites.

**Mutations in other areas**. Mutations in promoter sites can prevent or alter transcription rates; mutations within mRNA untranslated end regions can destroy ribosome recognition sites and alter mRNA stability.

## Gross changes

A number of larger changes to the genetic material can also have functional consequences.

**Chromosome segregation**. Whole chromosome mis-segregation at meiosis can lead to monosomy or trisomy and cause a range of conditions.

**Translocations**. Gross rearrangements can alter the 'dosage' of genes, or may result in loss of gene function or control of gene expression.

**Deletions**. Small deletions of all or part of a gene may destroy its function, leading to a 50% reduction in gene dose (a carrier state if 50% is adequate).

**Repeats**. Tandemly repeated nucleotide triplets are found normally in non-coding sequences, but are capable of increasing in number to form unstable repeats.

### Malformation syndromes

The majority of single congenital malformations have multifactorial inheritance and a relatively low rate of recurrence. The clinical approach to diagnosis and study of malformations and birth defects is known as *dysmorphology*. Not all *dysmorphic* syndromes are inherited.

A **syndrome** is a recognised pattern of clinical abnormalities that have a single cause, e.g Down syndrome.

A **deformation** is an alteration in the shape or structure of a part that has differentiated normally. This is often the result of an abnormal physical condition in utero. An example of this occurs with oligohydramnios. The fetus is squeezed and unable to turn; as a result, a breech presentation with deformation of the feet (talipes) may occur.

The term **disruption** is used for the destruction of a part that has previously developed normally. This may result from either physical severance (e.g. amputation of a digit by an amniotic band) or the interruption of the blood supply to a developing organ (e.g. gastroschisis, porencephaly).

By comparison, a **malformation** is a primary structural defect arising from a localised error in morphogenesis. Single malformations such as pyloric stenosis and cardiac septal defects tend to be multifactorial in origin.

**Multiple malformations** can occur as part of a syndrome, where the same malformations are seen consistently, and may be caused by a single gene change, chromosomal defects or teratogenesis.

The term **association** is used for non-specific malformations involving groups of organs. An example is the VATER association, where non-specific vertebral malformations are found to coexist with anal atresia, tracheo-oesophageal fistula and non-specific radial defects.

These conditions must be distinguished from a **sequence**, which refers to a series of events occurring after one initiating defect. In the Pierre–Robin sequence there is hypoplasia of the mandible. As a result the tongue is pushed posteriorly and interferes with the development of the soft palate. Consequently the child has micrognathia, cleft of the soft palate and glossoptosis.

## 9.2 Mendelian patterns of inheritance

### Learning objective

You should:

• know the different patterns of inheritance

## Autosomal dominant inheritance

An affected individual carries the abnormal gene on one pair of autosomes (chromosomes 1–22). The heterozygote, carrying one copy of the abnormal gene, manifests the condition, i.e. a single copy of the mutant gene is sufficient for expression of the disease phenotype. The affected person passes to each offspring either the normal or the abnormal allele. Each offspring has a 1 : 2 (50%) chance of inheriting the abnormal gene (Fig. 82). A family history is therefore highly predictive of these disorders. Occasionally an autosomal dominant condition may occur as the result of a new mutation, in which case there will be a negative family history. The gene may also be variably expressed (*incomplete penetrance*). For example, in a family with tuberous sclerosis the parent may only have skin abnormalities whereas the child, in addition, has neurological defects. Sometimes the effect of inheriting the abnormal gene (genotype) is not expressed in the phenotype, and this is referred to as *non-penetrance*. An example of this is otosclerosis, where only 40% of the gene carriers become deaf. Other examples of autosomal dominant conditions include achondroplasia, Marfan syndrome and neurofibromatosis.

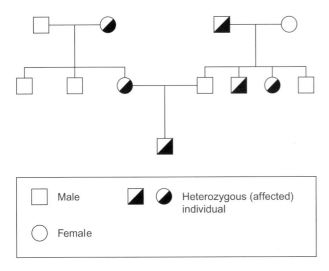

Fig. 82 Example of autosomal dominant inheritance.

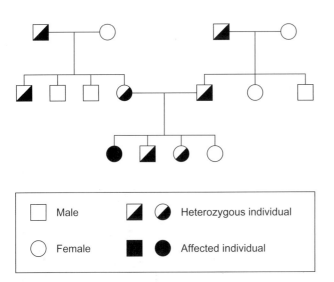

Fig. 83 Example of autosomal recessive inheritance.

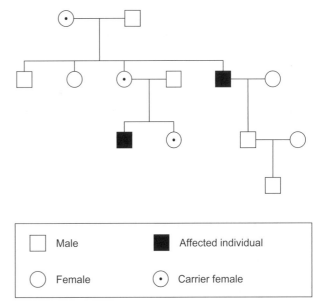

Fig. 84 Example of X-linked recessive inheritance.

## Autosomal recessive inheritance

Numerous disorders result from autosomal recessive inheritance, including cystic fibrosis, congenital adrenal hyperplasia, phenylketonuria and galactosaemia. Unlike autosomal dominant inheritance, the heterozygous (single abnormal allele) individual is healthy. The affected individual is one who is homozygous (both alleles are abnormal). In most instances, both parents are heterozygotes or carriers (though one or both may also be homozygous). The risk of each child of two carrier parents being affected is 25% (Fig. 83). Although the abnormal gene may be transmitted from one generation to the next, there is usually no positive history outside the sibship. This is because other members of the family will usually have non-carrier partners. In communities where *consanguinity* (marrying one's close relative) is practised there is an increased incidence of autosomally recessive diseases, and here the family history may be positive. Mostly, autosomal dominant conditions involve non-lethal structural defects, whereas autosomal recessive conditions often involve metabolic disorders resulting from enzyme deficiencies, and are more often life threatening. Where a number of different mutant alleles exist, individuals can be heterozygotes and express intermediate levels of enzyme activity, such as in β-thalassaemia.

**Co-dominance** is when both alleles are expressed in a heterozygote. For example, an individual who has inherited both A and B blood groups is blood group AB.

## Sex-linked inheritance

X-linked disorders are usually inherited in a recessive fashion. The abnormal gene is carried on the X chromosome. In the carrier female, the normal allele on her other X chromosome 'protects' her from disease. In the male, however, the abnormal allele on his X chromosome is not balanced by a normal allele and he manifests the disease. Daughters of affected males will be carriers, but sons will not be affected (Fig. 84). The family history is often negative, as many cases are a result of new mutations. Examples of X-linked recessive disorders include colour blindness, Duchenne and Becker muscular dystrophies, glucose 6-phosphate dehydrogenase deficiency, haemophilia A and B, and Hunter syndrome.

## X-linked dominant disorders

X-linked dominant inherited disorders such as vitamin D-resistant rickets are rare. No serious genetic defects, apart from some rare intersex conditions and a gene for azoospermia, are linked with the Y chromosome. After all, half the population lives very happily without a Y chromosome!

# Mitochondrial or cytoplasmic inheritance

There are rare metabolic disorders, such as the mitochondrial myopathies and Leber optic neuropathy, that are inherited as part of the mitochondrial DNA. Inheritance is not strictly mendelian: although the defect can only be maternal in origin, it is not related to the X chromosome.

## Trinucleotide repeats

A newly recognised class of unstable mutation is caused by expansion of trinucleotide repeat sequences inherited in a mendelian fashion. These include Fragile X, myotonic dystrophy, Huntington's disease, Friedreich's ataxia and spinocerebellar ataxia.

# Imprinting

Normally one allele each is inherited from either parent, and usually only one gene is active in a random fashion. In some cases genes only express the copy derived from a parent of a given sex, and this process is called imprinting. In some cases this is because both chromosomes of a pair are inherited from one parent (*uniparental disomy*). The classic examples of this are the Prader–Willi (learning difficulties, hypotonia, obesity) and Angelman (severe learning difficulties, ataxia, characteristic facies, epilepsy) syndromes, which are associated with deletion and uniparental disomy of chromosome 15. In Prader–Willi syndrome it is the paternally derived and in Angelman the maternally derived genetic information on chromosome 15 that is missing.

# Multifactorial inheritance

Multifactorial inheritance is a pattern of inheritance observed in several relatively common conditions that appear to result from the interactions of a genetic predisposition with environmental factors. The conditions vary from those seen in childhood, such as cleft lip/palate, congenital dislocation of the hip, neural tube defects, congenital heart disease and pyloric stenosis, to those seen in later life, such as asthma, depression, diabetes mellitus, hypertension and epilepsy. The concept of multifactorial inheritance is not entirely satisfactorily understood, but a few characteristic features are present.

- There is a similar rate of recurrence in first-degree relatives, and the risk declines sharply as the relationship with the affected person becomes more distant. For example, the risk of a neural tube defect in first-degree relatives is 4–5%; it is 1–2% in second-degree relatives, and in third-degree relatives is similar to that of the general population.
- The risk of recurrence is related to the incidence of the disease.
- The risk is higher if more than one first-degree relative has the defect. For example, if parents have two children with a neural tube defect the risk that the third child will be affected rises to 10–12%.
- The risk of recurrence may be greater when the disorder is more severe. An infant with long segment Hirschsprung disease has a greater chance of having an affected sibling than the infant who has short segment Hirschsprung disease.
- Some disorders have sexual predilection: pyloric stenosis is more common in males, whereas congenital dislocation of the hip is more common in females.
- The frequency of concordance in identical twins is 21–63%.

# 9.3 Chromosomal disorders

## Learning objectives

You should:

- know the clinical features of Down syndrome
- know the clinical features of Turner syndrome

Chromosomal abnormalities are either numerical or structural, occur in 0.4% of live births, and are an important cause of mental defects and congenital anomalies.

## Down syndrome (trisomy 21)

Down syndrome is the most common autosomal trisomy and the commonest genetic cause of severe learning difficulties. The incidence is 1 in 650 liveborn infants. Figure 85 shows the typical facies and Table 50 lists the characteristic clinical manifestations of children with Down syndrome. As shown in Table 51, the risk of Down syndrome is related to maternal age. In those at risk, either because of age or a previous child with Down syndrome, blood tests during pregnancy can be

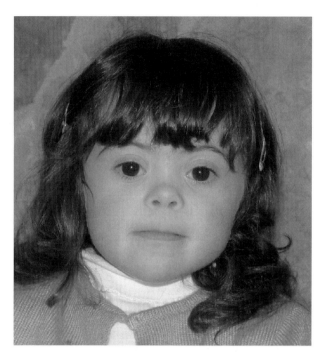

**Fig. 85** Child with epicanthic folds, slant to eyes, downturned mouth and other features of Down syndrome.

**Table 50** Clinical features of Down syndrome

| | Features |
|---|---|
| Head | Brachycephaly, low set hairline, flattened occiput |
| Face | Round face, epicanthic folds, Brushfield spots in the iris, protruding tongue, small low-set ears |
| Limbs | Single palmar (simian) crease, fifth finger clinodactyly, short stubby digits, abnormal dermatoglyphics, wide gap between first and second toes |
| Other | Generalised hypotonia, small stature, congenital heart defect (atrioventricular valve defects), anal and duodenal atresia |
| Later problems | Severe learning difficulties (IQ usually around 50), growth failure, recurrent respiratory infections, auditory and visual handicaps, hypothyroidism, Alzheimer disease, increased risk of leukaemia |

**Table 51** The risk of Down syndrome and maternal age

| Maternal age (years) | Risk of Down syndrome |
|---|---|
| All ages | 1 : 650 |
| 30 | 1 : 900 |
| 35 | 1 : 380 |
| 37 | 1 : 240 |
| 40 | 1 : 110 |
| 44 | 1 : 37 |

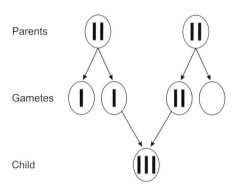

Chromosome 21

Parents

Gametes

Child

**Fig. 86** Non-disjunction in Down syndrome.

indicative of a Down fetus. In pregnancies where the fetus has Down syndrome, maternal serum levels of pregnancy-associated plasmaprotein-A, α-fetoprotein and unconjugated oestriol tend to be low, and inhibin and free β-hCG levels tend to be raised. Fetal ultrasound scanning in the first trimester can indicate an increased risk of DS where features suggestive (but not diagnostic) of DS are identified. The best-established of these features is a thickened nuchal fold at the back of the neck, referred to as *nuchal translucency* (NT). The definitive test is karyotyping of fetal tissue obtained from either chorionic villus biopsy or amniocentesis.

The commonest mechanism (~94%) by which an extra chromosome 21 is acquired is by *non-disjunction*. This results from an error at meiosis, when one pair of chromosome 21 fails to separate, so that one gamete has two chromosomes 21 and one has none (Fig. 86). In 80% of children, the extra 21 chromosome is maternal in origin. If females with trisomy 21 conceive, there is a 50% chance that they will have a baby with trisomy 21. Males with Down syndrome are generally infertile.

In about 5% of individuals there is a translocation involving chromosome 21 (Fig. 87). Half of the translocations arise de novo and half are inherited from a carrier parent. The majority of translocations are examples of fusion at the centromeres (robertsonian) of chromosomes 13, 14 and 15 with 21. As shown in Figure 87, parents who are carriers produce three types of live offspring, a normal phenotype and karyotype, a phenotypically normal translocation carrier, and a translocation trisomy 21. In practice, however, the risk of Down syndrome is 2–5% for a carrier male and 10–15% for a carrier female. Rarely, the parent carries a balanced 21q21q robertsonian translocation, and the risk of Down syndrome in the liveborn offspring is then 100%. About 1% of Down syndrome babies have *mosaicism*. This is the result of non-disjunction after the zygote has been formed, and occurs during mitosis.

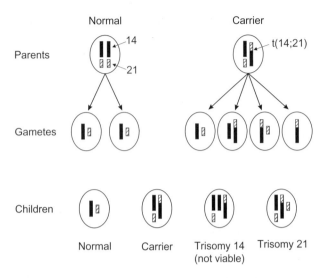

**Fig. 87** Down syndrome with an inherited t(14;21) translocation.

Variable proportions of cells in the body are of the normal karyotype, whereas others have trisomy 21. The phenotype is therefore often milder in mosaic Down syndrome.

## Other trisomies

### Trisomy 18

Trisomy 18 (Edward syndrome) affects approximately 1 in 3000 neonates. Intrauterine growth retardation is a common feature and 90% of the babies have congenital heart disease. Most die within the first year of life. The clinical features include mental retardation, prominent occiput, low-set dysplastic ears, small mouth and jaw, clenched hands with second and fifth fingers overlapping the third and fourth fingers, and rocker-bottom feet.

### Trisomy 13

Trisomy 13 (Patau syndrome) is rare and is characterised by a structural defect of the brain (holoprosencephaly), polydactyly, scalp defects, microphthalmia, and cardiac and renal anomalies. Survival beyond a few weeks is unusual.

### Klinefelter syndrome

Klinefelter syndrome occurs in approximately 1 : 1000 liveborn males. These children have a 47XXY karyotype and are usually phenotypically normal, though they may have mildly impaired verbal IQ. Adults are taller than average, with long limbs; 30% have gynaecomastia, and all are infertile.

---

**Box 56** Features of Turner syndrome

Short stature (100%)
Facial features
  Low-set hairline
  Micrognathia
  Prominent ears
  Epicanthal folds
  Ptosis
  High arched palate
Increased carrying angle
Multiple pigmented naevi
Dysplastic nails
Osteoporosis
Deafness
Widely spaced nipples (shield-shaped chest)
Congenital heart defects
  Bicuspid aortic valves (30%)
  Coarctation of the aorta (20%)
Renal anomalies (horseshoe kidney)
Primary amenorrhoea and infertility
Autoimmune diseases

## Turner syndrome

The incidence of Turner syndrome is 1 : 5000 of liveborn females, but it can be detected in 3–5% of abortus material, as most cases result in miscarriage. The affected individuals have a delayed maturation of the lymphatic system, which manifests as a cystic hygroma and puffy hands and feet in the neonate, and later on with residual neck webbing. The other common clinical features are shown in Box 56. Presentation in adult life is with primary amenorrhoea and infertility resulting from ovarian dysgenesis, although 20% will start puberty spontaneously. In 50% there is only one sex chromosome (45XO), which is maternal in origin. In the others there is either deletion of the short arm of one X chromosome or an isochromosome with two long arms and no short arm. Intellectual development is normal and the children benefit from growth hormone therapy during childhood, with oestrogen replacement therapy at puberty. Boys and girls with *Noonan syndrome* display the Turner phenotype, but the disorder is autosomally dominantly inherited and the classic cardiac malformation is that of peripheral pulmonary artery stenosis.

## 9.4 Inborn errors of metabolism

### Learning objective

You should:

* know the features and management of children with phenylketonuria and galactosaemia

## Disorders of amino acid metabolism

### Phenylketonuria (PKU)

This rare disorder is caused by deficiency of the enzyme phenylalanine hydroxylase (leading to classic PKU) or of the biopterin cofactor for this enzyme (resulting in atypical PKU, which is more difficult to manage). Untreated, it presents with infantile spasms and developmental delay in late infancy. There is a characteristic musty odour and many of the children are fair haired and blue eyed, with eczematous skin. Raised phenylalanine is detected once milk feeding has been established for 5–7 days, and in the UK most children are detected in the neonatal stage by the national screening programme. The latter entails blood spot collection on blotting paper (Guthrie cards) on day 5, which are then analysed for phenylalanine level, phenylalanine to tyrosine ratio and other screenable conditions, such as congenital hypothyroidism, galactosaemia, congenital adrenal hyperplasia etc. Treatment involves the restriction of dietary phenylalanine while ensuring that there is sufficient protein for optimal physical and neurological growth. The plasma phenylalanine level needs to be monitored regularly. The majority (75%) of patients on this regimen will be able to attend normal school, though there is a higher incidence of behavioural and learning difficulties. Dietary restrictions should be maintained lifelong, though this is often difficult to achieve in practice. Maternal PKU is devastating to the fetus (microcephaly, severe handicap) unless dietary restrictions have been strictly followed prior to conception. Other disorders of amino acid metabolism are listed in Table 52.

### The organic acidaemias

The organic acidaemias disrupt the catabolic pathways of several essential amino acids (the branched-chain amino acids leucine, isoleucine and valine, and the odd-chain amino acids, e.g. threonine) resulting in *maple syrup urine disease* (MSUD), *methylmalonic* and *propionic acidaemia* among others. MSUD most often presents in the neonatal period, with severe metabolic acidosis, hypoglycaemia and seizures. There is increased excretion of the branched-chain amino acids. The urine has a characteristic maple syrup odour. A delay in diagnosis leads to learning difficulties and neurological dysfunction, and there remains a high risk of death during any acute illness. The management of organic acidaemias centres on the restriction of dietary protein. During acute decompensation, catabolism is limited by a high-carbohydrate low-protein intake. Acidosis is corrected and the hyperammonaemia is treated by adequate hydration, avoidance of hypoglycaemia, vitamin cofactor infusions and, if necessary, peritoneal dialysis or haemoperfusion. The outcome is often guarded, with the likelihood of hypotonia and neurodevelopmental delay even in those who have not suffered crises with severe acidosis and/or hyperammonaemic encephalopathy.

### Urea cycle defects

Enzyme defects have been identified for all stages of the urea cycle. They tend to cause neonatal encephalopathy owing to high blood ammonia levels, but the onset can be delayed; if so, the child presents with coma and infection.

## Liver enzyme deficiencies

### Galactosaemia

Galactosaemia results from a deficiency in the enzyme galactose 1-phosphate uridyl transferase. The infant is unable to convert galactose to glucose and will therefore become hypoglycaemic while on a pure milk diet. The affected neonate feeds poorly, vomits, and develops jaundice and hepatomegaly and, ultimately, liver cell failure. Management is with a galactose-free diet. Untreated patients will develop chronic liver disease and cataracts.

**Table 52** Disorders of amino acid metabolism

| Disorder | Enzyme deficiency | Characteristics |
|---|---|---|
| Phenylketonuria | Phenylalanine hydroxylase and others | Infantile spasms, developmental delay, microcephaly, severe mental deficiency, convulsions |
| Tyrosinaemia | Fumarylacetoacetate hydrolase | Failure to thrive and acute hepatic failure in infancy, cirrhosis, renal tubular dysfunction, neuropathy in childhood |
| Homocystinuria | Cystathionine synthetase | Failure to thrive, developmental delay, marfanoid features, ectopia lentis, thromboembolic episodes |
| Albinism | Defects in the production and distribution of melanin | Oculocutaneous albinism, Chédiak–Higashi syndrome (neutrophil dysfunction), Hermansky–Pudlak (platelet dysfunction), piebaldism |

**Table 53** Glycogen storage disorders

| Type | Enzyme deficiency | Symptoms |
|------|-------------------|----------|
| I Von Gierke | Glucose 6-phosphatase | Growth failure, asymptomatic hypoglycaemia and enlarged kidneys; the prognosis is good and most children can be managed with dietary regimens such as frequent night-time feeding |
| II (Pompe disease) | Lysosomal enzyme | Lysosomal enzyme deficiency; excess glycogen is deposited in both liver and muscle, especially in cardiac muscle; most patients present in early infancy with marked hypotonia, poor feeding, severe cardiomegaly and congestive cardiac failure; the prognosis is poor |
| III | Debranching enzyme | Milder form of type I |
| V | Muscle phosphorylase | Muscle cramps |
| VI | Liver phosphorylase | Milder form of type I |
| VII | Phosphofructokinase | Muscle cramps |
| XI | | Rickets and renal tubular problems |

## Glycogen storage disorders

The glycogen storage diseases are mostly recessively inherited disorders that have specific enzyme defects which prevent the mobilisation of glucose to glycogen. Most enzymes are liver based, although some defects affect other tissues as well, and a few affect only muscle. There are 11 main enzyme defects (types I–XI), which all lead to an abnormal storage of glycogen in different tissues (Table 53).

## Hereditary fructose intolerance

Fructose intolerance arises from deficiency of aldolase B. Again, prompt recognition and action can be life saving. Ingestion of fructose results in the toxic accumulation of fructose 1-phosphate in the liver and other tissues. Once fructose-containing foods are started, the child presents with abdominal pain, nausea, vomiting, and symptoms of hypoglycaemia. In the long term, hepatomegaly, growth reduction and liver failure occur. Therapy involves eliminating all fructose-containing items from the diet.

## Defects in the conjugation of bilirubin

Hepatic glucuronyl transferase activity is deficient in the *Crigler–Najjar syndrome* and produces congenital, non-haemolytic non-obstructive unconjugated hyperbilirubinaemia. It is a rare cause of kernicterus. Low levels of unconjugated hyperbilirubinaemia are also seen in the benign *Gilbert syndrome*. Inherited conjugated hyperbilirubinaemia, a mild benign disorder, is seen in the *Dubin–Johnson* and *Rotor* syndromes.

## Deficiency in α₁-antitrypsin

Deficiency of the protease inhibitor (Pi) α₁-antitrypsin is associated with emphysema in adults and liver disease in infancy and childhood. There are more than 25 phenotypes of the Pi, coded for by a gene on chromosome 14. Liver disease is associated with the phenotype PiZZ. It is a cause of neonatal hepatitis and will ultimately progress to cirrhosis and portal hypertension. Replacement therapy using fractionated plasma α₁-antitrypsin and milk from transgenic sheep has been used in adults with emphysema, but its use in children with hepatitis is still experimental. The current therapeutic goal is to transplant the liver as the cirrhosis decompensates. This is also a disease that is a potential target for gene therapy.

## Lipid storage disorders

The lipid storage disorders are rare and have a predominantly fatal neurodegenerative presentation.

**Tay–Sachs disease** is a **gangliosidosis**. The enzyme hexosaminidase D is deficient and there is an increased deposition of GM2 ganglioside in the grey matter. The affected infant presents with developmental regression, an exaggerated startle response and visual inattention. Findings include severe hypotonia, a large head and a cherry-red spot on the macula.

**Gaucher disease** is caused by glucocerebroside deposition in the reticuloendothelial system and has an early-onset neuropathic and a late-onset non-neuropathic presentation. The former presents with feeding problems, stridor and spasticity. There is progressive enlargement of the liver and spleen, and Gaucher cells can be identified in the bone marrow. The late-onset variety presents with hepatosplenomegaly and bone disease.

**Niemann–Pick disease** causes an abnormal storage of sphingomyelin in the reticuloendothelial system. Of the four varieties, two resemble Tay–Sachs disease and are neuropathic, and the others present with a hepatitic picture with hepatosplenomegaly.

## Mucopolysaccharidoses

The mucopolysaccharidoses (MPS) are a group of mostly recessively inherited disorders caused by incomplete degradation and storage of acid mucopolysaccharides (glycosaminoglycans). Mucopolysaccharides are the major components of the intracellular substance of connective tissue. The clinical manifestations result from its accumulation in various organs and are listed in Table 54. There are various characteristic syndromes, but the most severe is *Hurler syndrome*, which is the only X-linked MPS that results from deficiency of α-L-iduronidase. The features of some of them are given in Table 55. Treatment is supportive according to the child's needs. Enzyme replacement by bone marrow transplantation has been performed for Hurler syndrome, which is also a target for gene therapy.

## Lipid metabolism

### Hyperlipidaemia

Hyperlipidaemia is one of the main risk factors for coronary heart disease. Identification and treatment of hyperlipidaemia in childhood may delay the onset of cardiovascular disease in later life. Children should be screened for hyperlipidaemia if there is a family history of coronary heart disease, peripheral vascular disease, cerebrovascular disease, or sudden death before 55 years of age.

### Familial hypercholesterolaemia

Familial hypercholesterolaemia is an autosomal dominant disorder of lipoprotein metabolism resulting from a defect in the low-density lipoprotein (LDL) receptor. About 1 : 500 are heterozygous and affected. The serum LDL cholesterol concentration is markedly raised (>3.3 mmol/L). The condition is associated with premature coronary heart disease, which occurs in 50% of patients by 50 years of age in males and 60 years of age in females. Skin and tendon xanthomata may be present, but are uncommon in childhood. Homozygous disease is very rare and much more severe, causing xanthomata in childhood and clinical cardiovascular disease in the second decade.

### Familial combined hypercholesterolaemia

Familial combined hypercholesterolaemia is an autosomal dominant condition associated with an increased risk of premature coronary heart disease in adult life. Management involves attention to accompanying risk factors, such as obesity, hypertension, diabetes mellitus and smoking.

### Management in lipid disorders

Diet remains the main component of lipid-lowering strategies. Anion-exchange resins such as cholestyramine are effective in lowering LDL cholesterol, but compliance is a problem. Pravastatin and simvastatin, inhibitors of hydroxymethylglutaryl (HMG) CoA reductase (the rate-limiting enzyme in cholesterol synthesis), have been shown to be clinically effective in lowering serum cholesterol levels.

**Table 54** Clinical features of mucopolysaccharidoses

|  | Features |
|---|---|
| Eyes | Corneal clouding, retinal degeneration, glaucoma |
| Skin | Thickened skin, coarse facies |
| Heart | Valvular lesions, cardiac failure |
| CNS | Developmental regression |
| Skeletal | Thickened skull, conductive deafness, broad ribs, claw hand, thoracic kyphosis, lumbar lordosis, carpal tunnel syndrome |
| Other | Umbilical and inguinal hernias, hepatosplenomegaly |

**Table 55** Types of mucopolysaccharidose

| Type | Inheritance | Cornea | Heart | Brain | Skeletal | Visceral |
|---|---|---|---|---|---|---|
| MPS IH (Hurler) | AR | +++ | ++ | +++ | ++ | +++ |
| MPS IS (Scheie) | AR | +++ | ++ | – | – | +/– |
| MPS II (Hunter) | XR | – | + | ++ | + | +++ |
| MPS III (Sanfilippo) | AR | +/– | – | + | + | +/– |
| MPS IV (Morquio) | AR | + | + | – | + | +/– |
| MPS VI (Maroteaux–Lamy) | AR | +++ | ++ | – | ++ | + |
| MPS VII | AR | +/– | – | ++ | ++ | ++ |

AR, autosomal recessive; XR, sex-linked recessive.

## 9.5 Immunodeficiency disorders

### Learning objective

You should:

- know the features in the clinical history that suggest an inherited immunodeficiency

Immunodeficiencies may be primary when there is an intrinsic, often inherited, defect in the immune system or, more commonly, they may be secondary to another phenomenon, such as malnutrition, malignant disease, immunosuppressive therapy, or infections such as HIV. Many of the primary immunodeficiency disorders are inherited in an autosomal recessive or X-linked fashion. There may be a family history of unexplained death, particularly in boys, and parental consanguinity. Children will usually present with a history of recurrent, persistent or unusual infections (Table 56), or with protein-losing enteropathy and failure to thrive. The management involves aggressive treatment of infections, antibiotic prophylaxis (e.g. co-trimoxazole for *Pneumocystis carinii* and penicillin for pneumococcal infections), replacement immunoglobulin for defects in antibody function, replacement of missing factors such as adenosine deaminase, and bone marrow transplantation for severe combined immunodeficiency (SCID). With the discovery that most of these disorders have a genetic defect they have become prime targets for gene therapy.

**Table 56** Immunodeficiency disorders of childhood

| Defect | Disorder | Characteristics |
|---|---|---|
| B cell | X-linked agammaglobulinaemia (Bruton's disease) | X-linked; caused by abnormal Bruton tyrosine kinase on Xq22, which leads to panhypogammaglobulinaemia |
| | | Presents with **bacterial** sinopulmonary infections |
| | Selective IgA deficiency | Autosomal inheritance, gene on 6p21 leads to selective deficiency of IgA |
| | | **Bacterial** infections of the renal, pulmonary and gastrointestinal systems |
| T cell | Thymic hypoplasia (DiGeorge syndrome) | 22q11 deletion, dysmorphogenesis of the third and fourth pharyngeal pouches; aplasia of parathyroids and hypocalcaemia; aortic arch, palatal and mandibular malformations |
| | | Predominantly **fungal**, **viral** and ***Pneumocystis carinii*** infections |
| | Hyper-IgM syndrome | X-linked, owing to abnormal CD40 on Xq26 in defective T cells; leads to defective signaling of B cells |
| | | Boys present with frequent **bacterial** otitis media, tonsillitis and pneumonia |
| B and T cell | Severe combined immunodeficiency (SCID) | Genetically diverse; some are X-linked (Xq13); absent T- and B-cell function from birth |
| | | Pulmonary, gastrointestinal, cutaneous and systemic infections |
| | Nezelof syndrome | Autosomal recessive, combined immunodeficiency |
| | Wiskott–Aldrich syndrome | X-linked |
| | Adenosine deaminase (ADA) deficiency | Adenosine deaminase gene on 22q13 |
| | Ataxia-telangiectasia | Autosomal recessive |
| Complement | Primary | Manifests as recurrent infections of capsulated bacterial organisms such as *Neisseria* and *Pneumococcus* or as autoimmune diseases such as systemic lupus erythematosus or glomerulonephritis |
| | Secondary | Nephrotic syndrome, sickle cell disease, cirrhosis, splenectomy |
| Phagocytic cells | Chronic granulomatous disease (CGD) | X-linked (50–60%): defective expression of the cytochrome *b* 91 kDa subunit (gene on Xp21) |
| | | Autosomal recessive: defective expression of 47 kDa and 67 kDa cytosolic factor |
| | | Chronic recurrent pyogenic infections with unusual organisms and granuloma formation in skin and viscera |

## 9.6 Diagnosis of genetic disorders and counselling

### Chromosomal analysis

Cells can be obtained from blood, bone marrow or fibroblasts and cultured, stimulated to divide, and the subsequent metaphases analysed by Giemsa staining. This G-banding process marks each chromosome with clearly identifiable dark and light bands, allowing the identification of abnormal chromosomes. This technique has been greatly refined by the identification of chromosomal region-specific DNA probes that can be fluorescently labelled. Fluorescent in situ hybridisation (FISH) is able to identify small deletions and can be used on uncultured cells to obtain a rapid diagnosis. It is now possible to obtain whole chromosome 'paints' specific to each individual chromosome. Using spectral division of colour and computer enhancement, complex chromosomal rearrangements, hitherto undetectable by G-banding, are being identified.

### Restriction analysis

**Restriction endonucleases** recognise typical DNA sequences at which they will cut DNA. A change in the nucleic acid sequence can alter the enzyme cutting sites and change the lengths of DNA produced when genomic DNA is digested with a restriction endonuclease. These are called *restriction fragment length polymorphisms* (RFLP) (Fig. 88). The figure shows a stretch of DNA that contains three enzymatic sites in the wild type (A) and the loss of the second enzymatic site in the mutant (B). The squiggle represents a radioactively labelled probe that recognises DNA at the site of the second restriction site. Restriction digestion will result in two similar size fragments in the wild type but only one larger fragment in the mutant. When these are electrophoresed on a gel, the smaller fragments will migrate faster. The separated fragments are then *denatured* (DNA is made single stranded), blotted onto a nylon membrane (*Southern blot*) and *hybridised* with the radioactively labelled probe. On autoradiography, in this instance the wild type is detected as two smaller bands and the mutant as a single larger band. The use of this procedure in clinical practice is illustrated in Figure 89. The mother clearly has one mutant and one normal *allele*

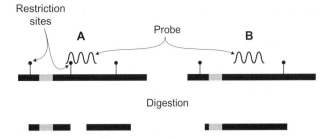

Southern blot, probe and autoradiograph

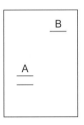

**Fig. 88** Restriction fragment length polymorphism. See text for details.

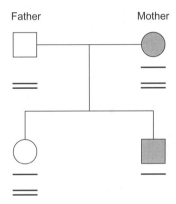

**Fig. 89** Pedigree showing segregation of a sex-linked recessive disorder by restriction analysis.

(gene), whereas the father is normal. In this case, the daughter has inherited the mother's genotype, but the son only has the mother's mutant gene. This is an example of an X-linked recessive disorder such as Duchenne muscular dystrophy or haemophilia A.

Another form of mutation is the expansion of tandemly repeated nucleotide triplets. Figure 90 illustrates the molecular diagnosis of such conditions. In the Fragile X syndrome, a CGG repeat occurs near the 5' end of the gene. The number of repeats ranges from 5 to 50 in the general population, from approximately 50 to 200 in asymptomatic carriers, and exceeds 200 in those with the Fragile X syndrome. To detect the abnormality, DNA is treated with a restriction enzyme that cuts at recognition sites flanking the CGG repeat. Hybridisation on a

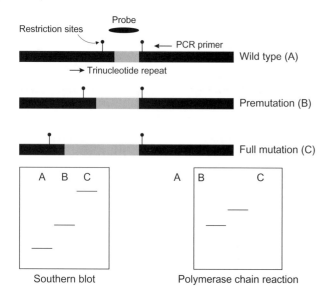

**Fig. 90** Molecular analysis of increased tandem repeats. See text for details.

**Box 57** Features of genetic counselling

*Establish the correct diagnosis*: History, examination and laboratory investigations
*Estimate the risk*: Based on diagnostic tests and pedigree information
*Communication*: Written as well as verbal
*Management and prevention options*: No further action; restrict family size; adoption; artificial insemination; ovum donation; preimplantation diagnosis

Southern blot with labelled DNA from the region of the gene reveals a single band in a normal male subject (wild type; A in Fig. 90). An asymptomatic male carrier will have a band of higher molecular weight (B), and a subject with a full mutation will have a very large, diffuse band because of the instability of the full-mutation allele (C). The normal and asymptomatic carrier alleles can also be detected by the *polymerase chain reaction* (PCR). This is a method that allows a small targeted DNA sequence to be amplified to assist in its analysis. The full-mutation allele cannot be amplified by PCR because it is too large (Fig. 90).

For genes where the mutation is known, direct *sequencing* can be performed for detection, as in cystic fibrosis patients with the δF508 mutation. A different strategy is to look for differences between the known DNA sequence and the patient's DNA, using techniques such as *single-stranded conformation polymorphism* (SSCP) or *high-performance liquid chromatography* (HPLC). These techniques are now all high throughput and semiautomated, allowing rapid and accurate diagnosis. Newer methods such as *single nucleotide polymorphism* (SNP) arrays will allow entire genome searches for individual patients in a matter of days.

## Genetic counselling

In England, each regional health authority has a regional genetic service that combines clinical and laboratory skills. Genetic counselling aims to provide parents with greater autonomy and choice in their reproductive decisions. In Cyprus prenatal screening for β-thalassaemia using *chorionic villus biopsy* or *amniocen-*

*tesis*, and termination of affected fetuses, has almost wiped out the disease within a generation. The administration of steroids to a mother carrying a fetus with congenital adrenal hyperplasia will prevent virilisation in a female fetus. The same principle applies to an increasing number of conditions, such as Duchenne muscular dystrophy, haemolytic anaemias, and inherited malignancies such as retinoblastoma.

Given the huge number of inherited conditions, the rarity of their occurrence and the clinical and molecular heterogeneity, a diagnosis may not always be possible. Counselling is directed at providing the family with information about the prognosis and chance or recurrence. It should be non-directive and compassionate. Counsellors need to be aware of psychological, ethnic, social and educational issues. Follow-up consultations are essential (Box 57).

## Gene therapy

Gene therapy is a technique for correcting defective genes responsible for disease development. There are a number of techniques: a normal gene may be inserted into a non-specific location within the genome to replace a non-functional gene, or the regulation of a particular gene can be altered. An abnormal gene can be swapped for a normal gene through homologous recombination, or repaired. In most gene therapy studies a normal gene is inserted into the genome via a 'vector' to replace a disease-causing gene. Currently, the most common vector is a virus that has been genetically altered to carry normal human DNA. The different viruses used include retroviruses, adenoviruses and herpes simplex viruses. Non-viral options include direct introduction of therapeutic DNA into target cells; the use of liposomes to carry DNA through the target cell's membrane; or chemically linking the DNA to a molecule that will bind to special cell receptors. Currently, gene therapy remains experimental, although there are a number of projects worldwide for treating children with conditions such as severe combined immunodeficiency disorder (SCID) or inborn errors of metabolism.

# Self-assessment: questions

## Multiple choice questions

1. Methods used to look for DNA that has been rearranged include:
   a. In situ hybridisation
   b. Southern blotting
   c. Polymerase chain reaction
   d. Northern blotting
   e. Fingerprinting.

2. With regard to diseases of autosomal recessive inheritance:
   a. A child of two heterozygotes has a 25% chance of being homozygous for the condition
   b. The frequency of the carrier state will be many times higher than those with disease
   c. It is the commonest form of inherited disease
   d. Most homozygotes will have affected children
   e. It is usually the result of a single gene mutation.

3. The following diseases and their mendelian inheritance are correctly matched:
   a. Glucose 6-phosphate dehydrogenase deficiency and X-linked recessive
   b. Cystic fibrosis and autosomal recessive
   c. Hereditary spherocytosis and autosomal dominant
   d. Vitamin D-resistant rickets and X-linked dominant
   e. β-Thalassaemia and autosomal co-dominance.

4. The following describe chromosomal anomalies:
   a. 90% of karyotypically abnormal conceptions do not survive pregnancy
   b. They occur in 50% of cases of primary amenorrhoea
   c. They are associated with 20% of cases with mental retardation
   d. They account for 10% of male sterility
   e. They are seen in approximately 10% of human conceptions.

5. Chromosomal breakage can be seen in children with:
   a. Congenital telangiectatic erythema and dwarfism
   b. Constitutional aplastic anaemia
   c. Louis–Bar syndrome
   d. Xeroderma pigmentosum
   e. Chickenpox.

6. Maternal serum α-fetoprotein may be altered when the fetus has:
   a. Trisomy 21
   b. Anencephaly
   c. Myelomeningocoele
   d. Died
   e. Congenital nephrotic syndrome.

7. Teratogenic drugs include:
   a. Diethylstilboestrol
   b. Thalidomide
   c. Warfarin
   d. Lysergic acid diethylamide
   e. Cocaine.

8. Metabolic acidosis is a feature of:
   a. Phenylketonuria
   b. Maple syrup urine disease
   c. Insulin-dependent diabetes mellitus (IDDM)
   d. Isovaleric acidaemia
   e. Galactosaemia.

9. Hepatosplenomegaly is seen in:
   a. Tay–Sachs disease
   b. Niemann–Pick disease
   c. I-cell disease
   d. Laurence–Moon–Biedl syndrome
   e. Hurler syndrome.

10. Hepatic failure may be seen in the following:
    a. Wilson's disease
    b. Gaucher's disease
    c. Tyrosinaemia
    d. Galactosaemia
    e. Von Gierke disease.

11. Hypoglycaemia can occur in:
    a. Glucose 6-phosphate dehydrogenase deficiency
    b. Galactosaemia
    c. Tyrosinosis
    d. Maple syrup urine disease
    e. Salicylate poisoning.

12. Secondary hyperlipidaemia is often seen in:
    a. Nephrotic syndrome
    b. Von Gierke disease
    c. Diabetes mellitus
    d. Hypothyroidism
    e. Use of oral contraceptives.

13. Cardiomyopathy is seen in:
    a. Pompe disease
    b. Primary carnitine deficiency
    c. Kwashiorkor
    d. Hunter syndrome
    e. Friedreich's ataxia.

14. Mental retardation is a feature of the following mucopolysaccharidoses:
    a. Hunter
    b. Hurler
    c. Scheie
    d. Maroteaux–Lamy
    e. Morquio.

15. An altered colour of fresh urine can be expected in:
    a. Porphyria
    b. Indicanuria
    c. Antituberculous therapy
    d. Alkaptonuria
    e. Congenital biliary atresia.

## Case history

A young Asian couple come to ask you for advice. They have been married for 3 years and have an 18-month-old son who was investigated for anaemia and has just been diagnosed to have β-thalassaemia. They have been planning to have another child but are now worried that the second child might also be affected.

Outline the steps you would take to help them with their dilemma.

## Short notes

Write short notes on the investigations required in a child with a suspected immunodeficiency

# Self-assessment: answers

## Multiple choice answers

1. a. **True**. For example fluorescent in situ hybridisation (FISH) is often used to detect known chromosomal rearrangements.
   b. **True**. The method used to detect a change in or differences between DNA samples.
   c. **True**. This is a highly specific technique that allows even point mutations to be detected.
   d. **False**. A method for RNA analysis.
   e. **True**. This is a restriction fragment length polymorphism (RFLP) technique, and an example of its use is in the establishment of paternity/maternity.

2. a. **True**. As there is a 1 : 4 chance that the offspring will inherit both affected alleles.
   b. **True**. As those who have only one affected allele are phenotypically normal.
   c. **False**. Multifactorial inheritance is the most common.
   d. **False**. Not unless the other partner is heterozygous, but all children will be carriers.
   e. **True**.

3. a. **True**. It is therefore more likely to cause haemolytic anaemia in boys.
   b. **True**. This is the commonest inherited condition in the caucasian population.
   c. **True**. Therefore there is no carrier state!
   d. **True**. It is a rare condition.
   e. **True**. This is because even those with one abnormal allele may show a phenotypic change; the number of alleles involved influences the severity of the clinical condition.

4. a. **True**. These are considered to be 'blighted' ova.
   b. **True**. Usually 45XO involved.
   c. **True**. This includes Down syndrome.
   d. **True**. This includes Klinefelter syndrome.
   e. **True**.

5. a. **True**. This is Bloom syndrome (short stature, malar hypoplasia, telangiectatic erythema of the face).
   b. **True**. This is Fanconi anaemia (radial hypoplasia, hyperpigmentation, pancytopenia).

   c. **True**. This is ataxia telangiectasia (ataxia, telangiectasia, lymphopenia, immune deficit).
   d. **True**. Increased sensitivity to sunlight occurs, atrophic and pigmentary skin changes, actinic skin tumours.
   e. **True**.

6. a. **True**. Lowered.
   b. **True**. Raised.
   c. **True**. Raised.
   d. **True**. Raised.
   e. **True**. Raised.

7. a. **True**. It causes carcinoma and adenosis of the vagina.
   b. **True**. It causes phocomelia.
   c. **True**. It causes abnormal facies.
   d. **False**.
   e. **True**. It causes prematurity and addiction.

8. a. **False**. PKU involves mental retardation, hypopigmentation, skin rashes, seizures.
   b. **True**. Neonatal onset of hypertonicity, convulsions, hypoglycaemia.
   c. **True**. It occurs in diabetic ketoacidosis.
   d. **True**. Neonatal onset of vomiting, lethargy and convulsions.
   e. **True**. Neonatal onset of liver cell failure, hypoglycaemia and convulsions.

9. a. **False**. Though it is seen in other gangliosidoses.
   b. **True**. Other findings include neurological and mental deterioration.
   c. **True**. Sufferers also have coarse facial features, congenital dislocation of hips, gum hypertrophy and psychomotor retardation.
   d. **False**. This syndrome includes retinal pigmentation, polydactyly and obesity.
   e. **True**. Patients also have coarse facial features, clouding of the cornea and progressive neurological and mental deterioration.

10. a. **True**. It is caused by copper deposition.
    b. **True**. This is rare in Gaucher disease and results from deposition of glucocerebroside.
    c. **True**. Intermediate metabolites of tyrosine are thought to be hepatotoxic.

d. **True**. Galactose 1-phosphate, which is not metabolised, is hepatotoxic.

e. **False**. Deposition of glycogen leads to hepatomegaly but not liver cell failure.

11. a. **False**. Glucose 6-phosphate deficiency (type I, glycogen disorder) is associated with hypoglycaemia.

b. **True**. The inability to metabolise galactose leads to hypoglycaemia in babies who are dependent on milk.

c. **True**. It occurs in addition to hepatic failure.

d. **True**. However, correcting the hypoglycaemia alone does not improve the clinical condition.

e. **True**. Usually occurs in the later stages along with dehydration, hypokalaemia and metabolic acidosis (which overrides the respiratory alkalosis).

12. a. **True**. Hypoproteinaemia also occurs.

b. **True**. It may present as xanthomas.

c. **True**. Hyperinsulinaemic states lead to lipogenesis.

d. **True**.

e. **True**. Ingestion of oestrogen-containing pills increases the production of very low-density lipoproteins.

13. a. **True**. This is a lysosomal storage disorder.

b. **True**. This is a lipid myopathy.

c. **False**. Fatty infiltration of the liver occurs.

d. **False**. Hurler syndrome includes cardiomyopathy (Hunter syndrome does not).

e. **True**. Ataxia, degeneration of the posterior columns and late-onset cardiomyopathy occur.

14. a. **True**.

b. **True**.

c. **False**.

d. **False**.

e. **False**.

15. a. **True**. Burgundy red urine caused by uroporphyrin; this is most common in congenital erythropoietic porphyria.

b. **True**. This is blue diaper syndrome.

c. **True**. Rifampicin alters urine colour (it turns pink).

d. **False**. Urine turns black only on standing.

e. **True**. Colour change is caused by the presence of conjugated bilirubin in the urine.

## Case history answer

The main aim in genetic counselling is to provide parents with greater autonomy over decision-making and a choice in reproductive decisions. The first step in this direction is to confirm the diagnosis. In this case, the diagnosis of β-thalassaemia at such an early age suggests that the child has thalassaemia major and will be transfusion dependent and have a shortened lifespan. This is an autosomal recessive or codominant condition, and it is likely that both the parents are carriers. The history needs to determine to at least three generations whether there is a family history of anaemia requiring transfusion, and early deaths. The parents need to be screened to determine whether they are anaemic (as carriers can be in this condition), and whether they have abnormal haemoglobins other than the thalassaemic β globin (such as HbE).

Once the carrier status is known, the next step is to explain to the parents what it means to have this disorder. Details of this disease are discussed in detail in Chapter 11. However, they include the fact that the child is producing an abnormal haemoglobin and has an increased breakdown of the red blood cells, for which there is no medical treatment currently available other than blood transfusion. The risks of frequent blood transfusions include iron overload and infections such as hepatitis. The child will need to be on a regular transfusion–chelation programme to allow normal growth, but in the end this will not be enough to provide a normal lifespan.

Explain the risk for the second child. Assuming that both parents are carriers, the risk estimation for the second child to be affected is 25%. Drawing the pedigree chart and explaining how the disease is transmitted is an essential part of counselling. Information should be presented in an unbiased way; for example, the impact of saying that the risk of recurrence is 1 in 4 may appear to be different from saying that the risk of no recurrence is 3 in 4. Both should be presented.

The final goal is to discuss the options. These include not having any more children, ignoring the risk, artificial insemination or ovum donation or antenatal diagnosis and, where available, termination of pregnancy of an affected fetus.

The counselling should be non-directive but should assist in the decision-making process. The counsellor should be aware of the psychological issues, such as denial, grief and anger, that are evoked by genetic illness, and of the ethnic, social, religious and educational backgrounds of the family. A compassionate and patient approach is required, and counselling should be carried out over several sessions with an adequate follow-up. The latter is essential, particularly where there has been a termination of pregnancy. In the UK, most regional health authorities have at least one clinical genetics centre where genetic counselling is carried out as a special service. As antenatal diagnosis becomes established for more genetic disorders, it will be important to develop a more coordinated approach to the community, which includes education of both the community and the medical profession about genetic issues, the setting up of comprehensive screening programmes, and the training of non-medical genetic counsellors.

## Short notes answer

The investigations are outlined in Table 57.

**Table 57** Investigations in suspected immunodeficiency

| Test | Measurements |
|---|---|
| Full blood count | Determine the white cell and differential count. Is there neutropenia or lymphopenia? Is there thrombocytopenia? |
| Lymphocyte subsets | Determines the number of T cells (and CD4/CD8 ratio), B cells, monocytes and natural killer cells |
| Immunoglobulins | Level of IgM, IgA, IgE and IgG (with subclasses) to determine whether there is deficiency of all or a single immunoglobulin class and to assess B-cell function |
| Antibody screen | Another test of B-cell function; antibodies to type A and B blood groups or childhood vaccines are the commonest used |
| Candida skin test | Intradermal candida antigen test; a positive reaction will rule out virtually all primary T cell deficiencies |
| T cell proliferation | Functional test of cell-mediated immunity with mitogens |
| Complement assay | Total haemolytic complement is a functional test for the complement system and, when suspected, individual complement components can also be looked for |
| Neutrophil function | Nitroblue tetrazolium (NBT): defective in chronic granulomatous disease (CGD)<br>Chemotaxis: decreased in leucocyte adhesion defects<br>Oxygen release: decreased in CGD, increased in neutrophil granule defects |
| Imaging | X-ray of the superior mediastinum to detect an absent thymus (DiGeorge syndrome), visceral ultrasonography (multiple pyogenic granulomas in CGD) |

# 10 Infectious diseases

**10.1** Introduction                                    207

**10.2** Symptoms and assessment              207

**10.3** Immunisation                                   212

**10.4** Bacterial infections                          214

**10.5** Viral infections                                218

**10.6** Miscellaneous conditions               221

Self-assessment: questions                       224

Self-assessment: answers                         228

## Overview

Every child will suffer a number of infections during childhood. Worldwide, acute respiratory infections and gastroenteritis are leading causes of death in childhood. However, the majority of childhood infections are minor self-limiting diseases. A diagnosis can often be made from the history and physical examination, and therefore it is important to understand the natural history of disease and know the presenting symptoms and signs. Prevention is the cornerstone of managing infections. Successful, universal immunisation programmes have led to a marked decrease in the incidence of serious infections worldwide. New challenges are being posed by human immunodeficiency virus (HIV), malaria, and the re-emergence of tuberculosis. A sophisticated armamentarium of antimicrobials equips the physician with tools to fight infection. Nevertheless, these must be used with caution as new, more resistant strains of organism continue to evolve.

## 10.1 Introduction

This chapter will deal with only the common systemic infections seen in children. Localised infections of organs such as the gastrointestinal tract, the urinary system and respiratory system are covered in their respective chapters.

## 10.2 Symptoms and assessment

### Learning objectives

You should:

- know how to assess a child with pyrexia of unknown origin
- be able to recognise the symptoms and signs of septic shock.
- know the management of a child with septic shock

### Fever

The commonest symptom of an infection is fever. Body temperature follows a circadian rhythm, being lowest in the morning and highest around 4–6 pm. An alteration of this normal homeostatic mechanism can be brought about by numerous clinical causes other than an infection, for example drugs, inflammatory disorders, tissue injury, malignancies and metabolic disorders. Regardless of the aetiology, the final pathway of most common causes of fever is the production of endogenous pyrogens that directly alter the hypothalamic temperature set point by increasing local production of prostaglandin $E_2$ ($PGE_2$). As a result, heat is both generated (increased cell metabolism, muscle activity and involuntary shivering) and conserved (vasoconstriction). The neonate, lacking muscle mass, is able to generate heat by the oxidation of brown fat (*non-shivering thermogenesis*). The diurnal variation of temperature is usually preserved in patients with febrile illnesses. Other than in specific infections such as malaria, the pattern of fever is of little diagnostic importance in children. In contrast, an associated rash may be indicative of the underlying diagnosis (Box 58).

Fever can be controlled with paracetamol, aspirin and other non-steroid anti-inflammatory agents (NSAIDs) (e.g. diclofenac, ibuprofen). These are all inhibitors of hypothalamic cyclooxygenase, and therefore inhibit $PGE_2$ synthesis. These drugs are equally effective, but because of the association of aspirin with Reye syndrome in childhood, paracetamol (10–

15 mg/kg every 4 hours) and ibuprofen (4–10 mg/kg every 6–8 hours) are the drugs of choice.

## The child with pyrexia of unknown origin

In most children with prolonged fever, the development of additional clinical manifestations over a relatively short period makes the infectious nature of the illness apparent. Therefore, pyrexia of unknown origin (PUO) is defined as persistence of documented fever in a child for more than 1 week with no apparent diagnosis 1 week after investigation has begun. There is an extensive list of causes of PUO in children, but in general most are caused by infections, connective tissue disorders, atypical presentations of common disease or malignancies.

### History

The evaluation of a child with PUO should start with the history (Box 59). The younger child is more likely to have genitourinary tract, respiratory or localised infection (e.g. osteomyelitis) or juvenile chronic arthritis. The adolescent is more likely to have tuberculosis, inflammatory bowel disease or an autoimmune process.

### Symptoms and signs

Symptoms and signs may provide a clue to the diagnosis (Table 58). Physical examination should include tapping over the sinuses and teeth and palpating the muscles, bones and joints. For example, point tenderness over a bone may suggest occult osteomyelitis or malignant infiltration, and tenderness over the trapezius provides a clue to a subdiaphragmatic abscess.

### Investigations

Initial laboratory investigations should include a full blood count and examination of the blood film for parasites; urine and blood cultures (repeated serially); chest X-ray; tuberculin skin testing; and measuring the C-reactive protein levels (CRP) and/or ESR.

Depending on the condition, other X-ray and ultrasonographic examinations may be necessary, as well as

---

**Box 58** Differential diagnosis of a child with fever and rash

| Type of rash | Infection |
|---|---|
| Vesicular | Chickenpox, herpes simplex, hand foot and mouth, zoster |
| Pustular | Impetigo (*Staphyloccoccus* or *Streptococcus*) |
| Desquamation | Kawasaki, Staphylococcal scalded skin, Stevens Johnson |
| Maculopapular | Measles, rubella, HHV6, HHV7, Enterovirus |
| Drug fever | |

---

**Box 59** Leading questions in PUO

Has the child been to the zoo or been in contact with domestic pets or wild animals recently? – **zoonosis**, including psittacosis, toxoplasmosis, cat scratch disease

Is there pica? – *Toxocara* **and** *Toxoplasma* **spp. infection**

Are their dietary habits unusual? – **brucellosis, tuberculosis, salmonellosis**

Have they or others in the family travelled recently? – **malaria,** typhoid, shigellosis, legionella)

Any outdoor activities? (rickettsial diseases, Lyme disease, leptospirosis)

Is the child on any medications (including eye drops)? – **drug fever**

What is the genetic background? – **nephrogenic diabetes, Riley–Day syndrome, anhidrotic ectodermal dysplasia**

Is anyone else in the family unwell?

---

**Table 58** Symptoms and signs of diagnostic importance in pyrexia of unknown origin (PUO)

| Symptom/sign | Possible cause |
|---|---|
| Absence of sweating | Nephrogenic diabetes insipidus, anhidrotic ectodermal dysplasia, atropine poisoning |
| Absent tears, absent corneal reflex | Riley–Day syndrome |
| Red, weeping eyes | Connective tissue disorder |
| Palpebral conjunctivitis | Viral infections |
| Bulbar conjunctivitis | Kawasaki syndrome, leptospirosis |
| Petechial conjunctival haemorrhages | Endocarditis |
| Oral candidiasis | Immune deficiency |
| Repetitive chill and temperature spikes | Systemic onset juvenile chronic arthritis, septicaemia |
| Fever blisters | Pneumococcal, streptococcal infection |
| Congested pharynx | Viral infection, Kawasaki syndrome, leptospirosis |

examination and culture of a bone marrow aspirate. Bone marrow cultures are often more sensitive for occult *Salmonella*, leishmaniasis, *Mycobacterium* and fungal infections. Serologic evidence may aid diagnosis in some viral and bacterial infections as well as in juvenile chronic arthritis (JCA). Radioactive scans are helpful in localising osteomyelitis and abdominal abscesses, and echocardiography in identifying endocarditis. On occasion, total body imaging with computed tomography (CT) or magnetic resonance imaging (MRI), radiolabelled white cell isotope scans, and ultimately biopsy via laparoscopy or endoscopy, may be required.

## Sepsis and shock

In children beyond the neonatal period, *Streptococcus pneumoniae*, *Haemophilus influenzae* type b, *Neisseria meningitidis*, *Salmonella* spp. and *Staphylococcus aureus* are the most common microorganisms causing bacteraemia. One potential consequence of bacteraemia is septic shock, a state characterised by inadequate tissue perfusion and frequently associated with endotoxaemia. Although this is more often seen with infections with Gram-negative organisms (*Pseudomonas aeruginosa* being a frequent culprit), it is also seen with Gram-positive (*Streptococcus pneumoniae*, *Streptococcus pyogenes* and *Staphylococcus aureus*), viral and fungal pathogens. A *systemic inflammatory response syndrome* (SIRS) is thought to occur as a result of tissue damage following host response to endotoxin from Gram-negative bacteria and the lipoteichoic acid–peptidoglycan complex from Gram-positive bacteria. SIRS is recognised to be a cytokine-mediated process involving tumour necrosis factor (TNF), interleukins (IL) 1, 6 and 8, platelet-activating factors and interferon-γ. Either alone or in combination, bacterial products and proinflammatory cytokines trigger physiological responses to stop microbial invasion (Box 60). These result in diffuse capillary leakage, reduced vascular tone, and an imbalance between tissue perfusion and the increased metabolic requirements of the tissues.

The primary symptoms and signs of septic shock are listed in Table 59. As shown in Figure 91, ultimately irreversible organ failure may occur.

Children with septic shock need to be treated in an intensive care unit where central venous and continuous intra-arterial monitoring is possible (Box 61). Broad-spectrum synergistic bactericidal antimicrobials should be started while awaiting the results of cultures. Shock should be managed by infusing IV fluids – 20 mL/kg body weight of crystalloid, and later, colloid – which can be repeated. If the blood pressure remains low, inotropic drugs such as epinephrine (adrenaline), dopamine and

**Box 60** Physiological responses to infection

Activation of the complement system
Activation of coagulation factor XII
Adrenocorticotropic hormone (ACTH) and β-endorphin release
Stimulation of the kallikrein–kinin system
Stimulation of neutrophils

**Table 59** Symptoms and signs of septic shock

|  | Symptoms and signs |
|---|---|
| Primary effects | Fever, shaking chills, hyperventilation, tachycardia, hypothermia, cutaneous lesions (petechiae, ecchymoses, echthyma gangrenosum, diffuse erythema, cellulitis), mental obtundation |
| Secondary effects | Hypotension, cyanosis, symmetrical peripheral gangrene (purpura fulminans), oliguria or anuria, jaundice, congestive cardiac failure, tissue hypoxia and lactic acidosis |

dobutamine may be used. Where there is bradycardia or a poorly contracting myocardium, epinephrine or isoprenaline are more effective. Sodium bicarbonate is only infused in severe acidosis (pH < 7.1), and glucose supplements may be required. Oxygen and ventilation may be required in the severely compromised child. The routine use of corticosteroids has not been shown to be of benefit except in the treatment of adrenal haemorrhage (Waterhouse–Friderichsen syndrome). A poorer prognosis is seen in those who are initially refractory to resuscitative measures and those with multiorgan failure.

## The immunocompromised child

A child with a defective immune system, whether caused by disease or by therapy, is at risk of infection with the usual pathogens and with organisms that would not normally be able to cause infection and disease. Opportunistic infections are generally caused by organisms indigenous to the host or commonly found in the environment. The skin and mucous membranes are important barriers to infections, and any breaches in these protective layers can predispose to infection by opportunistic organisms (Table 60).

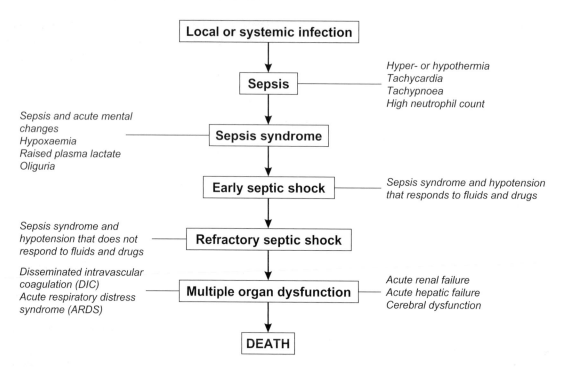

**Fig. 91** Progression from bacteraemia to sepsis to the systemic inflammatory response syndrome (SIRS) and its complications.

---

**Box 61** Management of the child with septic shock

**Assessment**

| | |
|---|---|
| Is the child conscious and coherent? | Sensorium |
| Is there pallor or central cyanosis? | Colour |
| Is the respiratory rate rapid? | Respiration |
| Are the peripheries cool and clammy? | Temperature gap, capillary return |
| Is the pulse thready and rapid? | Pulse |
| Is the capillary refill longer than 2 seconds? | Perfusion |
| Is the child hypotensive? | Check BP |
| Is the child oliguric? | Check urine output (catheter) |
| Is the child covered with a rash? | Consider meningococcal infection |

**Management**

| | |
|---|---|
| Airway | Secure airway with pharyngeal airway device or intubate if necessary |
| Breathing | Oxygen, bag and mask |
| | Ventilation |
| Circulation | External cardiac compressions if severely bradycardic |
| Drugs, fluids | Obtain venous or intraosseous access as soon as possible |
| | Take blood samples (CBC, U & E, glucose, X-match, cultures) |
| | Fluid bolus of 20 mL/kg of crystalloid, can be repeated to 60–100 mL/kg |
| | May require inotropes such as dopamine, dobutamine, adrenaline |
| Supportive | Empirical broad-spectrum antibiotics |
| | Glucose |
| | Bicarbonate |
| | Colloid or albumin infusion, blood products |

Table 61 shows some of the diseases in which a defect in immunity predisposes to certain kinds of infection. Children with cancer or those undergoing transplantation are at a particularly high risk, for four different reasons.

**Indwelling catheters.** Most of these children have an indwelling central venous catheter, which breaches the mechanical skin barrier. This increases the incidence of Gram-positive infections, especially with skin-dwelling commensals such as *Staphylococcus aureus* and *S. epidermidis*.

**Drug therapy.** Many cytotoxics are highly immuno-suppressive and can predispose to fungal, viral and protozoal (*Pneumocystis carinii*) infection.

**Neutropenia.** Most children receiving chemotherapy will go through periods when they are severely neutropenic. During these periods they are highly susceptible to both Gram-negative and Gram-positive infections.

**Mucositis and gut damage.** The side effects of most chemotherapy drugs and radiation include damage to the protective oral and intestinal mucosa. Not only does this produce considerable debility and malnutrition, it also allows colonisation of the gut with pathogens and systemic invasion of organisms normally restricted to the intestinal lumen.

## Prevention of infection

Prevention of infection in the immunocompromised child varies with the type and severity of the individual defect. Often simple measures such as improving personal hygiene and the use of non-touch techniques when inserting internal devices and attending to their routine maintenance are far more effective than the use of antimicrobial agents. The use of prophylactic co-trimoxazole has been extremely successful in decreasing the incidence of *Pneumocystis carinii* infections in children being treated for acute lymphoblastic leukaemia. Similarly, prophylactic antibiotics used in children with valvular or septal heart defects prevent endocarditis. Routine prophylactic antibiotics have not proved to be useful, and indeed may be detrimental, in children with immunodeficiency, immunosuppression and severe neutropenia. Therapy with broad-spectrum antibiotics is started empirically in these children when an infection is suspected. Often a combination of a third-generation cephalosporin and an aminoglycoside is given until symptoms subside or an organism is isolated, when more specific therapy can be instituted.

**Table 60** Common opportunistic infections associated with defective anatomic barriers

| Defects in anatomic barriers | Common opportunistic organism |
|---|---|
| Dermal sinus tracts | *Staphylococcus epidermidis*, diphtheroids |
| Cerebrospinal fluid shunts | *Staphylococcus epidermidis* and *Staph. aureus* |
| Intravenous catheters | *Staphylococcus*, *Pseudomonas* and *Candida* spp. |
| Urinary catheters | *Pseudomonas*, *Serrati* and *Candida* spp. |
| Burns | *Pseudomonas*, *Serratius*, *Candida* and *Staphylococcus* spp. |
| General surgery | *Staphylococcus*, *Pseudomonas* spp. |
| Cardiac surgery | *Staphylococcus epidermidis*, diphtheroids and *Candida* sp. |
| Congenital cardiac defects | Viridans streptococci, *Corynebacterium* and *Pseudomonas* spp. |

**Table 61** Opportunistic infections in immunodeficiency

| Predisposing cause | Common organisms isolated |
|---|---|
| Chronic granulomatous disease | *Staphylococcus* spp., Gram-negative enteric organisms |
| Job syndrome (Hyper-IgE) | *Staphylococcus aureus* |
| Complement deficiencies | *Streptococcus pneumoniae*, *Streptococcus pyogenes*, *Neisseria meningitidis* |
| Splenic insufficiency | *Streptococcus pneumoniae*, *Salmonella* spp. |
| Sickle cell disease and other haemoglobinopathies | *Streptococcus pneumoniae*, *Salmonella* spp., *Haemophilus influenzae* type b |
| Humoral immunodeficiency | Bacterial pathogens, *Pseudomonas* spp. |
| Cellular immunodeficiency | *Mycobacterium*, *Listeria*, *Candida* spp., cytomegalovirus (CMV), varicella zoster (VZV), *Pneumocystis carinii* |
| Cystic fibrosis | *Staphylococcus*, *Haemophilus*, *Pseudomonas* spp. |
| Diabetes mellitus | *Staphylococcus* spp., *Escherichia coli* |
| Nephrotic syndrome | *Streptococcus pneumoniae*, *Salmonella* spp. |

## 10.3 Immunisation

### Learning objectives

You should:

- know the current immunisation schedule
- know the relative and absolute contraindications for immunisation

Two hundred years ago, Edward Jenner was able to demonstrate that vaccination with material from cowpox provided protection against smallpox. At that time smallpox caused 20% of all deaths in Glasgow, and 90% of those who died were under the age of 5. In 1980, smallpox was eradicated worldwide. We are now poised to eradicate poliomyelitis, and hopefully measles will follow.

Many countries have an immunisation programme targeting children and intended to reduce the incidence of infectious diseases (Table 62).

Immunity can either be induced actively (long term) or provided by passive transfer (short term) against a variety of bacterial and viral agents.

### Active immunity

Using inactivated or attenuated live organisms or their products induces active immunity. Live attenuated vaccines include those for poliomyelitis (OPV), measles, mumps, rubella, varicella and Bacillus–Calmette–Guérin (BCG) vaccine. Whole-cell pertussis, whole-cell typhoid and inactivated poliomyelitis (IPV) vaccines contain inactivated organisms. Others, such as influenza, Hib, hepatitis B, acellular pertussis, meningococcal and pneumococcal vaccine, contain immunising components of the organisms. Tetanus and diphtheria vaccines contain toxoid, which is toxin inactivated by treatment with formaldehyde. A first injection of inactivated vaccine or toxoid in a subject without prior exposure to the antigen produces a slow antibody or antitoxin response of predominantly IgM antibody, called the *primary response*. Depending on the potency of the product and the time interval, further injections will lead to an accelerated response in which the antibody or antitoxin titre (IgG) rises to a higher level, called the *secondary response*. Following a full course, the antibody or antitoxin level remains high for months or years. Even if the level of detectable antibody falls, the immune mechanism has been sensitised and a further dose of vaccine reinforces immunity. Some inactivated vaccines contain adjuvants (substances that enhance the antibody response). Examples are aluminium phosphate and aluminium hydroxide, which are contained in adsorbed diphtheria/tetanus/pertussis vaccines and adsorbed capsular polysaccharides. Those younger than 2 years are unable to mount an effective response to polysaccharide antigens. To improve the immune response these vaccines are conjugated with carriers that elicit a T-cell response, and have been shown to be highly active in infants and young children. An example of such a carrier is $CRM_{197}$ (a non-toxic diphtheria mutant) used in both the Hib and the heptavalent pneumococcal vaccines.

### Passive immunity

Passive immunity results from the injection of human immunoglobulin. The protection afforded is immediate, but lasts only a few weeks. There are two types of immunoglobulin available. Human normal immunoglobulin (HNIG) derived from pooled plasma donors contains antibody to infectious agents currently prevalent in the general population. It is used, for example, to protect an immunosuppressed child against measles, or individuals against hepatitis A. Specific immunoglobulins for tetanus, hepatitis B, rabies and varicella-zoster are obtained from the pooled blood of convalescent patients or those recently immunised with the relevant vaccine. Each specific immunoglobulin therefore contains antibody at a higher titre than that present in normal immunoglobulin.

### Special risk groups

Some conditions increase the risk of complications from infectious diseases, and children and adults with those

**Table 62** The UK immunisation schedule (2004)

| Age | Immunisation |
|---|---|
| Birth | BCG[1] |
| 2 months | DTaP, IPV, Hib, Meningococcal C |
| 3 months | DTaP, IPV, Hib, Meningococcal C |
| 4 months | DTaP, IPV, Hib, Meningococcal C |
| 12–15 months | MMR |
| 3–5 years | Booster DTaP, IPV, MMR second dose |
| 10–15 years | BCG (can be given in infancy) |
| 13–18 years | Booster dT and IPV |

[1] BCG is given at birth to those with infected or previously infected family members, and immigrants from countries where TB is highly prevalent.
DTP, diphtheria/tetanus/pertussis; OPV, oral polio vaccine; Hib, *Haemophilus influenzae* type b; MMR, measles/mumps/rubella; BCG, Bacillus–Calmette–Guérin (tuberculosis); dT, low-dose diphtheria and tetanus toxoids used to immunise adults.

conditions should be immunised as a matter of priority. These conditions include asthma, chronic lung disease, congenital heart diseases, Down syndrome, HIV infection, small-for-dates babies and those born prematurely. The latter should be immunised according to the recommended schedule from 2 months of age, irrespective of the extent of prematurity.

Those children who, for a variety of reasons, have not been immunised, or for whom the immunisation history is unknown, should be immunised fully. For children under 10 years of age this should include the full primary immunisation schedule. *Haemophilus influenzae* type b (Hib) is only given up to the age of 4 years: three doses for those under 1 year and one dose for those aged 1–4 years. Children over the age of 10 should receive dT (low-dose diphtheria and tetanus toxoid).

Children with no spleen or with functional hyposplenism are at increased risk from the bacterial infections most commonly caused by encapsulated organisms. Such infection occurs most often in the first 2 years after splenectomy. The following vaccines are recommended in addition to the routine schedule: pneumococcal vaccine in those over 2 years of age; Hib vaccine irrespective of age; and influenza, meningococcal A and C vaccines. Where possible, immunisation should be completed 2 weeks before splenectomy.

Children on haemodialysis or those who have a hepatitis B virus (HBV) carrier in the family should be immunised against HBV. In addition, HBV vaccination is now being adopted as part of the routine schedule by many countries. The age of vaccination with HBV will depend on the 'risk level' of the individual country: it is given in the first few years of life in those countries with an incidence of HBV carriage in over 3% of the population. In these countries it is given as an accelerated course, including three doses starting from birth and spaced over 3 months. Otherwise, HBV vaccine is spread over three doses, generally 6 weeks and then 3–4 months apart. Recent evidence would suggest that immunity against hepatitis B may wane with time, particularly if given as an accelerated course. The same would appear to be the case for pertussis, especially if the less toxic acellular vaccine is used, and additional booster doses of these vaccines may be required at 18 months and again at 3 years of age.

## Indications and contraindications

HIV-positive children with or without symptoms should receive MMR (measles, mumps, rubella), DTaP (diphtheria, tetanus, pertussis), HBV and Hib. Injectable polio vaccine (IPV) may be used instead of oral vaccine (OPV) for symptomatic or immunosuppressed patients.

**Box 62** The following are *not* contraindications to immunisation:

Family history of epilepsy or any adverse reaction following immunisation
Previous history of pertussis, measles, rubella or mumps infection
Prematurity: immunisation should not be postponed
Stable neurological conditions such as cerebral palsy and Down syndrome
Contact with infectious disease
Asthma, hay fever, snuffles, diarrhoea, *afebrile* upper respiratory infections
Treatment with antibiotics or locally acting steroids (topical or inhaled)
Child's mother is pregnant or child is breastfed
History of jaundice at birth
Under a certain weight
Over the age recommended in the immunisation schedule

BCG should not be given, as dissemination of the bacillus can occur in these children.

Immunisation should not be carried out in individuals who have a definite history of severe local or general reaction to a preceding dose. A general reaction includes fever of at least 39.5°C within 48 hours of vaccination, anaphylaxis, bronchospasm, laryngeal oedema, shock, prolonged unresponsiveness, prolonged inconsolable or high-pitched screaming for more than 4 hours, convulsions, or encephalopathy occurring within 72 hours.

Children who are immunosuppressed through treatment for cancer or have undergone a bone marrow transplant should not be immunised until at least 6 months after stopping treatment. Children who have received prednisolone 2 mg/kg daily for at least 1 week or 1 mg/kg daily for 1 month should not have live vaccines until at least 3 months after stopping the steroids.

## Adverse effects of vaccines

Every now and then concern is raised about the so-called toxicities of vaccines. The truth is that they are among the safest 'drugs' known, but, like all medications, may possibly have side effects.

**DTaP**. Adverse effects include acute encephalopathy, shock and unusual shock-like state, and protracted inconsolable crying. There is little evidence to suggest that the whole-cell pertussis vaccine causes permanent brain damage or death. However, acellular pertussis vaccines contain just three or four bacterial proteins and produce adequate immunogenicity with fewer side effects, although they may need additional booster doses in early childhood. Combination vaccines, including Hib–DTaP, Hib–DTaP–IPV and Hib–DTaP–IPV–HBV, are now available.

**OPV/IPV.** OPV has been implicated in vaccine-induced paralysis. As IPV is a killed vaccine, it does not have this disadvantage. IPV, however, has to be given as an injection and produces less herd immunity, unlike OPV.

**MMR.** Although thrombocytopenia and anaphylaxis have been reported, this is one of the safest of the commonly used vaccines. There have been anecdotal reports linking the combined vaccine with infantile autism and inflammatory bowel disease. However, the scientific evidence would strongly suggest that there is no evidence to link MMR with the aetiology of these disorders, and indeed the risk posed by the wildtype infections is considerably greater.

## 10.4 Bacterial infections

### Learning objectives

You should:

- appreciate the different presentations of bacterial infections in childhood and understand the basis for antibiotic therapy

- know the clinical features and management of meningococcal disease

- know the clinical features and management of childhood tuberculosis

### Staphylococcal infections

*Staphylococcus aureus* is ubiquitous. Most neonates are colonised within the first week of life, and 20–30% of adults carry *Staph. aureus* in the anterior nares. It is the commonest cause of pyogenic skin infections (Box 63), and may cause furuncles, osteomyelitis, septic arthritis, lower respiratory infections, septicaemia, pericarditis, endocarditis and deep-seated abscesses. The organism releases exotoxins that can cause tissue necrosis. Exfo-

liative toxins can result in bullous impetigo or the scalded skin syndrome (Ritter disease). Enterotoxins A and B are associated with diarrhoea and vomiting and may cause food poisoning. TSS-1 is associated with toxic shock syndrome (TSS), which is related to menstruation and focal staphylococcal infections. Enterotoxins A and B can also cause non-menstrual TSS. Methicillin-resistant *Staphylococcus aureus* (MRSA) accounts for up to 40% of nosocomial staphylococcal infections in hospitals. Nasal and skin colonisation can occur in both patients and staff, and overcrowding, poor ward and clinical hygiene, and lack of simple disinfection (i.e. handwashing) contribute to the spread of this organism. As a result, most hospitals now have well established screening and prophylactic measures to prevent the spread of MRSA and other infections.

### Management

Staphylococcal infection is transmitted primarily by direct contact. Strict attention to handwashing techniques is the most effective measure for preventing the spread of staphylococci from one individual to another. Antibiotic therapy alone is rarely effective in individuals with undrained abscesses or foreign bodies. Loculated collections need to be drained, and foreign bodies such as cannulae and lines removed. Therapy should always be initiated with a penicillinase-resistant antibiotic, as over 90% of all staphylococci isolated are resistant to penicillin. In serious infections, parenteral therapy is employed along with an aminoglycoside. Sodium fusidate can also be used adjunctively in localised infections. The coagulase-negative staphylococci *Staph. epidermidis* and *Staph. haemolyticus* are nosocomial pathogens and can cause infections in immunosuppressed patients or those with indwelling foreign devices such as catheters, shunts and valves. The glycopeptide antibiotics vancomycin and teicoplanin are used where the organism is resistant to semisynthetic penicillins (e.g. MRSA). Enterococci and now staphylococcal strains are exhibiting resistance to glycopeptide antibiotics. However, newer agents such as linezolid are now available for the management of vancomycin-resistant organisms.

### Streptococcal infections

Streptococci are Gram-positive cocci classified according to their ability to haemolyse red blood cells. Complete, partial and non-haemolytic strains are classified as β-, α- and γ-haemolytic. They are further classified according to the carbohydrate components of the cell wall into A–H and K–V types (Lancefield groups). The β-haemolytic groups A and B are major pathogens in

---

**Box 63** Staphylococcal and streptococcal skin infections

Impetigo
Boils
Cellulitis
Scalded skin syndrome
Toxic shock syndrome
Postinfectious complications, e.g. glomerulonephritis

---

**Table 63** Common streptococcal infections of childhood

| Lancefield group | Species | Haemolysis | Site of colonisation | Common human diseases |
|---|---|---|---|---|
| A | *S. pyogenes* | β | Pharynx, skin, rectum | Pharyngitis, tonsillitis, erysipelas, impetigo, septicaemia, wound infections, cellulitis, rarely meningitis, toxic shock-like syndrome, rheumatic fever, glomerulonephritis |
| B | *S. galactiae* | β | Pharynx, vagina | Puerperal sepsis, chorioamnionitis, neonatal sepsis, pneumonia, meningitis, osteomyelitis, endocarditis |
| C–H, K–O | *Various* | β, α | Mouth, pharynx, skin, vagina | Puerperal sepsis, endocarditis, wound infections, nosocomial or opportunistic brain abscess |
| Non-typable[1] | *Viridans streptococci* | α | Pharynx | Endocarditis |
| Non-typable[1] | *S. mutans* | α | Pharynx | Endocarditis |
| Non-typable[1] | *Enterococcus (faecalis, faecium)* | α, β, NH | Large bowel | Endocarditis, urinary tract, biliary tract and intestinal infections, peritonitis, bacteraemia |

[1] These organisms have Lancefield D antigens but cannot be distinguished from *Enterococcus* spp.
NH, non-haemolytic.

children, affecting the skin, soft tissues, blood and respiratory tract (Table 63).

Clinically, it is difficult to distinguish streptococcal pharyngitis from that caused by other bacterial and viral pathogens. A mixture of staphylococcal and streptococcal infection often causes pyoderma. Similarly, streptococcal septicaemia, meningitis, arthritis etc. are diagnosed only on recovery of the organism from culture. Although direct culture of infected tissue is the best way to confirm the diagnosis of streptococcal infection, serological tests may also be of value. In 80% of children with untreated streptococcal pharyngitis within the first 3–6 weeks the antistreptolysin O (ASO) titre is more than 166 Todd units. In those with skin infections ASO is not a good test, but antideoxyribonuclease B (anti-DNAase B) provides the best serological test and is detectable 6–8 weeks after the start of the infection. Rheumatic fever is a late complication of streptococcal pharyngitis; a raised ASO (>330 Todd units) is one of the criteria used to establish a diagnosis. Poststreptoccal glomerulonephritis occurs after streptococcal skin infections; elevated anti-DNAase B titres (>170 units) help to confirm the diagnosis.

## Management

Therapy is directed at preventing suppurative and non-suppurative complications of the infection. In most cases the organism is exquisitely sensitive to penicillin. At least 10 days of therapy with oral penicillin or a single dose of long-acting intramuscular penicillin is required. In those allergic to penicillin, cefadroxil, erythromycin or clindamycin may be used. Those with severe infections require high doses of intravenous penicillin given every 3–4 hours (400 000 U/kg over 24 hours). Prophylactic use of penicillin is effective in preventing further attacks in those with a history of rheumatic fever. Many of the non-typable streptococci are only sensitive to the glycopeptide antibiotics (vancomycin, teicoplanin), though clinically significant strains of enterococci resistant to glycopeptide antibiotics are emerging.

## Pneumococcal infections

*Streptococcus pneumoniae* is a Gram-positive lancet-shaped encapsulated diplococcus. It is a normal inhabitant of the upper respiratory tract, but can also be an invasive pathogen. It is the most common cause of community-acquired bacterial pneumonia and otitis media, and the second most common cause of meningitis. Its frequency and severity are increased in those with functional or anatomic asplenia (splenectomy, sickle cell disease, after total body irradiation) and humoral and complement deficiencies. The signs and symptoms are related to the site of infection. The severity of disease is related to the virulence and number of organisms causing the infection. Pneumococcal septicaemia may have a fulminant onset with a high mortality unless promptly treated. In such children a high peripheral white cell count may be helpful in diagnosing pneumococcal septicaemia.

## Management

Resistance to penicillin and the third-generation cephalosporins is being reported. Currently it is advisable to use a third-generation cephalosporin or amoxicillin–clavulanic acid for the treatment of less serious infections and consider adding in vancomycin for serious infections. A pneumococcal vaccine containing purified polysaccharide from 23 pneumococcal serotypes responsible for more than 85% of infections is available, though its clinical efficacy is controversial. The conjugated pneumococcal vaccine has recently been shown to have better immunogenicity. Immunisation is currently recommended for those aged 2 years or older with functional or anatomic asplenia; chronic renal disease or nephrotic syndrome; cerebrospinal fluid leaks; chronic heart, lung or liver disease; diabetes mellitus; and those with immunodeficiencies or who are immunosuppressed, including those with HIV infection. Because the vaccine does not protect against all strains, these children will also require oral penicillin prophylaxis.

## *Haemophilus influenzae* infections

*H. influenzae* is a normal commensal of the respiratory tract in 60–90% of healthy children. Disease is caused mainly by serotype b, and invasive disease occurs primarily in those under the age of 2. Before the advent of an effective vaccine, *H. influenzae* was the leading cause of bacterial meningitis in young children. Another potential life-threatening complication was epiglottitis, which presents with acute upper airway obstruction. This has also become a rare disease with the advent of the vaccine. The organism is also an important pathogen in soft tissue infections. It is responsible for 10% of cellulitis in young children, and can present as orbital or preseptal cellulitis. Osteomyelitis, septic arthritis, pneumonia and pericarditis are other examples of invasive disease. Non-b serotypes are associated with acute otitis media, sinusitis and conjunctivitis.

## Management

Currently the third-generation cephalosporins and the fluoroquinolones are the antibiotics of preference. Children with invasive *H. influenzae* infections carry the organism in their upper airway. They and all close contacts need chemoprophylaxis with rifampicin if there are unvaccinated children in the group younger than 48 months. The goal of chemoprophylaxis is to prevent a susceptible child from acquiring *H. influenzae* type b from contacts by eliminating colonisation in all close contacts.

## Meningococcal infections

At least 13 serotypes of meningococcus have been identified, but groups A, B, C, W and Y account for most meningococcal disease. Heterogeneous groups of meningococcal serotypes cause endemic disease, whereas epidemics are caused by a single serotype. Individuals with primary or acquired complement deficiency have an increased risk of developing meningococcal disease. The spectrum of disease can vary widely, from occult bacteraemia to septic shock and death. Acute meningococcaemia can present with pharyngitis, fever, myalgias, weakness and headache. With widespread haematogenous dissemination the disease progresses rapidly to septic shock, characterised by hypotension, disseminated intravascular coagulation, acidosis, adrenal haemorrhage (Waterhouse–Friderichsen syndrome), renal failure, myocardial failure and coma. More often meningococcal disease manifests as acute meningitis. Less common manifestations include pneumonia, myocarditis, purulent pericarditis and septic arthritis. Uncommon manifestations include endocarditis, purulent pericarditis, pneumonia, osteomyelitis and septic arthritis. Chronic meningococcaemia is a rare disease manifested by fever, rash, arthralgias and headache.

## Management

An attempt to isolate the organism in any suspected case should include blood cultures, petechial skin scrapings, throat swabs, serological/antigen tests and, in those whose cardiorespiratory condition is not compromised, cerebrospinal fluid. Ceftriaxone and cefotaxime are currently the drugs of choice, with penicillin-resistant strains being reported. Despite the use of appropriate antibiotics, the mortality rate for disseminated meningococcal disease remains around 10% and the majority of patients will require intensive management. Poor prognostic features include hypothermia, hypotension, purpura fulminans, seizures or shock at presentation, leukopenia and thrombocytopenia. Close contacts of patients are at risk, and prophylaxis with rifampicin or ciprofloxacin/ceftriaxone for older children/adults is indicated as soon as possible for household and other close contacts.

## Pertussis

*Bordetella pertussis* is the sole cause of epidemic pertussis and the usual cause of sporadic disease, the other pathogens being *B. parapertussis* and *B. bronchiseptica*. In the unvaccinated population pertussis is endemic, with superimposed epidemic cycles every 3–4 years after the accumulation of a sizeable susceptible cohort. It is a highly contagious disease, with attack rates as high as 100% in susceptible individuals. However, with widespread use of pertussis vaccine there has been a dramatic decline in cases. In contrast, the dramatic increase in the number of cases when immunisation was halted attests to the protective efficacy of the vaccine. Pertussis is a lengthy disease (it was known in ancient China as the 100-day cough), divided into *catarrhal*, *paroxysmal* and *convalescent* phases. After a non-distinctive period of low-grade fever, sneezing, rhinorrhoea and lacrimation, the paroxysmal stage sets in. Coughing begins first as a dry intermittent hacking cough and then progresses to the full-blown paroxysms. The rapid bursts of coughing preclude an adequate inspiration, and often the child's face becomes suffused and cyanosed. The cycle is broken by a forced inspiratory gasp, often against a closed glottis, producing the characteristic whoop. The last is often absent in those younger than 3 months of age, who may either become cyanosed or vomit after paroxysms. The episode may end with the expulsion of a thick plug of inspissated tracheal secretions, and post-tussive emesis is common. However, not 'all that whoops' is pertussis. A paroxysmal cough can also result from lower respiratory tract infections with adenovirus, chlamydia, mycoplasma and respiratory syncytial virus. Diagnosis can be difficult, as isolation and identification of the organism is not always possible. Complications of pertussis infection include pneumonia (25%), seizures (4%), encephalopathy (1%), apnoea, physical sequelae of forceful coughing (Fig. 92), and death (1%).

## Management

The goals of therapy are to limit the paroxysms, to provide supportive care, and to maximise nutrition, rest and recovery without sequelae. Erythromycin or clarithromycin are almost always prescribed for their potential clinical benefit and to limit the spread of the organism.

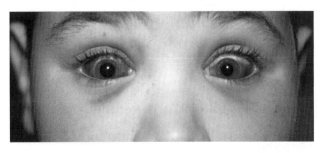

**Fig. 92** Bilateral traumatic conjunctival haemorrhages ('Dracula' eyes) due to forceful coughing in a child with pertussis paroxysms.

## Tuberculosis

*Mycobacterium tuberculosis* is spread from person to person by droplet infection and, rarely, by ingestion. Once inhaled, some bacilli remain at the site of entry and the rest are carried to the regional lymph nodes. The bacilli multiply at both sites, and the *primary focus*, along with the regional lymph nodes, is described as the *primary complex*. As the organism multiplies it can be disseminated via the bloodstream and lymphatic system. In about 4–8 weeks the body defence mechanisms react and the primary complex heals and disappears, or occasionally calcifies. Sometimes disease progresses either at the site of the primary complex or at a more distant site, such as the brain or spine. The greatest risk of dissemination occurs in the first year of infection. Particularly at risk are infants and those who are immunosuppressed as a result of malnutrition, infection with pertussis or measles, or because of immunosuppressive therapy. Figure 93 illustrates the natural history of untreated tuberculous infection in

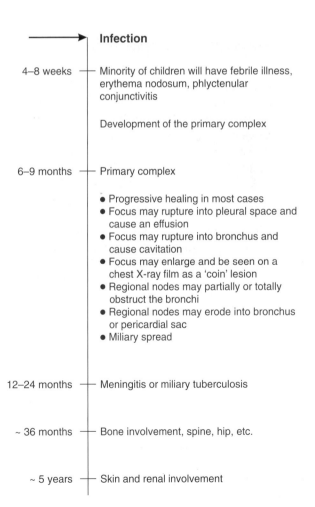

**Fig. 93** Evolution of untreated primary tuberculosis in children.

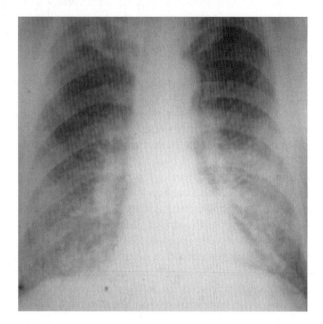

**Fig. 94** Radiological appearance of miliary mottling due to tuberculosis.

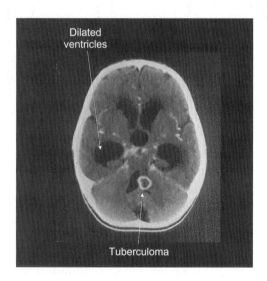

**Fig. 95** CT brain scan showing intracerebral tuberculoma.

children, along with some of the complications. The most serious complication is miliary or disseminated tuberculosis (Fig. 94), which involves the liver, the spleen and often the brain; choroidal tubercules can even be seen on fundoscopy. Central nervous system disease is characterised by an insidious onset of basal meningitis, which often results in acute hydrocephalus and cranial nerve palsies. Tuberculomas (Fig. 95) present as space-occupying lesions and are typically seen as ring lesions on a CT scan. A diagnosis of tuberculosis is considered on the clinical features. In progressive pulmonary disease or pleural effusion a

positive Mantoux tuberculin test (an induration of more than 10 mm 48 hours after an intradermal injection of 10 TU with Tween 80) is helpful. However, the Mantoux test is often unhelpful when other organs are involved, or with severe disease, when a false negative test may occur. Children do not cough up sputum but tend to swallow it, and culture and acid-fast staining of fasting gastric juice is often more helpful.

### Management

The current recommended treatment for pulmonary infection is isoniazid and rifampicin for 6 months, adding pyrazinamide with or without ethambutol for the first 2 months. For miliary or meningitic disease, three drugs should be used for the first 2 months and then isoniazid and rifampicin continued for 12 months. Adding dexamethasone for 1–2 months has been shown to reduce the incidence of complications in those with TB meningitis. Hospitalised patients whose sputum is Ziehl–Nielsen stain positive should be isolated in a negative-pressure room to avoid the spread of TB to other patients and healthcare workers. TB is a notifiable disease. It is essential to trace contacts of newly diagnosed patients and to perform a tuberculin test and chest X-ray. BCG vaccination appears to be protective against miliary spread and TB meningitis. However, its widespread use in immunisation programmes has been questioned, particularly as it is often given to sections of the population who are at least risk of TB (e.g. 12-year-olds), and its effectiveness wanes with time, rendering the vaccinated population non-immune when they are at greater risk (i.e. old age).

## 10.5 Viral infections

### Learning objectives

You should:

- know the differential diagnosis of a child with a viral exanthema
- know the clinical features and management of HIV infection in children

There are a number of illnesses that present with a rash, many of which are viral (Box 64).

## Measles

In the unvaccinated population measles is a common and highly contagious disease. It is characterised by an incubation period of about 10–12 days, after which there is a prodromal illness with fever, conjunctivitis, coryza and cough. General lymphadenopathy may be found as well as tiny grey-white dots surrounded by erythema on the buccal mucosa and soft and hard palate (Koplik spots). After 3–4 days the fever increases and a maculopapular erythematous rash spreads downwards from the head and neck to cover the whole body. The rash begins to fade by the third day, and by the fifth day after the rash first appeared the affected child is no longer infectious. The chief complications of measles are otitis media, pneumonia and encephalitis. A rare late complication occurring 4–10 years after an attack of measles is subacute sclerosing panencephalitis (SSPE). This is characterised by slow progressive dementia and deterioration. In developing countries measles tends to occur in infants and younger children, with a high morbidity and mortality. The mortality rate of measles correlates directly with the state of nutrition. An attack of measles in malnourished children results in a period of anergy, apathy, and often diarrhoea. This may result in severe and often intractable states of malnourishment such as marasmus and kwashiorkor.

## Management

Passive immunisation with measles-specific immunoglobulin is effective for the prevention and attenuation of infection in infants and immunocompromised children. In the USA and the UK, where measles immunisation is practically universal (>95%), the disease has been almost eradicated. The World Health Organization has included this in its Expanded Programme of Immunisation (EPI) and, with sufficient coverage, measles, like smallpox, can also be eradicated.

## Rubella

Rubella is a mild illness and often passes unrecognised. The incubation period is 14–21 days, and there may be no prodrome before the appearance [...] lopapular rash that generally lasts for [...] alised lymphadenopathy, especially i[...] suboccipital nodes, is a common finding. [...] erally shed 5–7 days before the appearance o[...] the disappearance of the rash. Complications [...] and include thrombocytopenia, encephalitis and [...] tis. The importance of this infection lies in the devastating effect on the developing fetus during the first trimester (see Chapter 2, Section 2.6). The state of immunity to rubella should be determined in all pregnant women. If a pregnant woman whose immune status is unknown is exposed to a person with rubella infection, she should have an antibody test performed as an emergency measure. If she has been infected during the first 3 months of gestation and is not willing to undergo a therapeutic abortion, human immunoglobulin may provide some protection.

## Mumps

With the advent of the MMR vaccine, mumps is now a rare disease. Painful enlargement of one or more parotid and occasionally submandibular glands usually follows a long incubation period (16–21 days). The swelling settles within 7–10 days. Aseptic meningitis is a common complication (60%), is often asymptomatic, and usually follows a benign course. Rare complications include sensorineural deafness and, in older children, epididymo-orchitis, which may result in male infertility and pancreatitis.

## Chickenpox (varicella)

Primary infection with the varicella-zoster virus causes chickenpox. The reactivation of dormant viral infection in the dorsal root ganglia manifests as zoster. In chickenpox, the rash appears first on the trunk after an incubation period of 14–16 days and little prodrome. The spots appear in crops, progressing rapidly from macule to papule to vesicle, and spread centripetally; they may appear in the mouth and mucous membranes. The pustules start drying by 48–72 hours after they first appear, and the child is no longer infective once all the lesions have scabbed. The commonest complication of chickenpox is secondary bacterial infections with either *Staphylococcus aureus* or *Streptococcus pyogenes*. Meningoencephalitis and acute cerebellitis are well-recognised neurological complications. Pneumonia can be either primary or secondary to varicella infection, and rarely the rash can be haemorrhagic, both conditions being associated with considerable morbidity. Progressive disease, sometimes with hepatitis, is seen in the immunocompromised. A live attenuated varicella vaccine is available and is part of the universal immu-

...tion programme in the United States, but not in the United Kingdom and most of Europe.

## Herpes zoster

Herpes zoster usually presents as a self-limiting vesicular rash in a dermatomal distribution, with prodromal symptoms of localised pain, hyperaesthesia and pruritus. It can follow an indolent or a recurrent course in the immunosuppressed.

### Management

For those at risk, an attenuated live virus vaccine is available along with zoster immunoglobulin. Aciclovir, either orally or parenterally, is the drug of choice in those who have progressive disease or are immunocompromised.

## Herpes simplex infections

Infection with herpes simplex is common and usually symptomatic in about 10% of those infected. Herpesvirus type 1 (HSV1) is spread by infected saliva and transmission requires close personal contact. Primary infection may affect the mouth, skin or eye. Herpes type 2 (HSV2) is a genital infection, usually spread by sexual contact. Neonatal infections with HSV2 occur during birth from the mother's genital tract, and with HSV1 during the postpartum period. Acute gingivostomatitis, keratoconjunctivitis and recurrent cold sores are common manifestations. Severe infections can occur in those with eczema (eczema herpeticum). The most feared complication is HSV1 encephalitis, which if untreated has a mortality rate of 70%. The drug of choice again is aciclovir.

## Infectious mononucleosis

Glandular fever is the best-known clinical syndrome caused by Epstein–Barr virus (EBV). It is characterised by systemic somatic complaints consisting primarily of fever and sore throat. There is an exudative tonsillitis, the lymph nodes are enlarged and the spleen is often palpable. A macular rash is often seen, particularly if ampicillin has been given. Complications are rare and include splenic rupture, airway obstruction, haemolytic anaemia, aplastic anaemia, myocarditis, interstitial pneumonia, and neurological manifestations such as ataxia, peripheral neuropathy, Guillain–Barré and Reye syndromes. A blood count will usually reveal raised white cells with an absolute mononuclear cytosis, and EBV IgM antibodies are raised in the acute phase, followed by IgG antibodies 10 days later.

## Poliomyelitis

Poliovirus is an enterovirus transmitted by the faeco-enteral route. The virus first multiplies in Peyer patches in the small intestine and then (about 10 days later) undergoes a viraemic phase. Most children are asymptomatic, though some can have non-specific flu-like symptoms. Some children can have myalgia with meningeal signs but no paralysis. In those children in whom anterior horn cells are destroyed, flaccid paralysis ensues. Life-threatening paralysis of the respiratory muscles occurs in those with high spinal, bulbospinal and bulbar poliomyelitis. Recovery is slow and can take as long as 18 months. Any residual paralysis after that is likely to be permanent, and affected muscles will atrophy and fibrose. Immunisation has eradicated the disease in many countries, and it is hoped to achieve worldwide eradication in the first decade of the new millennium. Vaccine-related paralytic poliomyelitis can occur with the oral rather than the injectable vaccine, and for this reason most countries have changed their immunisation programmes to incorporate IPV rather than OPV.

## Human immunodeficiency virus

Paediatric acquired immunodeficiency syndrome (AIDS) is caused by HIV types 1 (HIV-1) and 2 (HIV-2), the latter particularly in the African continent. Children are infected by vertical transmission, transfusion of contaminated blood products, intravenous drug usage or by sexual transmission. In the UK, almost all children with HIV-1 infection have acquired it from their mothers. Table 64 describes the clinical spectrum of HIV infection in children. The early diagnosis of infection in children born to HIV-positive mothers can be made by detecting viral nucleic acid by PCR. Approximately 93% of infants with HIV infection will be positive by 2 weeks of age. Vertical infection can be excluded if two HIV DNA PCR tests performed at 1 month and beyond, and a third at 4 months or older, are negative. Alternatively, an infant with two blood samples negative for HIV antibody obtained after 6 months of age and at an interval of at least 1 month, can also be considered not to be infected.

### Management

Antiretroviral therapy (ART) is indicated for most HIV-infected individuals. ART includes drugs that inhibit viral reverse transcriptase and protease. Reverse transcriptase inhibitors include nucleoside analogues (zidovudine, didanosine, lamivudine, stavudine, zalcitabine) and non-nucleoside analogues (efavirenz,

**Table 64** Clinical categories of paediatric HIV infection

| Category | Symptoms |
|---|---|
| N | Asymptomatic |
| A | Mildly symptomatic; at least two of: <br>Lymphadenopathy <br>Hepatomegaly <br>Splenomegaly <br>Parotitis <br>Rash, ear, nose and throat infections |
| B | Moderately symptomatic: <br>Single episode of a severe bacterial infection <br>Lymphocytic interstitial pneumonia <br>Anaemia, neutropenia, thrombocytopenia <br>Cardiomyopathy, nephropathy <br>Hepatitis, diarrhoea <br>Candidiasis, severe varicella-zoster or herpes simplex virus infection |
| C | Severely symptomatic (AIDS): <br>Two serious bacterial infections <br>Encephalopathy <br>Wasting syndrome <br>Opportunistic infections <br>Disseminated mycobacterial disease <br>Cancer (Kaposi's sarcoma, lymphoma) |

## 10.6 Miscellaneous conditions

### Learning objectives

You should:

- know the clinical features and management of malaria in children

- know the clinical features and management of Kawasaki disease

### Malaria

Malaria may well be one of the world's most deadly infectious diseases. Forty per cent of the world's population is exposed to the disease, and there are over 500 million episodes per year. About 3 million people are thought to die of the disease every year. In Africa, one in every five childhood deaths is attributed to malaria. For practical purposes malaria may be regarded as two disease entities, the more dangerous being that caused by infection with *Plasmodium falciparum*. The other is caused by *P. vivax*, *P. ovale* or *P. malariae*. The severity of clinical features correlates with the degree of parasitaemia.

Children with malaria typically develop fever, vomiting, headache and flu-like symptoms and have a palpable spleen. If untreated, the disease may progress rapidly (often within 24 hours) to convulsions, coma and death. Of the more than 500 000 African children who develop cerebral malaria (a severe form of the disease that affects the brain) each year, 10–20% die and approximately 7% are left with permanent neurological damage. Malaria is a major cause of anaemia in many parts of the world. Chronic anaemia may adversely affect a child's growth and intellectual development. Repeated episodes of malaria may lead to severe, life-threatening anaemia. Blood transfusions may save lives in these circumstances, but also expose the child to the risk of HIV and other bloodborne infections.

### Prevention and prophylaxis

Sleeping under insecticide-treated mosquito nets has been shown to decrease infections in young children, though the nets themselves are prohibitively expensive. All children travelling to areas endemic for malaria should receive chemoprophylaxis. Persuading young children to take antimalarial medications may be difficult because of the lack of paediatric formulations and the bitter taste of many drugs. Furthermore, some chemoprophylactic drugs are contraindicated in children. Chloroquine remains the drug of choice in areas

nevirapine, delavirdine). Protease inhibitors are a more powerful class of drugs and include ritonavir, saquinavir, indinavir, amprenavir, nelfinavir and lopinavir. Early studies using one or two drugs from the nucleoside analogue class showed some immunological and virological benefit, but the development of viral resistance to these drugs over time resulted in virological failure. More recently combination antiretroviral therapy or highly active antiretroviral therapy (HAART) has been shown to be more effective than monotherapy. Data indicate that good HIV suppression can be achieved with triple drug therapy including a protease inhibitor or a non-nucleoside reverse transcriptase inhibitor, indicating that at least three antiretroviral drugs should be given whenever possible. Suppression of virus to undetectable levels is the desired goal. Following adequate viral suppression, immunological recovery and immune restoration occurs, resulting in significant reductions in morbidity and mortality, particularly due to opportunistic infections. However, combination antiretroviral therapy requires high levels of adherence to prevent the development of drug resistance. These drugs are also associated with significant toxicity and side effects, particularly disorders of lipid metabolism and lipodystrophy. ART is also costly and therefore unavailable to the vast majority of HIV-infected individuals living in resource-poor countries.

where malaria remains sensitive to this drug, whereas mefloquine is the preferred agent in chloroquine-resistant areas. Chemoprophylaxis should be taken 1 week prior to travelling in an endemic area, and continued for 4–6 weeks after returning.

## Treatment

Most *P. vivax* infections are sensitive to chloroquine. As there is a latent hepatic (hypnozoite) stage of infection this may lead to disease recurrence and requires treatment with primaquine. *P. falciparum* infections are increasingly resistant to chloroquine and are currently treated with either quinine or atovaquone–proguanil.

Over the past decade, artemisinin compounds, such as artesunate, artemether and dihydroartemisinin are being used. These compounds produce a very rapid therapeutic response, are active against multidrug-resistant *P. falciparum* and are well tolerated. To date, no parasite resistance to these compounds has been detected. The WHO Roll Back Malaria Programme, which started in 2001, is using combination therapy of artemisin with other drugs as first-line treatment in areas highly endemic for the disease.

## Candidal infection

Thrush is a superficial mucosal infection with a *Candida* species that affects approximately 2–5% of newborns and is a causative agent of nappy dermatitis. Candidal vulvovaginitis will occur in as many as 75% of pubertal females.

## Management

Most candidal infections are superficial and can be treated with topical antifungals such as nystatin, clotrimazole or miconazole. Disseminated infection can occur in the immunocompromised child and may require treatment with fluconazole or amphotericin B.

## Mycoplasma infection

*Mycoplasma pneumoniae* is the only known human mycoplasmal pathogen. It is transmitted via droplet infection but is not a highly communicable disease. The peak incidence of infection occurs in the school-age group (5–15 years). Bronchopneumonia characterised by severe symptoms and a paucity of clinical signs is typical of early disease. X-ray findings are not pathognomonic, although unilateral dense infiltrates are seen mostly in the lower lobe. Bullous myringitis and infections of the skin, CNS, heart, blood and joints are rare complications. Diagnosis is based on rising titres of cold haemagglutinins and is often associated with a mild haemolytic anaemia that is Coombs' positive.

## Management

In general, mycoplasmal infection is a mild illness and patients rarely require hospitalisation. As the organism lacks a cell wall it is resistant to penicillin, and the macrolide antibiotics (i.e. erythromycin, clarithromycin) are the drugs of choice.

## Chlamydial infection

Chlamydiae are obligate intracellular bacteria. The recognised human pathogens include *Chlamydia trachomatis*, *C. pneumoniae* (TWAR) and *C. psittaci*. *C. trachomatis* is the causative agent of trachoma and lymphogranuloma venereum (LGV). Trachoma is the most important cause of preventable blindness in the world and is endemic in middle and southeast Asia. *C. trachomatis* is also responsible for a wide range of sexually transmitted infections in adults. Maternal cervical chlamydial infections can result in conjunctivitis in the neonate and pneumonia in early infancy. The TWAR agent is a major respiratory pathogen in school-aged children. As with *Mycoplasma pneumoniae*, it is known to trigger asthma and exacerbate pulmonary symptoms in those with cystic fibrosis. *C. psittaci* is the aetiological agent in psittacosis. Therapy is with either a macrolide antibiotic or a tetracycline.

## Kawasaki disease (mucocutaneous lymph node syndrome)

Kawasaki disease (KD) is an acute self-limiting multisystemic vasculitis of childhood of unknown cause. It is currently believed that KD involves an infectious trigger, and bacterial superantigens have been implicated as the cause. It affects children younger than 10 years, predominantly those under 3. The course of KD is divided into three clinical phases.

The **acute phase** is characterised by fever of more than 5 days' duration, conjunctival injection, mouth and lip inflammation, swelling and erythema of the hands and feet, rash, lymphadenopathy, aseptic meningitis, diarrhoea and hepatic dysfunction.

The **subacute phase** is a period when fever, rash and lymphadenopathy resolve but irritability, anorexia and conjunctival injection persist. Periungual desquamation of the fingers and toes, arthritis and arthralgia, myocardial dysfunction and thrombocytosis occur during this phase, which typically lasts from approximately 10 to 24 days of the illness. Other associated features include aseptic meningitis, hydrops of the gallbladder, otitis media, uveitis and extreme irritability in infants.

The **convalescent stage** begins when clinical signs disappear and continues until the erythrocyte sedimen-

**Box 65** Diagnostic criteria for Kawasaki disease

For a diagnosis of Kawasaki disease a child must have fever for at least 5 days and at least four of the features listed below:

1. Bilateral bulbar conjunctival injection without exudates
2. Erythematous mouth and pharynx, strawberry tongue and red, cracked lips
3. Polymorphous generalised erythematous rash
4. Induration of hands and feet with erythematous palms and soles or periungual desquamation
5. Acute non-suppurative cervical lymphadenopathy with at least one node of 1.5 cm in diameter

tation rate (ESR) returns to normal, usually 6–8 weeks after the onset.

## Diagnosis

As no confirmatory test exists the diagnosis is based on clinical criteria (Box 65), and clinicians must carefully exclude diseases that mimic KD. These include viral exanthems, drug reactions (e.g. Stevens Johnson syndrome), staphylococcal scalded skin syndrome, toxic shock syndrome and juvenile rheumatoid arthritis. In addition to the above clinical findings, KD causes aneurysm formation in medium-sized arteries, particularly the coronary arteries. These lesions are found in 25% of patients; they may persist, scar with stenosis, or resolve. Those who develop coronary thrombosis will require more aggressive treatment, including fibrinolytic therapy and angioplasty. Complications include myocardial infarction, which may occur during the acute illness or later, as a result of the coronary abnormalities.

## Management

An echocardiogram should be obtained early in the acute phase of the illness and 6–8 weeks later. Treatment consists of administering high-dose aspirin and intravenous immunoglobulin during the acute phase (until day 14 of the illness) and low-dose aspirin in the convalescent phase, with the goal of relieving acute illness and minimising sequelae. Although most respond rapidly, almost 10% of children do not improve clinically with treatment.

# Self-assessment: questions

## Multiple choice questions

1. Isolation is recommended:
   a. Until all lesions are crusted in chickenpox
   b. Until the fourth day of rash in measles
   c. Until 9 days after parotitis in mumps
   d. During the entire illness with respiratory syncytial virus infection
   e. Until 5 days of therapy are completed in pertussis.

2. The following drugs are useful in the management of Gram-negative organisms
   a. Gentamicin
   b. Vancomycin
   c. Pipercillin
   d. Linezolid
   e. Cefotaxime.

3. Rifampicin chemoprophylaxis is recommended for:
   a. Children with *Haemophilus influenzae* meningitis on discharge from hospital
   b. All household contacts of those with *H. influenzae* meningitis
   c. Close contacts of those with meningococcal meningitis
   d. Siblings of those with tuberculous meningitis
   e. Close contacts of those with lepromatous leprosy.

4. Coagulase-negative staphylococci are:
   a. The commonest cause of nosocomial bacteraemia
   b. The commonest pathogen involved in shunt meningitis
   c. Capable of causing native valve endocarditis
   d. Implicated in spontaneous peritonitis
   e. Best treated with glycopeptide antibiotics.

5. The following are true of the severe acute respiratory syndrome (SARS)
   a. It is caused by a DNA virus
   b. The commonest symptom is fever
   c. Ribavirin is the specific antiviral drug of choice
   d. The disease is spread by droplet infection
   e. The majority of those infected will have a fatal illness.

6. Viral infections associated with latent infections of the CNS include:
   a. Herpesviruses
   b. Measles
   c. Rubella
   d. Mumps
   e. Influenza.

7. Viruses capable of causing anterior horn cell disease include:
   a. Polioviruses
   b. Enterovirus
   c. Varicella
   d. Epstein–Barr virus
   e. Coxsackie virus A and B.

8. In HIV infection in children:
   a. The presence of antibody to HIV at 12 months of age is diagnostic
   b. A major cause of death in children is *Pneumocystis carinii* infection
   c. Measles, mumps and rubella vaccine is contraindicated
   d. All infants of HIV-positive mothers will contract the infection
   e. Persistent thrombocytopenia may be the first clinical sign.

9. Mosquito-borne illnesses include:
   a. Malaria
   b. Filaria
   c. Tularaemia
   d. Leishmaniasis
   e. Onchocerciasis.

10. Parvovirus infections can cause:
    a. Aplastic anaemia
    b. Congenital deformities
    c. 'Slapped cheek' disease
    d. Fetal hydrops
    e. Prodromal high fever prior to the appearance of a rash.

11. Primary pulmonary tuberculosis is often characterised by:
    a. A positive Mantoux test
    b. Pleural effusion
    c. Non-specific symptoms
    d. Paroxysmal productive cough
    e. Erythema nodosum.

12. The following are examples of inactivated vaccines:
    a. BCG
    b. Yellow fever
    c. Pertussis
    d. Rabies
    e. Oral typhoid vaccine.

13. Drugs used in chemoprophylaxis are:
    a. Rifampicin
    b. Chloroquine
    c. Penicillin
    d. Erythromycin
    e. Co-trimoxazole.

14. The following are often associated with human herpesvirus 6 infections:
    a. Roseola infantum
    b. Febrile seizures
    c. Neutropenia
    d. Gingivostomatitis
    e. Rapid resolution of symptoms with aciclovir.

15. The following agents are common causes of exudative tonsillopharyngitis:
    a. Coxsackie virus
    b. Epstein–Barr virus
    c. β-Haemolytic streptococci
    d. Adenovirus
    e. *Corynebacterium*.

16. Vesicular skin lesions are seen in the following infections:
    a. Varicella
    b. *Pseudomonas aeruginosa*
    c. Human herpesvirus 6
    d. Staphylococcal
    e. Coxsackie virus.

17. The following infections are correctly matched with the drug of choice:
    a. Tuberculosis and gentamicin
    b. Mycoplasmal pneumonia and tetracycline
    c. Scabies and miconazole
    d. Pediculosis and malathion
    e. Methicillin-resistant staphylococci and vancomycin.

18. Of the commonly seen fungal infections in childhood:
    a. Ringworm is best treated with griseofulvin
    b. Candidal vulvovaginitis is a very common infection
    c. Pulmonary aspergillosis is a problem of the immunosuppressed
    d. HIV infection is the most common predisposing factor for disseminated cryptococcosis
    e. Candidal paronychia is best treated with topical therapy.

## Case histories

### Case history 1

> A 3-year-old boy belonging to a community of travellers is brought to A&E with a history of fever, cough and coryza for 4 days, and anorexia for 2 days. On examination he is alert but tired-looking, with a temperature of 40°C, pulse rate 136/min and respiratory rate 52/min. You suspect measles.

1. What additional features in the history and examination will help you make this diagnosis?
2. What are the potential complications of measles virus infections?
3. The chest X-ray shows fine infiltrates bilaterally and the pulse oximeter shows a saturation of 92% in air. Explain these findings.
4. How will you manage this child?
5. On questioning there are a total of 30 people in this commune, comprising adults and children. What would you do to prevent any further cases of measles, and what are the potential side effects of immunisation?

### Case history 2

> For the case histories of children with fever listed below, select the most likely cause from the following:
>
> **Viruses**
> Coxsackie virus
> Herpes simplex virus
> Adenovirus
> Epstein–Barr virus
> **Bacteria**
> Streptococci
> Staphylococci
> Pertussis
> *Pneumococcus* sp.
> *Pseudomonas* sp.
> *Haemophilus influenzae*
> **Others**
> Kawasaki disease
> Malaria
> *Chlamydia*
> *Mycobacteria*

1. A 5-year-old child presents with fever and an abscess on the sole of his left foot. A thorn penetrated it 7 days ago while he was out in the garden, and since then the foot has become swollen and tender and today the puncture site has been discharging bluish-green pus.

2. A 12-year-old has a 2-week history of fatigue, fever and sore throat. On examination she has cervical lymphadenopathy and splenomegaly. The white cell count is $5 \times 10^9$/L, with many atypical mononuclear cells, and the serum aspartate aminotransferase (AST) is 200 U/L.

3. A 3-year-old presents with an acute onset of fever and dysuria. On examination of his urine there is macroscopic haematuria. There is antecedent history of an upper respiratory tract infection 1 week previously. He is otherwise well and normotensive. The full blood count is normal; urine culture is sterile and ASO (antistreptolysin O) and DNAase B titres are not elevated.

4. A 4-year-old presents with fever, puffy eyes and oliguria of 4 days' duration. Urine analysis is normal and the chest X-ray shows an enlarged heart.

## Case history 3

> A 10-year-old boy woke feeling slightly unwell with a low-grade fever, and stayed in bed. His mother looked in on him at 9.30 am and he seemed rather subdued, but by 11.45 am she had difficulty in waking him. He appeared to be delirious, with cold hands and feet despite a fever of 39.5°C. His mother phoned the family doctor urgently.

1. What additional information should the doctor ask for?
2. What advice should the family practitioner give over the phone?

> The boy is rushed to hospital shortly after the telephone conversation with the family doctor. In A&E the duty paediatric registrar finds a febrile, semiconscious boy with good pulses but cold peripheries, and records the diagnosis 'compensated shock' in the case file.

3. What other clinical signs would confirm or support this diagnosis of shock?

> On closer inspection the registrar notices several small-to-medium irregular reddish bruise-like macular lesions over the trunk and all four limbs (Fig. 96).

4. Where else may these lesions appear?
5. What diagnosis should be considered at this stage?

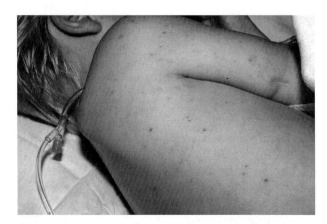

**Fig. 96**

> The boy's condition continues to deteriorate rapidly, with deepening unconsciousness and a disseminating rash, and 25 minutes after admission he develops a thready pulse and central cyanosis.

6. What process is evolving at this stage?
7. Briefly outline the plan of management for this boy.

## Short notes

Write short notes on the following:

1. A pregnant woman has been newly diagnosed to be HIV positive. What measures can you take to decrease the risk of vertical transmission?
2. The investigation of a child with pyrexia of unknown origin (PUO).

## OSCE questions

### OSCE 1
a. What is shown on Figure 97?
b. How would you treat this boy?

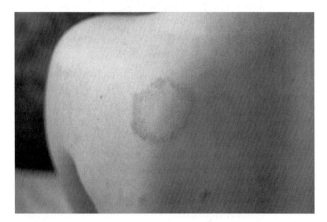

**Fig. 97**

## OSCE 2

a. What is shown on Figure 98?
b. What steps would you take in the management of this child?

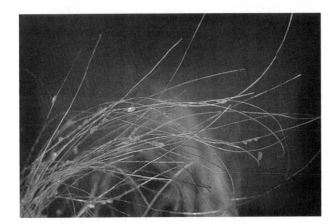

**Fig. 98**

## OSCE 3

a. Describe the rash shown in Figures 99 and 100 as accurately as possible.
b. What is the most likely diagnosis?
c. List three possible complications.

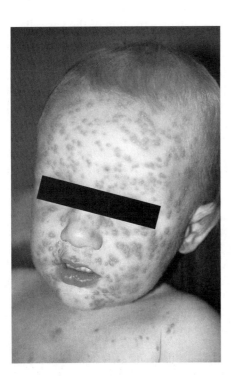

**Fig. 99**

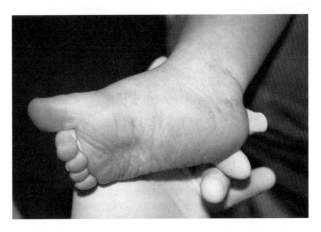

**Fig. 100**

## OSCE 4

a. What is the diagnosis/lesions shown in Figure 101?
b. What is the underlying pathological cause?
c. What is the natural history of this condition?

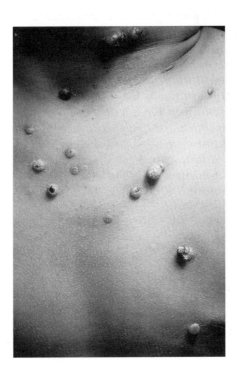

**Fig. 101**

# Self-assessment: answers

## Multiple choice answers

1. a. **True.** Moist lesions contain active virus.
   b. **True.** Infectivity is from the onset of the prodromal period until the fourth day of the onset of rash.
   c. **True.** Mumps is transmissible from several days before and after the classic swelling(s) appear.
   d. **True.** The most important preventive measure to prevent nosocomial infection is isolation of affected hospitalised children and infants.
   e. **True.** Antibiotics shorten the infectivity period but not the duration of illness.

2. a. **True.** Aminoglycosides (gentamicin, tobramycin, amikacin etc) are the mainstay in the treatment of Gram-negative infections.
   b. **False.** Vancomycin is a glycopeptide antibiotic and acts on the cell wall of Gram-positive organisms.
   c. **True.** Pipercillin is a class of penicillin compounds with activity against *Pseudomonas* species. It is usually used along with the β-lactamase inhibitor tazobactam.
   d. **False.** Linezolid is a new generation of antibiotics (oxazolidinone) active against Gram-positive organisms. It is primarily used for the treatment of glycopeptide-resistant organisms.
   e. **True.** Cefotaxime is a third-generation cephalosporin with a broad-spectrum activity against both Gram-positive and Gram-negative organisms.

3. a. **True.** Nasopharyngeal colonisation may not be successfully eradicated otherwise.
   b. **True.** Unvaccinated children under the age of 4 have a high risk of developing invasive disease.
   c. **True.** In epidemics, the secondary attack rate in household contacts may be as high as 5%.
   d. **False.** Meningitis is not an open infection and is not infectious; however, siblings and other contacts should be screened for tuberculosis (Mantoux and chest X-ray).
   e. **False.** Chemoprophylaxis in close contacts of leprosy has not been shown to be of any benefit.

4. a. **True.** This results from increased usage of percutaneous intravenous devices.
   b. **True.** Signs and symptoms may not be overt and diagnosis delayed.
   c. **True.** Though infection of a prosthetic valve is more common.
   d. **False.** This is associated with *Pneumococcus* spp.
   e. **True.** For example vancomycin, teicoplanin.

5. a. **False.** The causative agent is a coronavirus, SARS-associated coronavirus (SARS-CoV), which is an RNA virus.
   b. **True.** Other symptoms are headache and diarrhoea. Most people will develop pneumonia.
   c. **False.** Though this drug has been used empirically, there is no evidence to suggest that it is active against SARS-CoV.
   d. **True.**
   e. **False.** Although this is a serious and highly infectious disease, more than 90% of people will survive their illness.

6. a. **True.** Latent activation of the varicella-zoster virus in the geniculate ganglion produces facial palsy, loss of taste, tinnitus, vertigo and hearing loss (Ramsay–Hunt syndrome).
   b. **True.** Subacute sclerosing panencephalitis can occur.
   c. **True.** Progressive rubella panencephalitis can occur.
   d. **False.** It is a cause of acute CNS infections.
   e. **False.**

7. a. **True.** Poliovirus directly affects the anterior horn cells.
   b. **True.** It causes a non-polio paralytic illness.
   c. **False.** Though varicella infection is associated with a cerebellitis.
   d. **False.** This is not a neurotropic virus; it targets B lymphocytes.
   e. **True.** These are enteroviruses like poliovirus and can cause non-polio paralytic illness.

8. a. **False.** Antibody is seen only after 15 months of age.
   b. **True.** It causes a fatal pneumonia.
   c. **False.** Live viral vaccines can be safely given.
   d. **False.** Usually only 20–35% will become infected.

e. **True**. Isolated anaemia or neutropenia may also occur.

9. a. **True**. Bites from previously infected female anopheline mosquitoes.
   b. **True**. Both anopheline and culicine mosquitoes can infect, according to the geographic locale.
   c. **True**. Though it can be transmitted by other vectors as well.
   d. **False**. The vector is a sandfly.
   e. **False**. The vector is a blackfly.

10. a. **True**. It occurs particularly in those with chronic haemolytic anaemias.
    b. **True**. Infection in pregnancy more commonly may result in fetal hydrops, death and miscarriage.
    c. **True**. This is the first stage of the disease.
    d. **True**.
    e. **False**. This seen in exanthem subitum caused by human herpesvirus 6; fever is unusual in parvovirus infections in children.

11. a. **True**. It is usually positive 4–8 weeks after infection.
    b. **True**. This follows rupture of a subpleural focus into the pleural cavity.
    c. **True**. Symptoms such as fever, malaise and anorexia are often seen.
    d. **False**. A productive cough is unusual in primary tuberculosis.
    e. **True**. Usually occurs in the first 4–8 weeks of infection.

12. a. **False**. A live attenuated vaccine.
    b. **False**. A live attenuated vaccine.
    c. **True**. Whole-cell killed vaccines are now being replaced by acellular vaccines in some countries.
    d. **True**. Human diploid cell vaccine.
    e. **False**. A live attenuated vaccine.

13. a. **True**. It is used for close contacts of those with *H. influenzae* and meningococcal meningitis.
    b. **True**. It is used for those travelling to regions with endemic malaria.
    c. **True**. This is used as prophylaxis against streptococci in post splenectomy patients.
    d. **True**. It is used in non-immunised infants who have been exposed to pertussis.
    e. **True**. It is used to prevent *Pneumocystis carinii* infections in the immunocompromised host.

14. a. **True**. This is also known as exanthem subitum.
    b. **True**. Febrile seizures can occur in 15–35% of those with an acute febrile illness caused by HHV-6.
    c. **True**. Often occurs with lymphocytosis.
    d. **False**. Though it is commonly seen with herpes simplex virus infections.
    e. **False**. HHV-6 is only partially sensitive to aciclovir.

15. a. **True**. It causes a condition called herpangina.
    b. **True**. It occurs in the majority of infections related to EBV.
    c. **True**. This is the commonest bacterial cause.
    d. **True**. Acute febrile pharyngitis is the most common adenoviral infection of childhood.
    e. **True**. Though the membranous pharyngitis caused by *C. diphtheriae* is better known.

16. a. **True**. The lesions are a hallmark of chickenpox.
    b. **True**. It causes bluish fluid-filled vesicles called ecthyma gangrenosum.
    c. **False**. HHV-6 causes a macular rash.
    d. **True**. Bullous impetigo is fairly common.
    e. **True**. The lesions are a component of the hand–foot–mouth syndrome.

17. a. **False**. Although *M. tuberculosis* is sensitive to the aminoglycosides, the prolonged use of this group of drugs is not recommended and their use is restricted to organisms shown to be resistant to other drugs.
    b. **False**. The use of tetracycline is restricted in children, and erythromycin is the drug of choice in this case.
    c. **False**. Miconazole is a topical antifungal, and topical malathion is recommended.
    d. **True**.
    e. **True**. An alternative is teicoplanin.

18. a. **False**. It is best treated with topical antifungals such as clotrimazole and miconazole. Griseofulvin is reserved only for highly refractory or ungual cutaneous mycoses.
    b. **True**. It is seen in up to 75%.
    c. **True**. It is especially a problem in those with chronic neutropenia receiving a mixture of antibiotics for a length of time.
    d. **True**. Though otherwise normal individuals may develop meningitis or pneumonia.
    e. **True**.

## Case history answers

### Case history 1

1. Has the child been immunised? The uptake of immunisation is low in the traveller community. Has there been contact with other children with a similar history, or children with a rash, within the past 2 weeks (incubation period of measles)? Does the child have a rash that is maculopapular and localised mainly to the face and trunk? Are there Koplik spots (sand-like granules in the pharynx), and is there coryza and conjunctival inflammation?

2. Respiratory
   Otitis media
   Croup (laryngotracheobronchitis)
   Tracheitis
   Measles (giant cell) pneumonia
   Secondary bacterial pneumonia
   Conjunctivitis and keratitis
   Gastroenteritis
   Cancrum oris
   Meningoencephalitis
   Malnutrition, loss of appetite
   Haemorrhagic measles
   Subacute sclerosing panencephalitis (SSPE).

3. Viral interstitial pneumonia
   Secondary bacterial pneumonia
   Hypoxaemia secondary to a lower respiratory tract infection.

4. This child is unwell, with a lower respiratory tract infection. He is still contagious and will need admission into an isolation unit until at least 4 days after the appearance of the rash. He will need paracetamol or ibuprofen, oxygen, intravenous fluids and broad-spectrum antibiotics to cover secondary bacterial pneumonia. The diagnosis can be confirmed by a positive serological test for measles specific IgM antibody.

5. Consider immunising all children and adolescents with live attenuated MMR vaccine. In an outbreak, infants as young as 6 months may be immunised. All children should not be allowed to mix with others outside the commune until at least 2 weeks after the onset of rash in the last case of measles. The vaccine is usually well tolerated. Fever, transient rashes, transient thrombocytopenia and rarely meningoencephalitis are known complications. Prior testing for egg allergy is not required, and there is no evidence that MMR is associated with the aetiology of autism or inflammatory bowel disease.

### Case history 2

1. *Pseudomonas* sp. Whereas staphylococcal and streptococcal infections may also present in this fashion, *Pseudomonas* spp. are common garden commensals and are often found on decaying wood. They produce a green-blue pigment called pyocyanin that gives the pus its characteristic colour.

2. **Epstein–Barr virus**. Although adenovirus and streptococcal infections may present with a sore throat, the systemic features are atypical of these infections and the child is in the wrong age group for Kawasaki disease. The atypical large monocytes are, moreover, typical of the disease and give it the name of infectious mononucleosis.

3. **Adenovirus**. The most common infectious causes of haematuria are bacterial or viral cystitis and poststreptococcal glomerulonephritis. The last is associated with hypertension, raised streptococcal titres and painless haematuria. In the absence of a bacterial isolate, viral cystitis must be considered and adenovirus 11 is a common culprit.

4. **Coxsackie virus**. Although this child is in the right age group for Kawasaki disease and clearly has congestive cardiac failure, the onset is too acute and no other features of the disease are present. This child probably has viral myocarditis, and Coxsackie virus B1–4 are known to cause both myocarditis and pericarditis.

### Case history 3

1. He should ask about any recent infection, recent contacts and the presence of any rash.

2. Initiate temperature control, e.g. strip, cool, paracetamol, sponging; call for emergency ambulance.

3. Prolonged capillary return
   Temperature differential
   Weak pulses
   Tachycardia
   Decreased skin turgor
   Sunken eyes
   Decreased renal output
   *No to hypotension/altered consciousness in this case.*

4. The lesions may appear on mucous membranes, sclerae and retinae.

5. Meningococcal septicaemia (with or without meningitis) is the most important diagnosis. The rash is indicative of septicaemia, and a diagnosis of 'meningitis' alone is inadequate.

6. The clinical signs suggest a fall in blood pressure and are indicative of decompensated shock.

7. Resuscitate by securing ABC (**A**irway, **B**reathing and **C**irculation).
   Give high-flow oxygen and start ventilation if necessary.
   Set up IV infusion (ideally two or three large cannulae).
   Initiate rapid fluid replacement via boluses of 20 mL/kg of (initially) crystalloid and colloid.
   Start IV antibiotics (ideally ceftriaxone).
   Start inotropic support.

## Short notes answers

1. The risk of transmission of virus from a seropositive untreated mother to her infant is estimated to be 13–40%. In the non-breastfeeding population, 25–40% of transmissions occur in utero. The maternal viral load and CD4 counts are predictive for transmission and should be checked. Oral zidovudine should be given antenatally to pregnant women, beginning at 14 weeks' gestation and continued throughout pregnancy. Intravenous zidovudine should be given during labour and at delivery. The newborn should then receive the drug for the first 6 weeks of life. This can reduce perinatal HIV transmission by two-thirds. Postpartum transmission occurs through breastfeeding, and where possible this needs to be discontinued. Zidovudine may cause anaemia in the neonatal period and this requires monitoring. Other drugs that have been used to decrease perinatal transmission include lamivudine and nevirapine. In practice, most mothers in western countries will be on combination antiretroviral therapy. The potential effects of these combinations on the fetus are unknown, and the current recommendation is to continue the treatment, ensuring that zidovudine is part of it.

2. Ordering a large number of tests in every child with PUO is a waste of time and money. Diagnostic tests most likely to provide a prompt and definitive diagnosis should be used. The pace of evaluation should match the seriousness of the illness. Tests may be required more quickly in a seriously ill patient, whereas in a chronically ill child evaluation may proceed more logically and in an ambulatory setting. A detailed clinical history, which will need to be repeated as patients often remember important details on subsequent questioning, and regular thorough physical examination are the mainstay of diagnosis of PUO. A list of possible investigations is given in Table 65.

**Table 65** Investigative work-up for PUO

| Test | Diagnostic importance |
|---|---|
| **Blood, urine, skin tests** | |
| White cell count | Often elevated in bacterial infections |
| Platelets | Reduced with hypersplenism; raised with connective tissue disease |
| Blood smear | Malaria |
| Blood cultures (aerobic/anaerobic) | Very important and repeated, with best yield during temperature 'spikes' |
| Urine analysis/culture | Urinary tract infection |
| Tuberculin skin testing | Tuberculosis |
| | |
| **X-ray examination** | |
| Chest | |
| Sinuses, mastoid | |
| Bones | |
| | |
| **Bone marrow examination** | |
| Histology | Malignancies |
| Culture | Fungi, leishmaniasis, mycobacteria, salmonella |
| | |
| **Serology** | |
| Viral titres | Infectious mononucleosis, toxoplasmosis |
| Autoantibodies | Connective tissue disease |
| | |
| **Radioactive scans** | |
| CT or MRI imaging | Gallium or technetium scans for osteomyelitis, deep-seated abscesses |
| | |
| **Invasive** | |
| Biopsy | |
| Endoscopy | |

## OSCE answers

### OSCE 1
a. *Tinea corporis* or fungal skin rash or ringworm.
b. Topical antifungal cream for a prolonged period (usually around 10–14 days).

### OSCE 2
a. Head lice or nits.
b. Anti-louse shampoo for the child, any siblings and household members/contacts.
   Comb out dead lice/eggs.
   Advise on hair hygiene/regular washings.
   Inform school in order to screen and treat affected classmates.

### OSCE 3
a. Vesicular, erythematous, maculopapular vesicles/lesions over face, hair, trunk, soles, centripetal.
b. Chickenpox/varicella infection.
c. Meningitis or encephalitis.
   Haemorrhagic chickenpox.
   Chickenpox/giant cell pneumonia.

### OSCE 4
a. Molluscum contagiosum or viral warts.
b. Viral skin infection.
c. Self-resolution once body mounts adequate immunity after prolonged period (usually several years).

# Blood disorders and neoplasia

**11.1** Development of the haematopoietic system  233

**11.2** Anaemias  233

**11.3** Disorders of bleeding and coagulation  240

**11.4** The neoplastic disorders  244

Self-assessment: questions  251

Self-assessment: answers  255

## Overview

The assessment of a child with a haematological disorder involves taking a detailed history. You will need to know how to examine for pallor and lymph node enlargement as well as palpate the abdomen for hepatosplenomegaly. Diagnosis includes interpretation of common laboratory tests, and you will need to know the range of normal values, what the abnormal values signify, and what subsequent definitive diagnostic tests are indicated. As blood component therapy is part of the management of many paediatric disorders, you should also know the indications and drawbacks of administering blood products. Malignancy is rare in childhood, and although symptoms are often non-specific, you need to appreciate the scenarios that may suggest the presence of a malignant disorder, and to have a working knowledge of the more common types. Management of these disorders is complex and requires a multidisciplinary approach.

## 11.1 Development of the haematopoietic system

Developmental haematopoiesis occurs in three anatomic stages: mesoblastic, hepatic and myeloid. Mesoblastic haematopoiesis occurs in extraembryonic structures, principally in the yolk sac, and begins in the third week of gestation. By about 6 weeks of gestation the extraembryonic sites begin to ablate and hepatic haematopoiesis is initiated. By the 10th–12th weeks mesoblastic haematopoiesis ceases and a small amount of haematopoiesis is evident in the bone marrow. The liver remains the predominant organ until the last trimester of pregnancy.

The haemoglobin molecule is a tetramer made up of two polypeptide chains, each having an iron-containing haem group attached. The major haemoglobin (Hb) of the normal adult (HbA) is made up of one pair each of $\alpha$ and $\beta$ polypeptide chains. HbA is therefore represented as $\alpha_2\beta_2$. The $\alpha$ and $\beta$ chains differ in both the number and sequence of amino acids, and their synthesis is directed by separate genes. As shown in Table 66, six different haemoglobins can be detected in the blood cells of the embryo, fetus, child and adult. Some HbA can be detected even in the earliest embryos, and antenatal diagnosis of major $\beta$-chain haemoglobinopathies such as thalassaemia is therefore possible. Table 67 shows normal haematological values.

## 11.2 Anaemias

## Learning objectives

You should:

- know the causes and clinical features of anaemia in childhood

- know the diagnosis and management of iron deficiency anaemia

- know the differential diagnosis of a child with chronic anaemia and a splenomegaly

- know the aetiology, diagnosis and management of hereditary spherocytosis, sickle cell disease, thalassaemia syndromes and G6PD deficiency

### Blood loss

Anaemia is defined as a reduction of the red blood cell (RBC) volume or haemoglobin below the normal range. Anaemias can be classified on the basis of the size of the red blood cells, which may be large (macrocytic), small (microcytic) or normal-sized (normocytic) (Box 66). The normocytic anaemias can be differentiated

**Table 66** Haemoglobins present at different ages

| Hb type | Chains | Timescales |
|---|---|---|
| Embryonic haemoglobins | | |
| Gower – 1 | $\zeta_2\varepsilon_2$ | Disappears by 3 months |
| Gower – 2 | $\alpha_2\varepsilon_2$ | Disappears by 3 months |
| Hb Portland | $\zeta_2\gamma_2$ | |
| Fetal haemoglobin | | |
| HbF | $\alpha_2\gamma_2$ | Predominant haemoglobin at 8 weeks; 90% of haemoglobin at 6 months and 70% at birth. Less than 2% at 1 year of age and throughout life |
| Adult haemoglobins | | |
| HbA | $\alpha_2\beta_2$ | Detectable early in the fetus and forms 5–10% of haemoglobin at 6 months of gestation and 30% at birth |
| HbA$_2$ | $\alpha_2\delta_2$ | 2–3% during adult life, 1 : 30 ratio of HbA$_2$ : HbA |

**Table 67** Normal haematological values

| | Haemoglobin (g/dL) | MCV (fL) | White cell (×10⁹/L) | Platelets (×10⁹/L) |
|---|---|---|---|---|
| Cord blood | 13.7–20.1 | 110 | 9–30 | 150–450 at all ages |
| 3 months | 9.5–14.5 | 110 | 6–18 | |
| 6 months to 6 years | 10.5–14.0 | 70–74 | 6–15 | |
| 7–12 years | 11.0–16.0 | 76–80 | 4.5–13.5 | |
| Adult | 12.0–18.0 | 80 | 5–10 | |

**Box 66** Causes of microcytic and macrocytic anaemias

**Microcytic anaemia (MCV <75 fL)**
Iron deficiency
Thalassaemia syndromes
Lead poisoning
Chronic infections
Sideroblastic
Pulmonary haemosiderosis

**Macrocytic anaemia (MCV >100 fL)**
Folic acid deficiency
Vitamin B$_{12}$ deficiency
Orotic aciduria
Liver disease
Hypothyroidism
Drug-related damage

## Anaemia with decreased red cell production

Normally, a drop in the haemoglobin level and the accompanying 'anoxia' stimulates the production of erythropoietin (Epo). Red cell production by the marrow in response to Epo may expand several-fold to compensate for a mild-to-moderate reduction in the red cell lifespan (normally 120 days). In a variety of anaemias the bone marrow loses its usual capacity for sustained production and expansion of the red blood cell mass. In these instances there is a decrease in the number of erythrocyte precursors or reticulocytes in the blood. With elevated Epo levels the absolute number of reticulocytes should rise. A normal or low absolute reticulocyte count in anaemia is indicative of ineffective erythropoiesis or relative bone marrow failure.

### Physiological anaemia of infancy

The fetus lives in a relatively hypoxic environment and therefore has a higher haemoglobin and haematocrit than older children. From birth to 6–8 weeks there is a progressive decline in haemoglobin levels, termed the *physiological anaemia of infancy*. This is the result of several factors, including the rise in oxygen saturation to 95%, resulting in a drop in Epo levels while renal receptors mature. The need for an increase in the RBC production is further compounded by the rapid increase in body size, as well as the shorter fetal RBC lifespan of 90 days. In full-term infants, when the haemoglobin level has fallen to 9–11 g/dL at 2–3 months of age, erythropoiesis resumes. In contrast, because iron stores are largely acquired by the fetus in the third trimester, the decline in haemoglobin in preterm infants may be more extreme and rapid. In the latter group, RBC transfusions may be necessary to provide adequate oxygenation. Oral iron will only be useful after 4–8 weeks, as Epo is not active until then. In very low-birthweight infants recombinant human Epo (r-HuEpo, epoietin) has been used successfully in conjunction with iron from birth to decrease transfusion requirements.

by the reticulocyte count (immature red cells, normally comprising 1% of total red cells) and the Coombs' test (which detects rhesus antibodies on the surface of red cells) (Fig. 102). A decrease in the circulating haemoglobin leads to a decrease in the oxygen-carrying capacity of the blood. Physiological adjustments to anaemia include increased cardiac output and shunting of blood towards vital organs. The level of 2,3-diphosphoglycerol (2,3-DPG) increases in the red cell, with a resultant 'shift to the right' of the oxygen-dissociation curve and a more complete transfer of oxygen to the tissues. Pallor is manifest in the conjunctiva, mucous membranes and skin when the haemoglobin level falls to 7–8 g/dL. With increasingly lower levels, weakness, tachypnoea, tachycardia, dyspnoea, cardiac dilatation and, ultimately, congestive heart failure ensue.

## Iron-deficiency anaemia

Iron-deficiency anaemia is the most common haematological disease of infancy and childhood (Box 67). The newborn infant contains about 0.5 g of iron, whereas the adult content is estimated at about 5 g. Accordingly, to maintain a positive iron balance in childhood, about 1 mg iron must be absorbed each day.

As the high haemoglobin concentration of the newborn falls during the first 2–3 months of life, considerable amounts of iron are reclaimed and stored. These are usually sufficient for blood formation in the first 6–9 months of life. In term infants, anaemia caused solely by inadequate dietary iron is unusual before 4–6 months but becomes common at 9–24 months of age.

Thereafter, it is relatively uncommon. The usual dietary pattern observed in infants with iron-deficiency anaemia is the consumption of large amounts of cow's milk and of foods not supplemented with iron.

### Signs and symptoms

Chronic anaemia is remarkably well tolerated, with very few symptoms and signs. As the child becomes progressively iron deficient and the haemoglobin drops to below 8.0 g/dL, symptoms such as pica and tiredness may be seen and pallor observed on examination. At haemoglobin levels less than 5 g/dL the child may be irritable and anorexic and, in addition to pallor, examination may reveal tachycardia, signs of congestive cardiac failure, a flow murmur and koilonychia (spooning of the nails on the fingers and toes). The spleen is palpable in 10–15% of children with iron-deficiency anaemia.

### Laboratory diagnosis

Haemoglobinisation of the RBCs is affected and the cell is misshapen (poikilocytosis), small (microcytosis) and pale (hypochromic). The decrease in iron leads to a decrease in serum ferritin and iron and an increase in the iron-binding capacity. This is diagnostic of iron-deficiency anaemia. The absolute reticulocyte count indicates an insufficient response to anaemia, though nucleated RBCs can be seen in the peripheral smear. The white cells are normal, but thrombocytosis (600–1000 × 10^9/L) or thrombocytopenia may be present. The bone marrow is hypercellular, with erythroid hyper-

---

**Box 67** Aetiology of acquired aplastic anaemia

**Idiopathic (immune-related)** aplastic anaemia occurs in 70%

**Secondary** aplastic anaemia occurs in response to:
Drugs: chemotherapeutic agents, chloramphenicol, sulphonamide, phenylbutazone, quinacrine
Chemicals: DDT, parathione
Toxins: carbon tetrachloride, toluene, glue
Irradiation
Infections: HIV, hepatitis, rubella, cytomegalovirus, parvovirus
Premalignant conditions: preleukaemia
Graft-versus-host disease

---

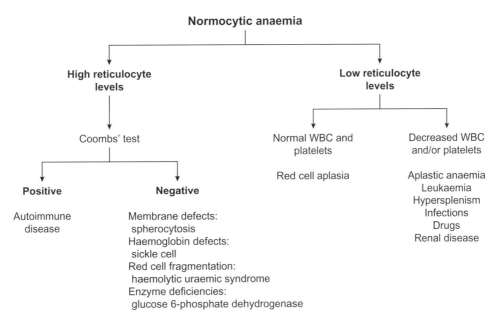

Fig. 102 Causes of the normocytic anaemias.

**Table 68** Treatment of folic acid or vitamin B$_{12}$ deficiency

| | Normal µg/24 h | Treatment |
|---|---|---|
| Folic acid | 100 | 50–100 µg daily for 2 weeks |
| Vitamin B$_{12}$ | 1–5 | 1 mg once |
| | | 1 mg for at least 2 weeks where there is neurological involvement |

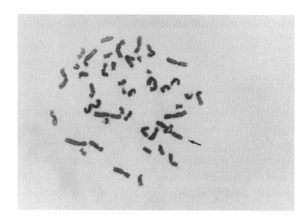

**Fig. 103** Metaphase spread in Fanconi anaemia showing bizarre triradial chromosomes.

plasia. The erythroid precursors (normoblasts), however, have scanty fragmented cytoplasm with poor haemoglobinisation.

### Treatment

Treatment is based on dietary regulation and iron supplementation. In those with intolerance to cow's milk protein, a decrease in the consumption of milk reduces the loss of blood iron from the gut and facilitates the intake and absorption of iron-rich foods. Iron supplementation must be in the ferrous form, and the dose should provide 6 mg/kg elemental iron per day. Iron absorption is improved when taken between meals, though this may cause nausea. Parenteral iron (iron dextran) can be used in those intolerant to cow's milk protein, but has no therapeutic advantage over oral iron.

## The megaloblastic anaemias

The megaloblastic anaemias have in common certain abnormalities of RBC morphology and maturation. Both folic acid and vitamin B$_{12}$ are cofactors required in the synthesis of nucleoproteins, and their deficiency results in defective synthesis of DNA and, to a lesser extent, RNA and protein. The arrest in development or the premature death of cells in the marrow results in ineffective erythropoiesis. In the peripheral blood, RBCs are larger (increased mean corpuscular volume (MCV) and oval, and are associated with hypersegmented neutrophils and giant platelets. In the marrow, macrocytosis is obvious, and although the red cells appear to have sufficient haemoglobin they still retain an immature nucleus.

Folates are abundant in green vegetables, fruits and animal organs (e.g. liver, kidney) and are absorbed from the small intestine as pteroyl monoglutamates. Vitamin B$_{12}$ is derived from cobalamins, mainly from animal sources or secondary to production by microorganisms. As vitamin B$_{12}$ is present in many foods, dietary deficiency is rare. It is seen in cases of extreme dietary restrictions where no animal products are consumed (e.g. strict vegetarian, 'vegans'). Treatment of folic acid and vitamin B$_{12}$ deficiency is described in Table 68.

## Bone marrow failure

### Congenital hypoplastic anaemia (Diamond–Blackfan syndrome)

Congenital hypoplastic anaemia is a rare condition presenting between 2 and 6 months of age. One-third of infants have congenital anomalies, such as dysmorphic facies or defects of the upper extremities, including triphalangeal thumbs. These children present with macrocytic anaemia, reticulocytopenia, and a deficiency or absence of RBC precursors in an otherwise normally cellular bone marrow. Bone marrow cultures show markedly reduced numbers of colony- and blast-forming erythrocytes (CFU-E and BFU-E).

**Management.** About 50% will respond to long-term corticosteroid therapy and 14% will undergo spontaneous remission. Others are transfusion dependent and death is ultimately related to transfusion-related haemosiderosis. Allogeneic bone marrow transplantation is curative.

### Congenital anaemias

Fanconi anaemia (FA) is characterised by the progressive onset of bone marrow failure in late childhood. Associated congenital anomalies include increased skin pigmentation, *café-au-lait* spots, short stature, microcephaly, microphthalmia, abnormalities of the ear, thumb, radius and long bones, as well as renal and cardiac anomalies. In 25–50% of patients there is a normal phenotype. Chromosomal studies reveal increased breakages and structural abnormalities (Fig. 103). Supportive treatment includes blood component therapy, steroids and androgens. Only allogeneic bone marrow transplantation is curative.

In cases of acquired aplastic anaemia, the aetiology may be a deficiency of pluripotent cells (type I) or suppression of the proliferating stem cells (type II). This suppression may be immune mediated.

The presenting features are usually a gradual onset of anaemia, with pallor, fatiguability, weakness and anorexia, thrombocytopenia with petechiae, nose and gastrointestinal bleeding, and granulocytopenia with an increased susceptibility to infections.

Examination of the bone marrow shows trilineage depression or absence of haematopoietic cell precursors. Poor prognostic features include:

- Absolute neutrophil count of $<0.5 \times 10^9$/L
- Platelet count of $<20 \times 10^9$/L
- <20% of haematopoietic cells in the marrow
- Older age
- The presence of haemorrhagic manifestations
- Infections.

**Management**. This is supportive, with blood products and the removal of the offending agent, if known. Infections must be treated aggressively and often in an empirical fashion. Methylprednisolone, antilymphocyte globulin and ciclosporin A may be effective in those with an immune-mediated suppression of proliferating stem cells. In those refractory to therapy, allogeneic bone marrow transplantation is the only option.

### Transient erythroblastopenia of childhood

Transient erythroblastopenia of childhood (TEC) is a disease of unknown aetiology that occurs between 6 months and 3 years of age. Reticulocytes and erythroid precursors alone are decreased.

**Management**. Recovery is spontaneous within 1–2 months and treatment includes RBC transfusions when anaemia is severe.

### Aplastic anaemia

Aplastic anaemia is the failure of the bone marrow to produce all three components of blood, i.e. RBCs, granulocytes and platelets. The causes can be congenital or acquired (Box 68).

| **Box 68** Causes of iron-deficiency anaemia | |
|---|---|
| **Mechanism** | **Causes** |
| **Deficient intake** | Poor diet |
| **Increased demand** | Low birthweight, prematurity, congenital heart disease |
| **Increased loss** | |
| Gut | Cow's milk related, Meckel diverticulum, gastro-oesophageal reflux, polyps with bleeding, hookworm infestation |
| Lung | Pulmonary haemosiderosis |
| Impaired absorption | Chronic diarrhoea, inflammatory bowel disease |

## Anaemias with red blood cell destruction

The haemolytic anaemias result from the increased destruction of RBCs. They can arise as a result of:

- Membrane defects
- Enzyme deficiencies
- Abnormal haemoglobin.

### Membrane defects

Membrane defects occur in spherocytosis, elliptocytosis, pyropoikilocytosis, stomatocytosis and paroxysmal nocturnal haemoglobinuria. The commonest example is hereditary spherocytosis (Box 69).

### Enzyme deficiencies

Enzyme deficiencies causing RBC destruction include pyruvate kinase, glucose 6-phosphate dehydrogenase (G6PD) and related deficiencies.

#### Glucose 6-phosphate dehydrogenase

There are over 300 distinct enzyme varieties of G6PD deficiency, an X-linked condition. The commonest are G6PD B+ and the G6PD A+ present in the African-American population.

There are four distinct clinical syndromes based on the type of enzyme defect:

- Oxidative stress-induced haemolysis (caused by drugs, infection, other illnesses)
- Favism (sensitivity to a chemical in fava beans)
- Neonatal jaundice
- Chronic congenital haemolytic anaemia.

The drugs implicated are mainly the sulphonamides and the antimalarials. Favism, as the name implies, is seen in certain individuals who experience haemolysis when exposed to fava (broad) beans (either by ingestion or by inhaling the pollen). The diagnosis is established by estimating the G6PD level. This is checked a few weeks after the acute haemolytic episode, as enzyme levels may be high in young red cells and could result in spurious high levels if tested at the time of presentation.

**Management**. The prevention of haemolysis is the most important aspect of management. Individuals from high-risk groups should be screened and, once identified, educated to avoid precipitating agents.

### Abnormal haemoglobin: the haemoglobinopathies

#### The sickle cell syndromes

Sickle haemoglobin (HbS) has glutamic acid instead of valine in position 6 of the β chain, a result of a point

**Box 69** Hereditary spherocytosis

**Aetiology**
Mutations in the genes encoding ankyrin, Band 3, $\alpha$ and $\beta$ spectrin or pallidin, which are proteins that exist on the red cell membrane, lead to a defective red cell membrane. The RBC is unable to maintain its biconcave shape, and becomes spherical and susceptible to mechanical stress while traversing the spleen and capillaries. It is commonly inherited in an autosomal dominant fashion.

**Clinical features**

| | |
|---|---|
| Jaundice | For those with severe disease this may present as haemolytic disease of the newborn. Commonly intermittent episodes of haemolytic jaundice occur through childhood. |
| Anaemia | Usually mild (in most cases haemolysis is compensated by bone marrow turnover), but may be more severe with intercurrent illnesses (due to splenic hyperfunction) |
| Splenomegaly | Mild to moderate increase in size as it is the main organ of red cell destruction. May be the earliest presenting feature in an otherwise asymptomatic child. |

**Complications**
Haemolytic disease of the newborn – requiring phototherapy or exchange transfusion
Pigmentary gallstones – due to increased bilirubin excretion
Aplastic crises – transient marrow suppression with parvovirus $B_{19}$ or other viral infections
Megaloblastic anaemia – unmet folic acid needs due to high red cell turnover

**Diagnosis**
Blood film shows spherocytes, mean corpuscular haemoglobin concentration (MCHC) >35 g/dL, red cell distribution width (RDW) >14
Negative Coombs' test (Coombs'-positive autoimmune haemolytic anaemia may also show spherocytosis in the peripheral blood)
Decreased osmotic fragility or cryohaemolysis test
Analysis of specific membrane protein defects

**Management**
Daily folic acid
Transfusions during haemolytic episodes
Splenectomy is the treatment of choice. It should be postponed until the child is 5 years old if possible, and pneumococcal vaccine is given prior to splenectomy. Post splenectomy, penicillin prophylaxis and immunisation with Hib and meningococcal C vaccine are continued lifelong.

mutation. When deoxygenated, this haemoglobin polymerises to rigid crystal-like rods that give the cell the characteristic sickle shape. This also provides the cell with resistance to parasitisation with *Plasmodium falciparum* (malaria), as any infected cell will promptly sickle. This is an autosomal codominant condition. Clinical manifestation usually occurs in later infancy as HbS gradually replaces HbF (Box 70). The clinical features are usually the result of arterial blockage by sickled cells, with resultant hypoxia and infarction of the affected tissue. Severe symptoms are associated with the homozygous state and sickle cell disease (HbSS), but are also seen with HbS-$\beta^0$-thalassaemia and HbSC disease.

The definitive diagnosis, distinguishing sickle haemoglobin from the sickle cell variants, is made by electrophoresis in an acidic pH and haemoglobin solubility. In high-risk families, antenatal diagnosis is possible.

**Management.** Almost all children with HbSS will have pain on a nearly daily basis. Paracetamol, anti-inflammatory agents, narcotics and, on occasion, epidural analgesia may be required. During a crisis, maintenance of hydration is absolutely essential. Blood transfusions are given only when necessary. In those with severe complications, such as cerebrovascular disease, chronic long-term transfusion regimens will avert crises, but these children will also require iron chelation to prevent haemosiderosis. In acute emergencies top-up transfusions may help stabilise a patient, and in some cases an exchange transfusion is the only way to prevent organ damage. As there is functional hyposplenism, prompt treatment of suspected/proven infections is a must, as is prophylaxis with penicillin and pneumococcal vaccination. Hydroxyurea increases fetal haemoglobin (HbF) and has been found to benefit some patients with sickle cell disease without significant side effects. It is usually recommended for patients older than 3 years who suffer from severe complications of sickle cell disease, including frequent pain crises and a history of acute chest syndrome. Bone marrow transplantation is usually reserved for patients with more severe sickle cell disease, including frequent pain crises requiring prolonged hospitalisation, multiple acute chest syndromes, and a history of stroke.

**Box 70** Clinical manifestations of sickle cell disease

| | |
|---|---|
| **Anaemia** | Moderate with clinically detectable jaundice from chronic haemolysis |
| **Painful crises** | Hand–foot syndrome (dactylitis) – symmetrical swelling of hands and feet owing to ischaemic necrosis of small bones; occasionally may develop sympathetic effusions; avascular necrosis of the head of femur |
| | Abdominal crises |
| **Acute chest syndrome** | Constellation of infection, infarction, embolism and pulmonary sequestration. Presentation is with fever, chest pain, cough, restricted chest movement and hypoxaemia. The chest X-ray may show pulmonary infiltrates. |
| **Haemolytic crises** | Usually seen in those with a concomitant G6PD deficiency |
| **Aplastic crises** | Maybe life threatening, due to parvovirus $B_{19}$ or other viruses |
| **Splenic sequestration crises** | Hypersplenism and acute splenic sequestration are more common in infants and young children. Present with collapse and acute enlargement of the spleen |
| **Infections** | Autoinfarction of the spleen occurs by late childhood and in these children leads to hyposplenism and infections with *Pneumococcus*, *Haemophilus* and *Salmonella* spp. |
| **Growth retardation** | |
| **CNS complications** | 10% of children will have cerebrovascular occlusion; proliferative sickle retinopathy |
| **Renal complications** | Progressive renal damage with diffuse glomerular and tubular fibrosis and occasionally papillary necrosis |
| **Priapism** | |
| **Leg ulcers** | In later life, indolent leg ulcers may pose problems |
| **Gallstones** | Due to increased bilirubin production |
| **Cardiac failure** | From chronic anaemia and iron overload |

**Table 69** The thalassaemias

| Type of thalassaemia | Globin gene expression | Anaemia | Clinical expression | Haemoglobin findings |
|---|---|---|---|---|
| **β-Thalassaemia** | | | | |
| β⁰ homozygous | $β^0/β^0$ | Severe | Thalassaemia major | HbF >90%; no HbA |
| β⁺ homozygous | $β^+/β^+$ | Moderately severe | Thalassaemia intermedia | HbF 60–80%; HbA 20–40% |
| β⁰ heterozygous | $β/β^0$ | Mild to moderate | Splenomegaly, icterus | Increased HbA₂, HbF |
| β⁺ heterozygous | $β/β^+$ | Mild to moderate | Normal | Increased HbA₂, HbF |
| β silent carrier | $β/β^+$ | Normal | Normal | Normal |
| **α-Thalassaemia** | | | | |
| α silent carrier | α/αα | Mild or normal | Normal | Normal |
| α trait | α/α or /αα | Mild or normal | Normal | Newborn: Hb Barts 5–10% |
| HbH disease | /α | Moderate to severe | Thalassaemia intermedia | Hb Barts (γ4), 20–30% |
| α hydrops | $α^0$ | Severe | Hydrops | Hb Barts >90% |

### The thalassaemia syndromes

*Aetiology* Thalassaemia major is an autosomal codominant condition. Two sets of genes, located on chromosome 16, code for the α polypeptide chains. The genes for β, γ and δ chains are closely linked on chromosome 11. The underlying genetic defects include total or partial deletions of globin chain genes, and nucleotide insertions, substitutions and deletions. A decrease, absence or functionally defective mRNA results, and the haemoglobin polypeptide chain synthesis is decreased or suppressed. The abnormal haemoglobin precipitates in the red cell and the abnormal cell is destroyed in both the marrow and the spleen. Thus the anaemia is a result of inefficient erythropoiesis as well as increased destruction. Depending on the amount of HbF and HbA present there are varying degrees of severity at presentation. Homozygous β⁰-thalassaemia presents in infancy as HbF levels decline (Box 71, Table 69).

In the absence of regular blood transfusions, these children become anaemic and develop features of extramedullary haematopoiesis. Massive expansion of the marrow of the face (malar hyperplasia) and skull (frontal bossing) produces the 'chipmunk' facies. Pallor, haemosiderosis and jaundice produce a greenish-brown complexion. Abdominal distension is due to liver and

**Box 71** Clinical features of thalassaemia

This varies with the severity of the disease and the regularity of transfusion. Those with mild forms or on regular transfusion programmes will have very little in the way of clinical signs and symptoms.

**Failure to thrive**
**Anaemia**
**Jaundice**
**Skeletal**      Compensatory extramedullary hypertrophy leads to the classic 'chipmunk' facies (bossing of the skull with maxillary overgrowth)

**Complications**
These are mainly complications of excessive and ineffective haematopoiesis in untreated children. In transfused children the problems are mainly of iron overload, which can be avoided by effective chelation.

*Ineffective haematopoiesis and red cell destruction*
Splenomegaly – can be massive
Folic acid deficiency
Delayed puberty
Infection
Hyperuricaemia and gout
Bleeding tendency – associated with thrombocytopenia

*Iron overload*
Cardiac      Enlargement, cardiomyopathy
Hepatic      Cirrhosis
Pancreas      Diabetes
Endocrine      Delayed puberty, growth hormone deficiency
Skin      Hyperpigmentation
*Transfusion*      Viral infections, may require permanent venous access, transfusion reactions
*Chelation*      Poor tolerance to multiple skin punctures; sensorineural hearing loss; retinopathy; bony abnormalities; growth retardation

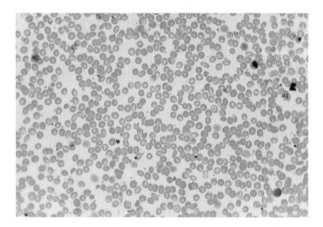

**Fig. 104** Target cells, anisocytosis, poikilocytosis and normoblasts in thalassaemia major.

splenic enlargement. As there is a large erythrocyte turnover, with or without transfusion, haemosiderosis occurs, damaging the liver, kidneys, pancreas and heart. As in sickle cell anaemia, indolent leg ulcers may be a problem. Mild forms (Table 69) are often mistaken for iron-deficiency anaemia, but a blood film would show additional target cells, anisocytosis, poikilocytosis and normoblasts reflecting enhanced marrow turnover (Fig. 104).

**Management**. Haemoglobin electrophoresis confirms the diagnosis. Hypertransfusion protocols aimed at keeping the haemoglobin above 9.5 g/dL permit normal activity and prevent bone and marrow changes in thalassaemia major. Transfusions are usually necessary once every 4–5 weeks. Regular chelation with desferrioxamine is essential to prevent haemosiderosis. This is usually given as a continuous subcutaneous infusion at night. Splenectomy can be offered to older children with hypersplenism to help to decrease the transfusion requirement. Allogeneic bone marrow transplantation can be offered in severe cases.

## 11.3 Disorders of bleeding and coagulation

### Learning objectives

You should:

- appreciate the mechanisms of coagulation and the laboratory tests that are used to diagnose bleeding and coagulation disorders

- know the aetiology, diagnosis and management of idiopathic thrombocytopenic purpura

- know the aetiology, diagnosis and management of Henoch–Schönlein purpura

- know the aetiology, diagnosis and management of haemophilia

A series of biochemical and physiological events is initiated to stop the flow of blood when a blood vessel is injured (Fig. 105). The vascular component is involved in constricting the damaged vessel; the platelets plug the defect, and the clot is formed and stabilised by plasma coagulation factors. Defects in any one of these components can lead to prolonged bleeding from minor injuries. The common causes are listed in Box 72.

The spontaneous onset of petechiae and bruising in an otherwise well child is a relatively common symptom. Because purpura/petechiae result from extra-vasation of blood into the skin, the lesions will not blanch with pressure.

## Henoch–Schönlein purpura

In *Henoch–Schönlein purpura* there is a characteristic distribution of petechiae and bruises over the anterior aspect of the shins, the extensor surfaces of the forearms and the buttocks, and the rash is often palpable. Other symptoms include arthritis (75%), usually polyarticular and involving the large joints; gastrointestinal (50%) with colicky abdominal pain, occult or frank haemorrhage and, rarely, intussusception; and renal (25–50%) with haematuria, nephrotic syndrome and, rarely, chronic renal failure. The diagnosis is based on the clinical findings, as the platelet count is normal. The bleeding is a result of IgA-mediated systemic vasculitis of small vessels. Resolution within a few weeks is the norm, though there may be subsequent exacerbations and remissions.

**Management.** The treatment is supportive for the symptoms of arthritis and abdominal pain. Steroids may be given when there is extensive disease.

## Idiopathic thrombocytopenic purpura

Idiopathic thrombocytopenic purpura (ITP), as the name suggests, is a disease of unknown aetiology that often presents a few weeks after a viral infection. It is the commonest cause of thrombocytopenia in childhood. It presents with spontaneous onset of petechiae and bruising, which have no particular distribution. Mucosal bleeding is not uncommon and nosebleeds may be quite difficult to stop. The platelet count is often less than $20 \times 10^9/L$ (normal $>150 \times 10^9/L$) and nearly all children have increased levels of platelet-bound IgG.

The diagnosis is based on the clinical features and platelet count. In 90% the disease will remit spontaneously within 3 months. Only children with platelet counts of less than $10 \times 10^9/L$ and significant mucous membrane bleeding require treatment.

**Management.** Therapy, for those who require it, is with a course of corticosteroids or, when the bleeding is problematic or refractory, intravenous immunoglobulin. Prior to commencing steroid therapy, most experts would recommend confirmation of ITP on a bone marrow aspirate, which would show a normocellular marrow with normal or increased megakaryocytes and, most importantly, will exclude acute leukaemia. In those children where the condition persists for longer than 6 months, splenectomy will allow the platelet count to rise. Transfused platelets are rapidly destroyed and are only of use in life-threatening emergencies.

---

**Box 72** Causes of purpura in childhood

**Platelet related**

| | |
|---|---|
| Increased consumption | Immune thrombocytopenic (ITP) – commonest |
| | Alloimmune neonatal thrombocytopenia |
| | Secondary to SLE, drugs, viral infections |
| | Disseminated intravascular coagulation (DIC) |
| | Haemolytic uraemia syndrome (HUS) |
| | Thrombotic thrombocytopenic purpura |
| Decreased production | Marrow infiltration e.g. malignancies such as leukaemia |
| | Marrow failure e.g. aplastic anaemia |
| | Wiskott–Aldrich (also associated with increased destruction) |
| | Thrombocytopenia with absent radii (TAR syndrome) |
| Sequestration | Giant haemangioma (Kasabach–Merritt syndrome) |
| Defective platelets | Glanzmann disease |
| | Von Willebrand disease (also coagulation abnormality) |
| | Bernard-Soulier syndrome |
| | Storage pool disorders |
| Drugs | Aspirin, NSAIDs |

**Vascular (non-thrombocytopenic)**

| | |
|---|---|
| Congenital | Connective tissue disorders e.g. Marfan, Ehler–Danlos |
| Infections | Meningococcal, enterovirus, TORCH etc. |
| Immune | Henoch–Schönlein, SLE |
| Drugs | Penicillin |

## Marrow failure

Marrow failure syndromes, including aplastic anaemia and acute leukaemia, can also present with a history of bleeding. In these cases, the blood count will reveal pancytopenia.

## Platelet/coagulation factor defects

Whereas platelet deficiency/dysfunction presents as petechiae, bruising and mucosal bleeds, coagulation factor deficiencies tend to present with deep-seated and joint bleeding. The coagulation factors are shown in Table 70 and their pathway of activation in Figure 105.

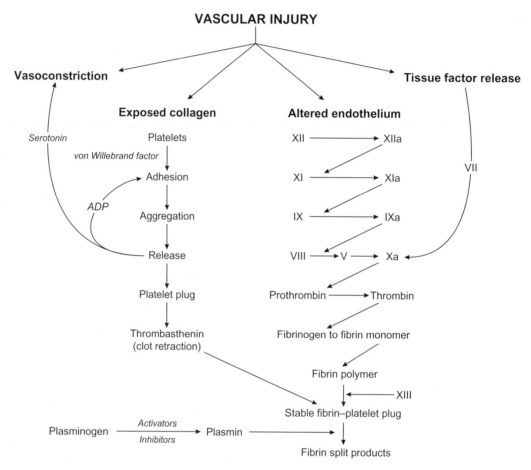

**Fig. 105** The coagulation cascade.

**Table 70** The coagulation factors

| International numbers | Synonyms | Description |
|---|---|---|
| I | Fibrinogen | Congenital deficiency: afibrinogenaemia |
| II | Prothrombin | Congenital deficiency is reported |
| III | Thromboplastin | |
| IV | Calcium | |
| V | Labile factor, proaccelerin | Congenital deficiency: parahaemophilia, Owren disease |
| VI | Activated labile factor, accelerin | Same as factor V |
| VII | Stable factor, proconvertin, SPCA | Congenital deficiency is known |
| VIII | Antihaemophilic factor | Congenital deficiency: haemophilia A |
| IX | Christmas factor, plasma thromboplastin | Congenital deficiency: haemophilia B component (PTC) |
| X | Stuart–Prower factor | Congenital deficiency is known |
| XI | Plasma thromboplastin antecedent (PTA) | Congenital deficiency is known |
| XII | Hageman factor | Asymptomatic congenital deficiency |
| XIII | Fibrin-stabilising factor | Congenital deficiency is known |

A careful history is essential in children with bleeding disorders. The initial screening tests must include a platelet count, prothrombin time, the partial thromboplastin test, bleeding time and, where relevant, levels of factor VIII and IX.

## Haemophilia

The dramatic effect of haemorrhages in the European Royal dynasties and the devastating role of therapeutic concentrates in the transmission of AIDS have made *haemophilia A* the subject of great medical and public scrutiny. The gene coding for factor VIII lies on the tip of the long arm of chromosome X. In one-third of patients with haemophilia there is a recent mutation and there is no family history. Clinically indistinguishable but rarer is *haemophilia B* (Christmas disease), which is caused by factor IX deficiency and is also transmitted on the X chromosome.

Factor VIII circulates in the plasma in a non-covalent complex with von Willebrand factor (vWF). vWF enhances factor VIII synthesis, protects it from proteolysis and concentrates it at sites of active haemostasis. The diagnosis of haemophilia is suspected whenever unusual bleeding is encountered in a boy. As shown in Table 71, the suspicion is supported by the presence of an abnormal activated partial thromboplastin time (APTT) with a normal prothrombin time and a normal platelet count. Factor assay is required to confirm the

diagnosis and distinguish between factor IX and factor XI deficiency. It is essential to distinguish patients with severe haemophilia A (<1% of factor VIII) from patients who have moderate (1–4%) or mild (5–25%) disease. Mild or moderate haemophilia is rarely complicated by spontaneous haemarthroses. The hallmark of severe disease is the occurrence of apparently unprovoked bleeding into joints when the child begins to walk. Untreated, haemarthroses are painful and result in limitation of joint mobility. The inflammatory response to an intra-articular bleed leads to synovitis and ultimately permanent joint damage. Bleeding also occurs at other sites, for example into muscles, or as intracranial haemorrhages.

Patients with *von Willebrand's disease* also have factor VIII deficiency as an indirect consequence of a qualitative or quantitative change in the vWF. There are at least four different varieties, and inheritance is either autosomal dominant or recessive. The diagnosis is usually confirmed by measuring the vWF antigen or ristocetin cofactor activity. The latter measures the ability of the vWF to support platelet aggregation in the presence of ristocetin.

## Management

The advent of factor VIII replacement revolutionised the management of children with haemophilia A until the AIDS epidemic. Highly refined viral inactivation

**Table 71** The diagnosis of bleeding disorders

| Disorder | Inheritance | Prothrombin time | Activated partial thromboplastin time | Platelets | Bleeding time | Specific test |
|---|---|---|---|---|---|---|
| Haemophilia A (factor VIII) | XR | N | E | N | N | Factor VIII |
| von Willebrand's disease | AD/AR | N | E/N | N | E/N | von Willebrand factor antigen or ristocetin cofactor activity; Factor VIII |
| Haemophilia B (factor IX) | XR | N | E | N | N | Factor IX |
| Haemophilia C (factor XI) | AD | N | E | N | N | Factor XI |
| Vitamin K-dependent factors (II, VII, IX and X) (>50% reduction in factors) | AR | E | E | N | N | |
| Idiopathic thrombocytopenic purpura | – | N | N | D | E | Blood count, bone marrow |
| Glanzmann | AR | N | N | N | E | Platelet function tests |

XR, sex-linked recessive; AD, autosomal dominant; AR, autosomal recessive; N, normal; E, elevated; D, decreased.

techniques and recombinantly synthesised factor VIII have now decreased the risk of transfusion-related virus transmission. Desmopressin (DDAVP) increases the plasma levels of factor VIII and vWF and can be used for the non-transfusional treatment of patients with mild or moderate haemophilia and von Willebrand's disease. Tranexamic acid can also be used to stabilise the clot. Factor replacement is necessary for those with severe haemophilia and an ongoing bleed. For those with minor bleeds, the replacement is aimed to achieve an increment of factor VIII of about 15%; for haemarthroses replacement is aimed at maintaining levels at 50% until resolution of symptoms. For surgery and intracranial bleeds, levels of 100% may be required. Additional hormonal manipulation (e.g. low-dose contraceptive pill) may be required in girls with vWD and problematic menorrhagia.

Certain countries have successfully introduced a prophylactic regimen for severe haemophiliacs. The infusion of factor VIII three times a week can prevent spontaneous haemarthroses. However, the financial implications of such a programme are considerable. About 10–20% of children with haemophilia unfortunately develop antibodies to factor VIII. The management of these children is complex, and includes the use of porcine factor VIII, prothrombin complex concentrates and factor VII infusions (which bypass the need for factor VIII) and, in severe cases, removal of the inhibitor by exchange plasmapheresis or the use of protein A–sepharose columns.

## 11.4 The neoplastic disorders

### Learning objectives

You should:

- know the types of cancer commonly seen in children

- know the common symptoms and signs related to childhood cancer, especially those relating to acute lymphoblastic leukaemia

Cancer is a rare disease of childhood with an incidence of approximately 1.4 per 10 000 total population. The malignancies of childhood tend to be different from those that occur in adults (Fig. 106). They usually originate in a primitive cell, are aggressive, and metastasise early. However, great strides have been made with childhood cancers and often – sometimes in excess of 70% of patients – it is possible to achieve a cure.

Overall, the prognosis for childhood cancer has improved since the mid-1970s. More importantly, the

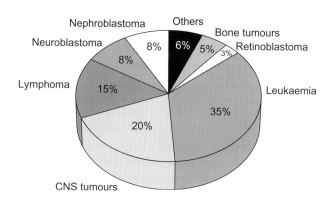

**Fig. 106** The common childhood malignancies.

majority of children cured can be expected to lead normal lives, hold jobs and raise a family.

## Approach to therapy

The improved survival rates in childhood cancers have been made possible by the development of specialised paediatric oncology units. A wide range of health professionals used to dealing with the problems of a child with cancer should be based in these centres, which can offer a multidisciplinary approach. The treatment of most childhood malignancies is multimodal, using a combination of chemotherapy, radiotherapy and surgery. In most cases, an indwelling central venous line is inserted to facilitate management. Various drugs act at different sites in the cell, and also at different times in the cell cycle (Fig. 107). Combination chemotherapy (using drugs with different mechanisms of action at the same time) ensures that the malignant cell is targeted in more than one fashion. Ideally, this enables cancer cells to be attacked at different phases of the cell cycle, avoids the toxicity that would occur from the dose required by a single agent, and prevents the emergence of a drug-resistant clone. In practice, all these targets are not always achieved.

### Side effects

The side effects of these drugs are varied and common. In general, most of the drugs cause bone marrow suppression, alopecia and mucositis. Therefore, all children receiving chemotherapy pass through a neutropenic period, during which they are prone to infections, which can be bacterial, fungal or viral. The empirical treatment with broad-spectrum antibiotics in children with febrile neutropenia has been effective in decreasing mortality and morbidity. In children with acute lymphoblastic leukaemia who are immuno-suppressed for prolonged periods, prophylactic co-trimoxazole has reduced the incidence of *Pneumocystis*

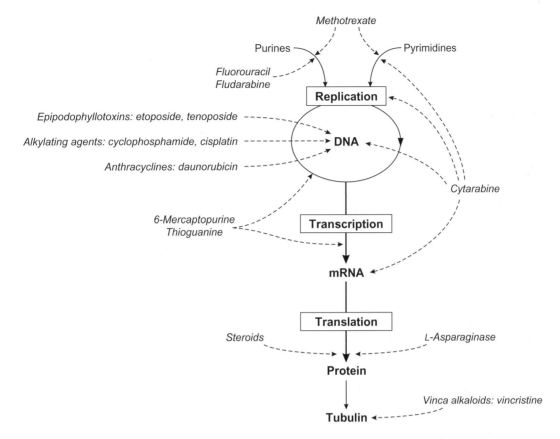

**Fig. 107** Sites of action of common chemotherapeutic agents.

*carinii* infection. Long-term toxicities include anthracycline-induced cardiotoxicity and epipodophyllotoxin-induced secondary leukaemias. Radiation may damage the pituitary or the gonads, leading to endocrine deficiency and infertility.

## Acute leukaemia

The commonest malignancy of childhood is *acute lymphoblastic leukaemia* (ALL). The incidence peaks in the 2–6-year age group, unlike *acute myeloid leukaemia* (AML), which is relatively more common in infancy. The presenting symptoms for both ALL and AML are very similar (Box 73).

The blood count usually shows a pancytopenia, though the white cell count (WCC) may be elevated, and often reveals the presence of peripheral immature white cells, referred to as 'blasts'. The diagnosis is confirmed by a bone marrow aspiration. The cerebrospinal fluid is examined to look for CNS disease.

The morphological appearances of the blast cell are classified according to the FAB (French–American–British) classification: lymphoblasts are classified as L1, L2 or L3. AML are classified from M0 to M7. Further characterisation of the malignant clone is done by

**Box 73** Signs and symptoms of leukaemia in childhood

| | | |
|---|---|---|
| Bone marrow infiltration | Anaemia | Pallor and lethargy |
| | Thrombocytopenia | Bruising, petechiae, nose bleeds |
| | Neutropenia | Fever, infection |
| Organ infiltration | | Hepatosplenomegaly |
| | | Lymphadenopathy |
| | | Testicular enlargement |
| | | Bone pains, painful swollen joints |
| | | Skin deposits (rare, usually in AML) |
| | | Superior mediastinal syndrome (usually in T-cell ALL) |
| Others | CNS involvement | Meningeal signs, cranial nerve palsies, raised intracranial pressure |
| | DIC | Rare, seen in AML (FAB type M3) |

**245**

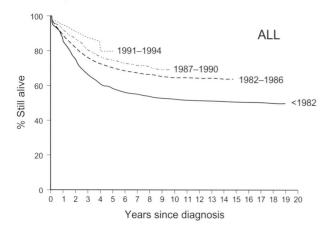

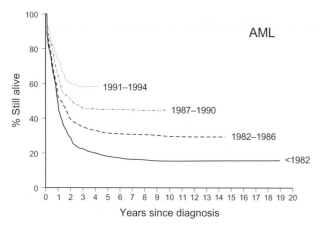

**Fig. 108** Actuarial survival curves showing improvement in survival for childhood ALL and AML.

**Table 72** Risk stratification in childhood ALL

| | |
|---|---|
| Standard risk: | Age < 10 years and presenting white cell count <50 × 10$^9$/L |
| Intermediate risk: | Age > 10 years or presenting white cell count >50 × 10$^9$/L |
| High risk: | Slow early response to treatment (within 2 weeks of induction) |
| Chromosomal changes: | t(9;22), t(4;11), near-haploidy and amplification of RUNX1 |

immunophenotyping. This is based on the identification of cells by cell surface molecules that are detected by specific monoclonal antibodies and numbered according to the cluster of differentiation (CD). The commonest ALL is of B-cell origin, is usually CD10 positive, and is often referred to as common-ALL. T-cell leukaemias tend to present with mediastinal masses, high WCCs and CNS involvement at diagnosis.

## Management of ALL

In the 1970s, survival in children with ALL was less than 1%. With modern methods of management it is now as high as 70% (Fig. 108). The treatment is stratified according to risk criteria, as shown in Table 72. The treatment regimen for standard risk children is shown in Figure 109. Intermediate and high-risk patients have a more intensive consolidation and a delayed intensification phase. Co-trimoxazole is given throughout treatment as prophylaxis against *Pneumocystis carinii* infection. The risk of relapse is highest in the first 24 months after stopping therapy and virtually negligible 60 months after

stopping therapy. Bone marrow transplantation is only recommended for some of the high-risk category and for children who relapse.

## Management of AML

Children with AML are treated for a shorter duration but with very intensive pulses of therapy. In the period since the mid-1980s this approach has resulted in a greater than 60% survival.

## Chronic myeloid leukaemia (CML)

Chronic myeloid leukaemia is a rare cancer of childhood. It is characterised by the t(9;22) chromosomal translocation, which results in the fusion of the gene *BCR* on chromosome 22q11 with the gene *ABL* on chromosome 9q34. The fusion results in an increase in the ABL tyrosine kinase, and this is thought to be critical to the disease process. Until recently, this was curable only by an allogeneic bone marrow transplant. Recently the drug imatinib mesylate, which specifically blocks ABL tyrosine kinase activity, has been shown to successfully induce remission in the majority of patients with CML.

## The lymphomas

The lymphomas include *Hodgkin's disease* (HD) and *non-Hodgkin's lymphoma* (NHL). NHL is more common in the UK and tends to be of T-cell, B-cell or large-cell origin.

Lymphomas present as localised enlargement of lymph nodes or other reticuloendothelial organs. T-cell disease usually presents with dyspnoea resulting from mediastinal compression caused by involvement of the thymus and mediastinal nodes and/or pleural effusion. In severe cases this may result in superior vena caval obstruction. Large-cell lymphomas tend to present with peripheral tissue masses in the skin and bone, or cutaneous infiltration. *Burkitt's lymphoma* usually presents with a mass in the jaw and is endemic in Africa.

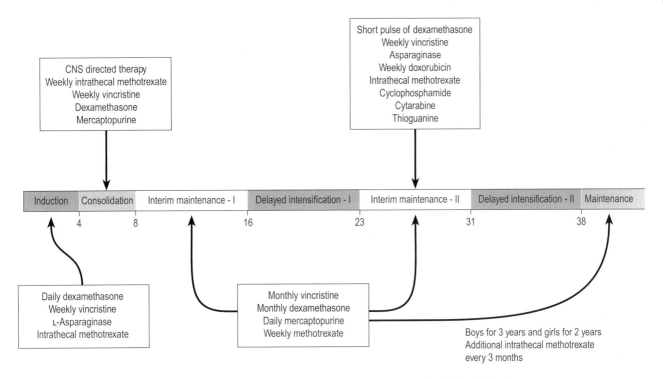

**Fig. 109** Management scheme for standard risk acute lymphoblastic leukaemia in the United Kingdom.

**Box 74** Features of childhood lymphomas

| Type | Site | Treatment | Prognosis |
|---|---|---|---|
| Hodgkin | Cervical lymph nodes | Short, moderately intensive multiagent chemotherapy, | Good |
| | Mediastinum | radiotherapy | |
| | Abdomen | | |
| T-cell NHL | Mediastinum | As for ALL | Intermediate |
| B-cell NHL | Bulky abdominal | Very intensive short course multiagent therapy | Good |
| Large cell anaplastic | Skin, bones | Very intensive short course multiagent therapy | Good |

Sporadic B-cell NHL tumours often present as an intra-abdominal mass, occasionally with associated malabsorption or intussusception. In all cases there may be additional involvement of the bone marrow. The treatment for T-cell malignancies is similar to that for ALL. B-cell and large-cell disease are rapidly growing tumours and can double in 24–48 hours. They are also highly chemosensitive, and once treatment has started may be complicated by the *tumour lysis* syndrome. This is a triad of hyperuricaemia, hyperkalaemia and hypercalcaemia (with hypophosphataemia) that can lead to renal failure and cardiac arrhythmias. This can be prevented by the use of hyperhydration and either allopurinol or a urate oxidase inhibitor (Rasburicase) prior to and along with chemotherapy. HD in childhood is commonly of either the nodular sclerosing or the lymphocyte-predominant type. Therapeutic modalities for children are not greatly different from those used in adults, and consist of combination therapy and/or localised radiotherapy. The precise regimen used depends on the histological grade and extent (i.e. stage) of disease (Fig. 110 and Tables 73 and 74).

## CNS tumours

CNS tumours form a heterogeneous group of conditions. The presenting symptoms are those of raised intracranial pressure (ICP), including *lethargy*, *headaches* and early morning *vomiting*, which may be projectile in nature. Cerebellar dysfunction is manifest by *altered gait* (ataxia), and occasionally diplopia and nystagmus. *Papilloedema* is a late clinical finding. Any child who presents with these symptoms and signs should be considered to have raised ICP due to a mass in the posterior fossa, and

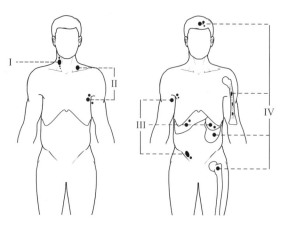

**Fig. 110** Staging of lymphomas. Stage I, single node/clump in one anatomical drainage site; stage II, two or more nodes in two sites on the same side of the diaphragm; stage III, two or more nodes on opposite sides of the diaphragm and hepatosplenomegaly; stage IV, extranodal sites, including brain, bone, bone marrow and kidneys.

**Table 73** Clinical staging of Hodgkin's disease

| Stage | Extent |
|---|---|
| I | Involvement of a single lymph node (I) or a single extralymphatic organ or site (I$_E$) |
| II | Involvement of two or more lymph node regions on the same side of the diaphragm (II) or localised involvement of an extralymphatic organ or site and one or more lymph node regions on the same side of the diaphragm (II$_E$) |
| III | Involvement of lymph nodes on both sides of the diaphragm (III), which may be accompanied by splenic involvement (III$_S$) or by localised involvement of an extralymphatic organ or site (III$_E$) or both (III$_{SE}$) |
| IV | Diffuse or disseminated involvement of one or more extralymphatic organs or tissues with or without lymph node involvement |

The presence or fever, drenching night sweats, or unexplained loss of weight is denoted by the suffix B, all others by the suffix A.

a CT or MRI scan of the head should be performed with urgency. The tumour can be benign (e.g. cerebellar astrocytoma) or malignant (e.g. medulloblastoma). Other brain tumours include pinealomas, gliomas, malignant astrocytomas etc. These tend to present with isolated cranial nerve palsies and long tract signs. Therapy includes surgical removal if possible, radiation and chemotherapy. Medulloblastomas seed early along the spine, and in general the prognosis for malignant CNS tumours is poor, only about 20–30% surviving at 5 years (Fig. 111).

**Table 74** Clinical staging of non-Hodgkin's lymphoma

| Stage | Extent |
|---|---|
| I | Single tumour or single anatomic area, excluding mediastinum or abdomen |
| II | Single tumour with regional node involvement on same side of the diaphragm; primary gastrointestinal tumour with or without mesenteric node involvement and grossly completely resectable |
| III | On both sides of the diaphragm; primary intrathoracic tumour; unresectable abdominal disease; paraspinal and epidural tumours |
| IV | Any of the above with initial CNS or bone marrow involvement |

### Neuroblastoma

Neuroblastoma is neuroectodermal in origin and usually arises in the abdomen (65%), especially from the adrenal gland (35%), and often crosses the midline (Fig. 112). It typically presents in a young child or infant as an abdominal mass. Metastatic disease at diagnosis is usual, the skeletal system and bone marrow being the most common sites. The primary tumour can present in a wide variety of tissues, as paraspinal (dumb-bell) tumours and in skin. It also occurs as rare but well-described paraneoplastic phenomena, such as the opsoclonus–myoclonus syndrome, and as intractable diarrhoea. The diagnosis is based on histopathology, as in other solid tumours. Additionally, 90–95% of the tumours synthesise sufficient catecholamines to result in increased urinary excretion. Poor prognosis is seen in stage IV disease, the loss of the small arm of chromosome 1, deletion of the long arm of chromosome 17 and the amplification of the gene N-*myc* in tumour cells.

**Management**. Therapy for advanced-stage disease centres on platinum compounds in high-dose therapy with autologous bone marrow/peripheral blood stem cell rescue. Refractory cases have been treated palliatively with radioactive iodine in the compound [[131]I]-labelled MIBG. Therapeutic progress remains moderate in this disease, with survival at 25–30% for advanced-stage disease.

### Nephroblastoma

Nephroblastoma is also called Wilms' tumour and arises from the kidney. It generally presents as an asymptomatic abdominal mass that rarely crosses the midline and is occasionally associated with haematuria. A CT scan will show a large mass, usually encapsulated, distorting a thin rim of normal renal tissue (Fig. 113). The tumour tends to invade the renal vein and inferior vena cava and metastasises to the lung. Associated features include aniridia, genitourinary abnormalities (WAGR

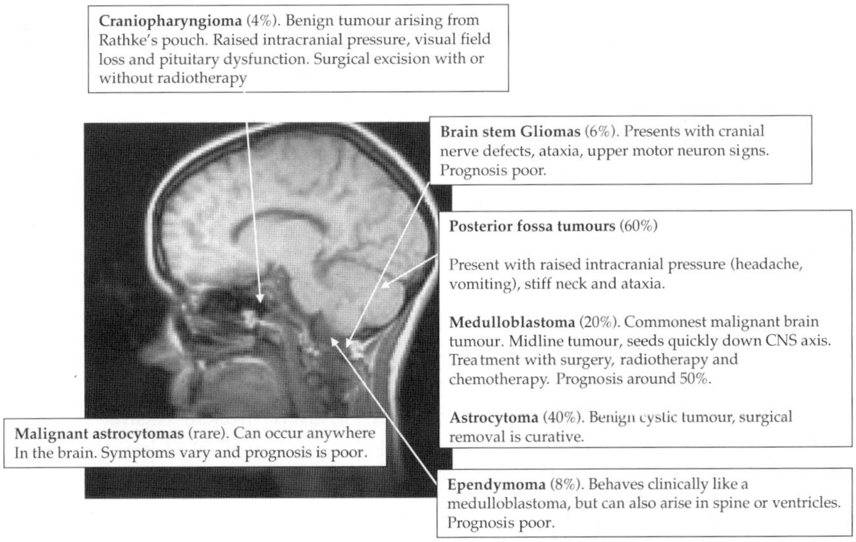

**Craniopharyngioma** (4%). Benign tumour arising from Rathke's pouch. Raised intracranial pressure, visual field loss and pituitary dysfunction. Surgical excision with or without radiotherapy

**Brain stem Gliomas** (6%). Presents with cranial nerve defects, ataxia, upper motor neuron signs. Prognosis poor.

**Posterior fossa tumours** (60%)

Present with raised intracranial pressure (headache, vomiting), stiff neck and ataxia.

**Medulloblastoma** (20%). Commonest malignant brain tumour. Midline tumour, seeds quickly down CNS axis. Treatment with surgery, radiotherapy and chemotherapy. Prognosis around 50%.

**Astrocytoma** (40%). Benign cystic tumour, surgical removal is curative.

**Malignant astrocytomas** (rare). Can occur anywhere in the brain. Symptoms vary and prognosis is poor.

**Ependymoma** (8%). Behaves clinically like a medulloblastoma, but can also arise in spine or ventricles. Prognosis poor.

**Fig. 111** Brain tumours of childhood.

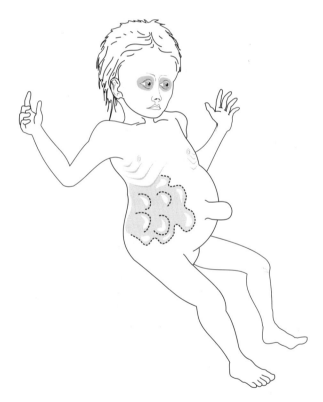

**Fig. 112** Abdominal neuroblastoma, resulting in a large, firm irregular mass extending from the right flank beyond the midline, abdominal distension with an umbilical hernia, generalised wasting (cachexia), and bilateral periorbital metastases with bruising ('panda eyes').

syndrome), nephrotic syndrome (Denys–Drash), hemi-hypertrophy and the Beckwith–Wiedemann syndrome. Histology is diagnostic and will classify the tumour into a favourable or unfavourable (undifferentiated) type.

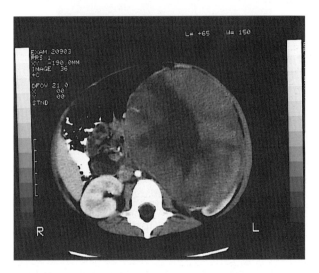

**Fig. 113** CT scan showing left-sided Wilms' tumour obliterating most of the kidney (seen as a thin rim of contrast-enhanced tissue toward the lower part of the scan).

## Management

Treatment is based on surgery and chemotherapy (vincristine alone or in combination with actinomycin and adriamycin in advanced disease), with radiotherapy to pulmonary metastases and to the abdomen in tumours that have seeded into the peritoneal cavity. For stage I (localised disease) the prognosis is >95% and for stage IV (disseminated disease) about 50–60%.

## Bone tumours

The two most common primary tumours of bone are Ewing's tumour (ET) and osteogenic sarcoma. ET is of

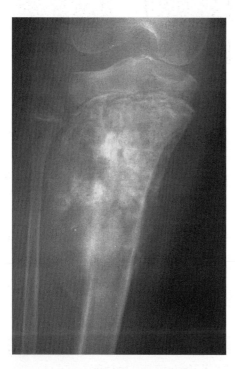

**Fig. 114** Osteosarcoma involving the upper tibial metaphysis.

**Table 75** Indications for bone marrow transplantation

| Malignant | Non-malignant |
| --- | --- |
| Relapsed and high-risk acute lymphoblastic leukaemia | Aplastic anaemia |
| Relapsed and high-risk acute myeloid leukaemia | Inborn errors of metabolism |
| Chronic myeloid leukaemia | SCID |
| Juvenile chronic myelocytic leukaemia | Hemophagocytic lymphohistiocytosis (HLH) |

neuroectodermal origin and often arises in the rib, pelvis, femur, tibia, fibula or ankle bones. Bulky tumours and intrathoracic or pelvic tumours carry a bad prognosis. Combination chemotherapy using ifosfamide/cyclophosphamide is used to shrink the tumour, which is then excised with a wide margin. Amputation of the affected bone or limb may be necessary. Where surgery is not feasible, local radiotherapy is used.

Osteogenic sarcoma often occurs at the upper end of the tibia (Fig. 114), the lower end of the femur and the pelvis. Treatment includes surgical removal of the bone whenever possible, and high-dose chemotherapy.

## Other tumours

Rhabdomyosarcoma, as the name implies, is an undifferentiated soft-tissue tumour arising from primitive striated muscle tissue. It can arise in the pelvis, orbit, limbs and bladder. It tends to be locally invasive but can also metastasise to other tissues, mainly the lung and bone. Therapy is similar to that for Ewing's tumour.

Retinoblastoma is a rare eye tumour. All bilateral tumours are thought to be hereditary, as are about 20% of unilateral cases. The gene responsible, Rb, is located on chromosome 13. The two most common presentations are the replacement of the normal red-eye reflex (commonly seen on a photograph taken with a flash) with a white-eye reflex (leukocoria) and the development of a squint. All such children must have a slit-lamp examination. Enucleation, radiotherapy and chemotherapy are modalities of treatment.

## Bone marrow transplantation

Some indications for bone marrow transplantation are given in Table 75.

Bone marrow transplants are performed to replace non-functioning marrow or malignant host cells with donor cells. There are a variety of donors and they need to be HLA matched to the recipient. Donors can be matched family or unrelated (from the bone marrow registry). Currently mismatched cord blood is being used, as it is less immunogenic and a complete match is not required. Techniques for performing mismatched and haploidentical transplants are still being perfected.

# Self-assessment: questions

## Multiple choice questions

1. The differential diagnosis of a child with hypochromic microcytic anaemia includes:
   a. Lead poisoning
   b. Pulmonary haemosiderosis
   c. Zinc deficiency
   d. Thalassaemia trait
   e. Sideroblastic anaemia.

2. The following statements describe oral iron therapy in a child with iron deficiency:
   a. Subjective improvement can occur within 24 hours
   b. Reticulocytosis peaks 3 weeks after starting iron
   c. It may cause a temporary staining of the teeth
   d. Iron absorption is improved by drinking tea
   e. The haemoglobin level will return to normal within a month.

3. The following are causes of folic acid deficiency:
   a. Tetrahydrofolate synthetase deficiency
   b. Orotic aciduria
   c. Surgical resection of the small intestine
   d. Pregnancy
   e. Treatment of epilepsy with phenytoin.

4. The following are features of vitamin $B_{12}$:
   a. Its absorption is dependent on intrinsic factor, secreted by the duodenum
   b. The bound vitamin is absorbed in the distal ileum
   c. Deficiency may result in hyperpigmentation
   d. Deficiency is also associated with neuronal degeneration
   e. The congenital absence of transcobalamin I leads to vitamin $B_{12}$ deficiency.

5. The following agents may precipitate a haemolytic crisis in those with glucose 6-phosphate dehydrogenase deficiency:
   a. Co-trimoxazole
   b. Aspirin
   c. Naphthalene
   d. Cheese
   e. Port or red wine.

6. Pancytopenia can be seen in:
   a. Sickle cell disease
   b. Aplastic anaemia
   c. Leukaemia
   d. Neuroblastoma
   e. Idiopathic thrombocytopenic purpura.

7. The following are features of bleeding disorders:
   a. The bleeding time is normal when the platelet count is normal
   b. The failure of the activated partial thromboplastin time (APTT) to correct after the addition of normal plasma indicates the presence of a circulating inhibitor
   c. The prothrombin time (PT) is prolonged in a child with haemophilia C
   d. Factor XIII deficiency is characterised by an abnormal prothrombin and APTT
   e. Fibrinogen deficiency can be corrected by the use of fresh frozen plasma.

8. Thrombocytopenia is a feature of:
   a. Wiskott–Aldrich syndrome
   b. Hypersplenism
   c. Kasabach–Meritt syndrome
   d. Aspirin ingestion
   e. Henoch–Schönlein purpura.

9. The following associations are characteristic of childhood malignancies:
   a. Nephroblastoma and raised urinary catecholamines
   b. Acute myeloid leukaemia and bleeding gums
   c. Ewing sarcoma and an 'onion peel' appearance on X-ray film
   d. An abdominal neuroblastoma tumour that crosses the midline
   e. Cerebellar astrocytoma and spinal metastases.

10. Recognised side-effects of cytotoxic agents include:
    a. Cardiomyopathy after vincristine
    b. Peripheral neuropathy after anthracyclines
    c. Mucosal ulceration after methotrexate
    d. Deafness after carboplatin
    e. Anaphylaxis after asparaginase.

11. The following congenital conditions and associated malignant diseases are correctly matched:
    a. Neurofibromatosis and gliomas
    b. Ataxia telangiectasia and lymphoma

c. Down syndrome and neuroblastoma
d. Beckwith–Wiedemann and nephroblastoma
e. Tuberous sclerosis and medulloblastoma.

12. The following describe neutrophils:
    a. Neutrophilia may occur with glucocorticoid administration
    b. A shift to the left may be seen in severe infections
    c. A deficiency is characteristic of the Schwachman syndrome
    d. Severe neutropenia is usually treated with granulocyte infusion
    e. Leukaemoid reaction can be differentiated from leukaemia by the nitro blue tetrazolium test.

13. The following describe autoimmune haemolytic anaemias:
    a. They are usually characterised by a reticulocytopenia
    b. Thrombocytopenia is common
    c. Drugs such as penicillin are aetiological agents
    d. Steroids are the mainstay of therapy
    e. The Coombs' test is positive.

14. The following are recognised associations:
    a. Acute haemolysis with the use of antimalarials
    b. Hookworm infection and megaloblastic anaemia
    c. Chronic haemolytic anaemia and folate deficiency
    d. Autoimmune haemolytic anaemia and severe bacteria infections
    e. Aplastic anaemia and the use of oral chloramphenicol.

## Short notes

Write short notes on:
1. Bone marrow transplantation
2. The indications and use of blood component therapy.

## Case history

1.

A 5-year-old boy with known HbSS disease comes to A&E with a 2-day history of fever, cough and right-sided chest pain. His temperature is 40°C, respiratory rate 66/min, pulse rate 110/min and oxygen saturation 88% in air. A full blood count has been taken and shows an Hb of 5.5 g/dL, and white cell count of $24 \times 10^9$/L with 60% neutrophils.

a. What is the most likely diagnosis, and what other investigations would you like to carry out?
b. Outline how you will manage this acute episode.
c. Once he has begun to settle you discover that this is his fourth episode in 6 months. His elder brother, who is 9 years old, has a right-sided hemiparesis. His mother wishes to know what can be done to prevent this from happening.

2.

A 4-year-old child is taken to his general practitioner with a 2-week history of progressive lethargy and nose bleeds. She notices multiple bruises and petechiae all over the skin and moderate cervical lymphadenopathy.

a. What additional information should the GP seek at this point?
b. Where else should she look for petechiae, apart from the skin?

The GP refers the boy to hospital, where he is examined thoroughly in A&E by the paediatric registrar, who confirms the family doctor's findings and also notes significant pallor and abdominal distension.

c. What are the likely causes for the abdominal distension?

The boy is admitted for further assessment, and on admission to the ward is noted to be miserable, with a fever of 38.5°C, and promptly develops epistaxis.

d. What is the differential diagnosis at this stage?

The registrar orders some initial baseline investigations, including a full blood count, clotting screen, serum electrolytes and chest X-ray. These reveal a haemoglobin of 7.5 g/dL, a white cell count of $45 \times 10^9$/L, platelets of $6 \times 10^9$/L, INR of 2.4, and normal electrolytes and normal chest X-ray.

e. What additional investigations are indicated:
   i. in view of the fever? and
   ii. in order to confirm the diagnosis?

f. What treatment is required in the first instance in order to stabilise the patient before curative therapy can commence?

## Viva voce question

A 17-month-old boy is brought to you with a history of pica, listlessness and failure to thrive. His mother comments that his stomach looks full, and she feels that he looks pale. In view of these symptoms, what questions would you ask of the mother, and describe your management.

## OSCE questions

### OSCE 1

You are shown a 6-year-old boy with ITP who has a generalised petechial–purpuric rash but is otherwise well (Fig. 115a and b). You are asked to inspect the rash and perform an appropriate examination. You may be expected to say why you do not think this is non-accidental injury.

b

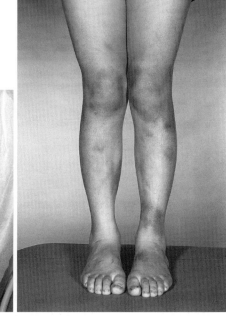

a

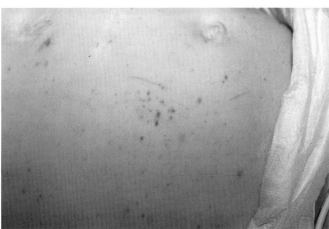

**Fig. 115**

### OSCE 2

You are shown a 4-year-old boy with hereditary spherocytosis, who is generally well (Fig. 116). You are asked to examine this child's face, hands and abdomen. You would be expected to mention the most likely diagnosis (hereditary spherocytosis) and the potential differential diagnosis. You may be expected to say why this is not sickle cell anaemia or G6PD.

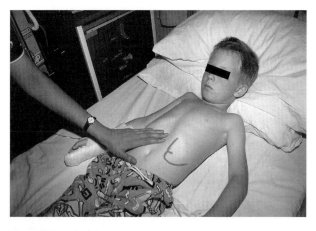

**Fig. 116**

**OSCE 3**

a. What is shown on this X-ray of a long bone (Fig. 117)?

b. What immediate step is required in this child's management?

c. What investigation is required to confirm a diagnosis?

**OSCE 4**

a. What is shown on Figure 118?

b. List THREE complications associated with this device.

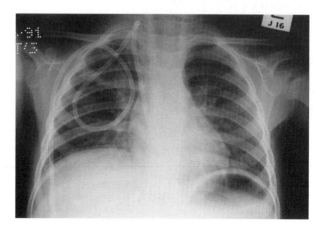

**Fig. 118**

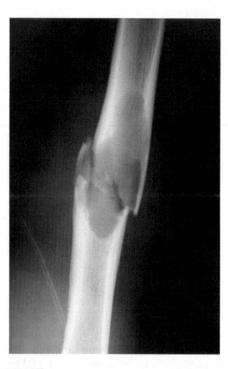

**Fig. 117**

# Self-assessment: answers

## Multiple choice answers

1. a. **True.** The red cells may also have basophilic stippling.
   b. **True.** It is associated with haemoptysis.
   c. **True.** It may result in an iron-deficiency state.
   d. **True.** It is the most common differential diagnosis for iron-deficiency anaemia.
   e. **True.** It is diagnosed by the presence of ringed sideroblasts in a marrow aspirate.

2. a. **True.** For example an improvement in mood and appetite.
   b. **False.** Reticulocytosis peaks at 5–7 days.
   c. **True.** It will disappear after stopping the medication.
   d. **False.** It can decrease iron availability and absorption.
   e. **True.** It may do so even earlier.

3. a. **False.** It is caused by dihydrofolate reductase deficiency.
   b. **False.** It results in megaloblastic anaemia independent of folic acid deficiency.
   c. **True.** Resection results in decreased absorption of folic acid.
   d. **True.** Malabsorption can occur.
   e. **True.** Though the deficiency rarely results in a clinically significant megaloblastic anaemia.

4. a. **False.** Intrinsic factor and R proteins, required for the absorption of vitamin $B_{12}$, are produced in the stomach.
   b. **True.** A $B_{12}$ deficiency can occur if the terminal ileum has been resected.
   c. **True.** Glossitis and neurological manifestations can also occur.
   d. **True.** It may occur in the absence of overt anaemia.
   e. **False.** Transcobalamin II is the physiologically important transporter.

5. a. **True.** Drugs that have oxidant properties, such as sulphonamides, aspirin and antimalarials, precipitate haemolysis in these individuals.
   b. **True.** Aspirin is an oxidant drug.
   c. **True.**
   d. **False.**
   e. **False.**

6. a. **True.** Aplastic crises are often associated with parvovirus infections.
   b. **True.** Pancytopenia defines trilineage deficiency in the peripheral blood.
   c. **True.** Marrow suppression results from malignant infiltration.
   d. **True.** Marrow infiltration suppresses cell production.
   e. **False.** There is only a decrease in the platelet count, which occurs because of peripheral destruction.

7. a. **False.** In Glanzmann disease (thrombasthenia), where there is a platelet function defect, the platelet count is normal but the bleeding time is prolonged.
   b. **True.** The addition of normal plasma should correct for the presence of any deficient factors; an inability to do so suggests the presence of a circulating inhibitor.
   c. **False.** Factor XI as well as VIII and IX deficiencies are phase I disorders and characterised by an abnormal APTT and normal PT.
   d. **False.** The fibrin-stabilising factor deficiency is characterised by normal PT and APTT and an abnormal clot solubility in 5M urea.
   e. **True.** Though fibrinogen concentrates or cryoprecipitate is a more substantial source.

8. a. **True.** Thrombocytopenia, atopic dermatitis and immunodeficiency occur.
   b. **True.** Consumption of cells can also lead to pancytopenia.
   c. **True.** Rapidly enlarging haemangioma, thrombocytopenia and acute or chronic consumption coagulopathy occur.
   d. **False.** Though aspirin can prevent platelet adhesion.
   e. **False.** This is a vasculitis without a thrombocytopenia.

9. a. **False.** This is seen in 90–95% of neuroblastomas.
   b. **True.** It is commonly seen in M3 and M4 types of AML.
   c. **True.** It is caused by repeated periosteal lifting and new bone formation.
   d. **True.** Unlike nephroblastoma, which usually does not cross the midline.

e. **False**. This is a benign tumour. Medulloblastomas, ependymomas and retinoblastomas tend to spread down the spinal axis.

10. a. **False**. Peripheral neuropathy occurs after vincristine and cardiomyopathy after anthracyclines.
   b. **False**. Cardiomyopathy is a side effect of anthracyclines.
   c. **True**. Marrow depression also occurs.
   d. **True**. Renal toxicity also occurs.
   e. **True**. There is also local reaction and hypercoagulable conditions.

11. a. **True**. As well as acute myeloid leukaemia.
   b. **True**. Either B cell or T cell.
   c. **False**. Leukaemia is more common in this condition.
   d. **True**. Usually due to deletions of chromosome 11p15.
   e. **False**. Gliomas, rhabdomyomas.

12. a. **True**. Lymphopenia also occurs.
   b. **True**. Particularly apparent in the neonatal period.
   c. **True**. Dwarfism, neutropenia and pancreatic insufficiency occur.
   d. **False**. Though granulocyte colony-stimulating factor (G-CSF) may be useful.
   e. **True**. Normal neutrophils contain superoxide, which will turn the normally yellow nitro blue tetrazolium to blue and appears as insoluble dark blue pigments on normal neutrophils.

13. a. **True**. As more immature red cells escape into the circulation to compensate for the haemolysis.
   b. **False**. Only rarely is immune thrombocytopenia associated with haemolytic anaemia (Evans syndrome).
   c. **True**. Though the most common cause is primary autoimmune haemolytic anaemia, which is idiopathic in nature.
   d. **True**. Red cell transfusion may be necessary; if no compatible blood can be found then the least incompatible should be given.
   e. **True**. It is also called the direct antiglobulin test (DAT), which identifies antibodies and complement components on the surface of circulating erythrocytes.

14. a. **True**. This occurs in individuals with glucose 6-phosphate dehydrogenase deficiency.
   b. **False**. Iron deficiency occurs and hence microcytic anaemia, though fish tapeworm

(diphyllobothriasis) infestations colonise the lower intestine and may produce megaloblastic anaemia through $B_{12}$ deficiency.
   c. **True**. There is increased red cell turnover.
   d. **False**.
   e. **True**. This is thought to be an idiosyncratic reaction.

## Short notes answers

1. Bone marrow transplantation (BMT) is the infusion of donor marrow or stem cells into a recipient.

   **Sources of haematopoietic stem cells for transplantation**:

   - Allogeneic BMT using HLA-matched sibling
   - Allogeneic BMT using HLA, DR-matched or partially mismatched family members (other than sibling donors) or unrelated donors
   - Syngeneic BMT from an identical twin
   - Autologous BMT: the patient's own marrow is cryopreserved and then reinfused (purged or unpurged) after high-dose chemotherapy and/or radiation therapy to treat the underlying malignancy
   - Peripheral blood stem cells: the number of circulating stem cells can be vastly increased before apheresis with haematopoietic growth factors such as the granulocyte colony-stimulating factor (G-CSF)
   - Umbilical blood stem cells from an unrelated donor
   - Fetal liver stem cells from an unrelated donor.

   In all cases, the marrow is infused back by a peripheral/central vein. Pluripotential stem cells settle in the marrow stroma, proliferate, and repopulate the ablated bone marrow.
   **Principles of therapy**. The philosophy with allogeneic or syngeneic transplantation is to replace the host immune–reticuloendothelial system, which is presumably diseased, with that of the donor. To facilitate this, the recipient is heavily immunosuppressed and receives marrow-ablating therapy (either drugs such as cyclophosphamide or busulphan, or total body irradiation). In those with leukaemia, the donor immune system then eradicates the leukaemic cells (graft-versus-leukaemia effect). The use of peripheral stem cells is becoming an increasingly popular source of pluripotential stem cells. The relative immunological naiveté and the high numbers of pluripotential cells in cord blood make this an attractive source of stem cells in those patients without a matched sibling donor.

**Indications for BMT:**

- Malignancy: acute lymphoblastic leukaemia in second or third remission, acute myeloid leukaemia in first or second remission, chronic myeloid leukaemia
- Non-malignant conditions: congenital immunodeficiencies (e.g. severe combined immunodeficiency (SCID)), inherited metabolic disorders (e.g. Gaucher disease, Lesch–Nyhan etc.), haematological disorders (e.g. thalassaemia, Fanconi's anaemia, congenital neutropenia etc.).

**Acute complications:**

- Infections as a result of immunosuppression and prolonged period of neutropenia
- Acute graft-versus-host disease
- Veno-occlusive disease.

**Chronic complications:**

- Chronic graft-versus-host disease
- Growth failure
- Multiple endocrine problems
- Second malignancies
- Sterility.

2. Blood component therapy
   **Red blood cells.** These are the most frequently transfused component and are given to increase the oxygen-carrying capacity and maintain tissue oxygenation (Box 75). There is no standard haemoglobin level at which one should transfuse, as children with chronic anaemia tolerate lower levels of haemoglobin and children with iron deficiency anaemia will respond adequately to oral iron.

   In the neonatal period the haemoglobin may drop to around 9.0 g/dL at 9–12 weeks. This is physiological. Transfusion is not required and may in fact blunt the normal neonatal erythropoietin drive. Usually 10–15 mL/kg are transfused over 2–6 hours. This will increase the haemoglobin by approximately 2.5 g/dL. In children who have severe chronic anemia or are in congestive cardiac failure, transfusion rates need to be slow (2 mL/kg/h).

   **Platelets.** Platelets are generally given when the platelet count is $<50 \times 10^9$/L *and* the child is bleeding or about to undergo a surgical procedure. Similarly, platelet transfusions are indicated in children with platelet function disorders such as Glanzmann syndrome. There is evidence to suggest that children with a very low platelet count tend to bleed spontaneously. Therefore, in children with thrombocytopenia due to marrow failure, platelet transfusions may be given when the count drops to below $10–20 \times 10^9$/L. In ITP, platelet transfusions are only of use in life-threatening situations. Pooled platelet concentrates (PC) contain about $5.5 \times 10^{10}$ platelets per unit. Therefore 1 PC per 10 kg body weight will raise the platelet count by $50 \times 10^9$/L. Some children, especially those who have received platelet transfusions before, may be refractory to pooled platelets. These children may benefit from ABO-matched platelets from a single donor, or require HLA-matched platelet transfusion.

   **Plasma** or fresh frozen plasma (FFP) contains coagulation factors and is often used in situations such as DIC or where coagulation factors have been diminished because of treatment with vitamin K inhibitors (e.g. warfarin). It is also used in haemolytic uraemic syndrome, severe liver disease, where massive transfusions are to be given, or in congenital coagulation deficiencies where a safer and more appropriate product is not available. A dose of 10–20 mL/kg will raise the coagulation factors by 20%.

   **Granulocyte** transfusions are very rarely used and their use is contentious.

   **Cryoprecipitate** is rich in factor VIII, fibrinogen, fibronectin, von Willebrand factor and factor XIII. With the advent of virus-inactivated plasma concentrates and recombinant factor products, the use of cryoprecipitate is limited to fibrinogen deficiency or where factors are unavailable.

## Case history answer

1. a. **Diagnosis**: Acute chest syndrome in sickle cell anaemia,
   **Investigations**: Chest X-ray and percentage of sickle cells on blood film.

---

**Box 75** Indications for red blood cells in children

| Children >4 years | Indications for those <4 months old |
|---|---|
| Acute blood loss >25% of the circulating blood volume | Hb <13.0 g/dL and moderate lung disease |
| Hb <13.0 g/dL in severe cardiopulmonary disease | Hb <13.0 g/dL and severe cardiac disease |
| Hb <9.5 g/dL in thalassaemia major (elective) | Hb <10.0 g/dL and major surgery |
| Hb <8.0 g/dL in marrow failure | Hb <8.0 g/dL and symptomatic anaemia |
| Hb <8.0 g/dL in the perioperative period | |

b. Admit this child.
He is hypoxaemic and in respiratory distress and will require oxygen.
He is in acute pain and requires analgesia. Pain control is best achieved with a sliding scale starting with NSAIDs; however, as he is unwell a morphine infusion is preferable, with parent-/nurse-controlled analgesia if he is unable to do this for himself. Give hydration fluids to decrease sickling and broad-spectrum antibiotics to treat possible pneumonia. A top-up transfusion will help decrease the sickle cell percentage and improve tissue oxygenation, and if the symptoms do not improve then an exchange transfusion maybe considered.

c. It is very likely that he will require more hospital admissions and there is a risk of a cerebral stroke. This child may benefit from a regular transfusion programme. The main drawback is that he will also require chelation therapy. Another possibility is to try hydroxyurea to increase fetal haemoglobin. If these measures are not successful, then bone marrow transplantation is an alternative.

2. a. **Ask about:**
Fever
Symptoms of infection (e.g. cough etc.)
Weight loss
Drugs/medication
Blood in urine
Blood in stool
Recent travels
Pets/animal contacts/bites

b. **Look at:**
Mucous membranes
Fundi

c. **Distension:**
Hepatomegaly
Splenomegaly
Ascites
Lymphadenopathy
Tumour mass
*Haemorrhage*

d. **Differential diagnosis:**
Acute leukaemia or ALL or AML
Septicaemia
Severe viral infection
Leishmaniasis

e. i) In view of fever:
Blood cultures
Viral titres
*Mycoplasma* titres
Urine cultures

Bone marrow culture
CRP/ESR
*Lumbar puncture*

ii) For diagnosis:
Bone marrow aspiration

f. **Treatment includes:**
Platelet transfusion
Blood transfusion
Transfusion of fresh frozen plasma
Broad-spectrum antibiotics
Rehydration/fluid replacement
Allopurinol

## Viva voce answer

The most common cause for these symptoms is iron-deficiency anaemia. In a child with anaemia, the history is often diagnostic. A broad guideline is given below.

**Birth history.** Was the child born prematurely or with low birthweight? This could be a contributing factor. Was there prolonged neonatal jaundice suggestive of congenital haemolytic anaemias?

**Diet history.** Was he breastfed? Artificially fed? Was weaning carried out appropriately, and if he required vitamin and mineral supplements did he receive them?

**Family history.** Is there a family history of anaemia or jaundice? What is the ethnic origin of the child?

**Recent history.** Is the child on any medication or 'fad' feeds that could precipitate a haemolysis?

**System review.** Are there any sources of obvious blood loss, i.e. blood in the stools or urine, a previous bout of pneumonia (pulmonary haemosiderosis)? Is there any neurological involvement (megaloblastic anaemia)?

**Examination.** The child should be examined for pallor and icterus (conjunctiva, oral mucosa, fingernails and palms). Palpate the abdomen gently, as a slightly enlarged spleen in children tends to be quite soft and easily missed. The additional presence of mucosal ulcers (neutropenia), petechiae (thrombocytopenia) and lymph node enlargement will suggest that the diagnosis is more sinister (e.g. acute leukaemia). In chronic iron deficiency the fingernails may be concave (koilonychia), and a blue line on the gums is occasionally seen in lead poisoning. Megaloblastic anaemia is often associated with hyperpigmentation, particularly of the buccal mucosa.

**Investigation.** The diagnosis is confirmed by examination of the blood film and reticulocyte count (see Fig. 88).

**Management.** Treatment of even severe iron deficiency is successful with oral iron given over a period of 3 months.

## OSCE answers

### OSCE 1

You would be expected to examine for pallor (conjunctivae, palms and nails); jaundice (sclerae); and petechiae (skin, mucosae, retinae). Run your hands over the purpuric spots (are they palpable?), note their distribution, could they have been caused by injury? Are the bruises of different ages? Indictors for ITP rather than acute leukaemia would include his general wellbeing, normal growth, absence of lymph nodes or pallor, and no liver or spleen enlargement.

The symmetrical distribution of the rash, absence of other bruises of widely different ages and absence of other injuries would mitigate against non-accidental injury.

### OSCE 2

Examine for pallor (conjunctivae, palms and nails), jaundice (sclerae), and peripheral signs of liver cell failure (oedema, palmar erythema, flap, leukonychia, spider naevi, gynaecomastia). Complete an examination of the abdomen to assess for liver and spleen enlargement.

You would be expected to mention the most likely diagnosis (hereditary spherocytosis), and a potential differential diagnosis that would include other forms of haemolytic anaemias and acute leukaemia. Splenomegaly would militate against sickle cell anaemia or chronic G6PD.

### OSCE 3

a. A pathological fracture OR a fracture through a bone cyst/abnormal bone
b. Reduction of the fracture
c. Biopsy of the bone cyst

### OSCE 4

a. Chest X-ray with central/Hickman line in situ
b. Line infection, septicaemia, local/tract infection, line rupture, line blockage/thrombosis, line dehiscence resulting in embolic foreign body.

# 12 General surgery, orthopaedics, ENT and dental problems

**12.1** Introduction 261

**12.2** Congenital surgical abnormalities 261

**12.3** Acquired surgical abnormalities 269

**12.4** Orthopaedic disorders 273

**12.5** Disorders of the ears, nose and throat 280

**12.6** Dental problems 281

Self-assessment: questions 284

Self-assessment: answers 288

## Overview

Surgical problems constitute a significant workload for any paediatric unit and the undergraduate will be expected to appreciate those symptoms suggestive of surgical disease, particularly those relating to bowel obstruction. Similarly, the student should have an understanding of basic surgical resuscitative measures, the operative approach for common surgical problems, and postoperative management. This chapter outlines the most important orthopaedic, ENT and dental problems that commonly present in childhood.

## 12.1 Introduction

Although paediatric surgery is a highly specialized field, some surgical problems are sufficiently common and a basic awareness of their presenting symptoms and signs is required. Significant morbidity in surgical patients results from delayed diagnoses, disregard of surgery-related complications and ignorance in postoperative care. The undergraduate is therefore expected to know the preoperative resuscitation and postoperative management of common conditions.

Orthopaedic disorders, ear, nose and throat (ENT) and dental disorders may also require surgical intervention.

## 12.2 Congenital surgical abnormalities

### Learning objectives

You should:

- be aware of the common presentations of upper and lower intestinal obstruction in the neonatal period
- know the presentation and management of tracheo-oesophageal fistula, duodenal stenosis, meconium ileus, Hirschsprung disease and diaphragmatic hernia

Many congenital anomalies requiring surgical repair are detected on routine antenatal ultrasound screening. If so, arrangements should be made for the delivery to take place in a specialist centre with facilities for neonatal surgery and neonatal intensive care.

### Gastrointestinal atresia

Gastrointestinal obstruction is a common surgical problem, particularly in the newborn. The symptoms and signs vary depending on the site of obstruction: upper gastrointestinal lesions present with early onset of vomiting, whereas lower lesions initially result in abdominal distension and constipation and later vomiting. *Bile stained vomiting* in the newborn must be taken to represent gastrointestinal obstruction until proven otherwise. Abdominal tenderness and bowel signs may be difficult to assess, especially in neonates.

#### Oesophageal atresia

Failure of canalisation of the oesophagus and its connection with the stomach results in high gastrointestinal obstruction in 1 in 4000 live births. In 86% of cases with oesophageal atresia, a tracheo-oesophageal fistula (TOF) connects the distal, blind-ending oesophagus and the trachea (Fig. 119). Air is therefore able to enter the stomach, producing a characteristic X-ray appearance with a blind upper oesophagus and a large gastric gas

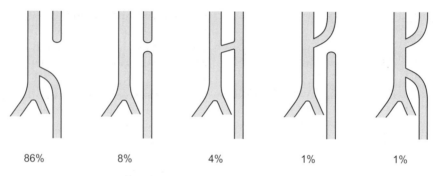

86%          8%          4%          1%          1%

**Fig. 119** Oesophageal atresia with tracheo-oesophageal fistula.

---

**Box 76** Oesophageal atresia

**Signs and symptoms**

| | |
|---|---|
| Antenatal (ultrasound) | Polyhydramnios |
| | Small or empty fetal stomach |
| | Dilated oesophageal pouch |
| Early neonatal | Frothy secretions |
| | Choking and cyanosis on feeding |

**Diagnosis**
Failure to pass nasogastric tube
Chest X-ray shows nasogastric tube in oesophagus

**Management**
Withhold all feeds
Pass large-bore nasogastric tube into upper oesophagus and put on continuous suction
Intravenous fluids and nutrition
Broad-spectrum antibiotics
Cross-match
Urgent closure of fistula and reanastomosis of oesophageal ends

---

**Box 77** Duodenal atresia

**Signs and symptoms**

| | |
|---|---|
| Antenatal (ultrasound) | Polyhydramnios |
| | Double bubble appearance |
| Neonatal period | Vomiting on first day of life |
| | Often bile stained vomitus |
| | Abdomen is not distended |

**Diagnosis**
X-ray showing 'double-bubble' appearance in an otherwise gasless abdomen (Fig. 120)

**Management**
Withhold all feeds
Pass large-bore nasogastric tube and put on continuous suction
Intravenous fluids and nutrition
Broad-spectrum antibiotics
Cross-match
Repair of the duodenum – Kimara Diamond anastomosis
Correct malrotation if present
Divide Ladd bands
Duodenoduodenostomy if there is an annular pancreas

---

bubble. Up to 50% of patients with tracheo-oesophageal (TE) abnormalities will have other anomalies, involving the vertebrae, anus, cardiovascular system, renal system and radii (VACTER), and these must be investigated appropriately in all cases.

All types of oesophageal atresia, barring the H-type, present in the newborn period. The H-type variant presents with recurrent aspiration and chest infections in later infancy and childhood.

Occasionally, the gap between the two ends of the oesophagus is too wide to close, and a gastric pull-up procedure is performed when the child is 6 months old. In the meantime, an oesophagostomy and feeding gastrostomy are fashioned. Late complications include tracheomalacia, gastro-oesophageal reflux and oesophageal stenosis. The prognosis depends on the preoperative condition and the severity of associated anomalies (Box 76).

## Duodenal atresia

At 5 weeks of embryonic life the lumen of the duodenum is obliterated by proliferating epithelium. The patency of the lumen is usually restored by the 11th week and failure of vacuolisation may lead to stenosis or atresia. Duodenal obstruction can also be caused by compression from the surrounding annular pancreas or by peritoneal fibrous bands (Ladd's band). The obstruction itself is often distal to the opening of the common bile duct. Duodenal atresia arises in 1 in 10 000 births: 30% of cases occur in children with Down syndrome, but it is common in association with other anomalies of the gastrointestinal tract (e.g. malrotation, oesophageal and anal atresia) and cardiovascular and renal systems (Box 77).

## Small-bowel atresia

Intestinal obstructions are either intrinsic or extrinsic. Intrinsic lesions result from absent (atresia) or partial (stenosis) recanalisation of the intestine. In cases of atresia, the two segments of the gut may be either completely separated or connected by a fibrous cord. In cases of stenosis, the lumen of the gut is narrowed or the two intestinal segments are separated by a septum with a central diaphragm. Apple-peel atresia is characterised by the absence of a vast segment of the small bowel, which can include distal duodenum, the entire jejunum and proximal ileus. Extrinsic obstructions are caused by malrotation of the colon with volvulus, peritoneal bands, meconium ileus, and agangliosis (Hirschsprung disease). The most frequent site of small bowel obstruction is distal ileus (35%), followed by proximal jejunum (30%), distal jejunum (20%) and proximal ileus (15%). In about 5% of cases obstructions occur in multiple sites. Anorectal atresia results from abnormal division of the cloaca during the 9th week of development. Antenatally, a diagnosis of obstruction is usually made quite late (after 25 weeks), as dilatation of the intestinal lumen is slow and progressive. On ultrasound, jejunal and ileal obstructions are imaged as multiple fluid-filled loops of bowel in the abdomen. In the neonatal period, jejunoileal atresia presents with bile-stained vomiting, abdominal distension and failure to pass meconium. Distended bowel loops are evident on a plain X-ray film and fluid levels on a lateral decubitus film. Contrast studies will delineate the level of obstruction. An NGT should be passed and left on free drainage, and antibiotic prophylaxis and intravenous hydration commenced. Surgical correction is planned when the condition is stable, and involves resection of non-viable bowel and, ideally, end-to-end anastomosis in the first instance. Following multiple resections, and when bowel distension is severe, a defunctioning ileostomy with distal mucus fistula is preferable, with reversal of the stoma 3–4 months later (Fig. 121).

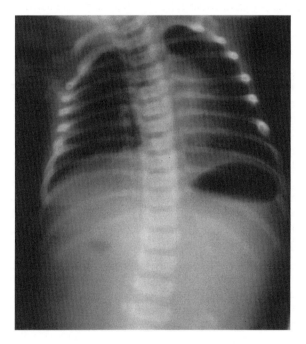

**Fig. 120** X-ray showing double-bubble appearance of duodenal atresia.

## Meconium ileus

Meconium ileus is a manifestation of intestinal and pancreatic dysfunction that results in the accumulation of a sticky and inspissated intraluminal meconium and is mostly a manifestation of cystic fibrosis. This is the earliest manifestation of disease, and up to a sixth of patients with cystic fibrosis develop meconium ileus. Pellets of viscid meconium obstruct the colon and terminal ileum *in utero* (Box 78).

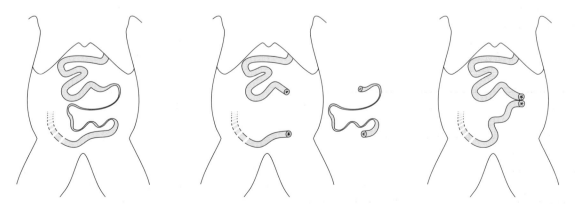

**Fig. 121** Primary ileostomy and late correction in small-bowel atresia.

---

**Box 78** Meconium ileus

**Signs and symptoms**

| | |
|---|---|
| Antenatal (ultrasound) | Intra-abdominal echogenic area |
| | Dilated bowel loops |
| | Ascites |
| Neonatal period | Abdominal distension |
| | Failure to pass meconium |
| | Bilious vomiting |

**Diagnosis**

| | |
|---|---|
| X-ray | Hazy, ground-glass appearance of bowel caused by air bubbles trapped in inspissated meconium |
| | Patchy calcification |

**Management**

Gentle enemas (e.g. Gastrografin with detergent) every 8–12 hours may reduce the impaction in 50% of patients

Consider irrigation of bowel via an ileostomy with mucolytic agents (e.g. acetylcysteine)

Meconium peritonitis or ischaemic complications may require bowel resection

May require long-term intravenous feeding

Screening for cystic fibrosis

---

## Anorectal anomaly

Anal atresia is a manifestation of maldevelopment of the cloaca. Hence an imperforate anus is often associated with lower urogenital defects, especially a fistula to the perineum, urethra, bladder or female vestibule. Additionally, anal atresia may be associated with sacral agenesis, other bowel atresias and heart defects. The diagnosis relies on the absence of an anal orifice on routine examination at birth, and failure to pass meconium. The level of the atresia and the presence of a fistula should be determined preoperatively. After the first 24 hours the infant is placed prone for half an hour with the buttocks supported over a small towel. A radio-opaque marker is placed on the anal dimple and a lateral X-ray film taken. If the distance between the rectal gas shadow and the marker is greater than 1 cm, this is suggestive of a high atresia and an indication for a colostomy. Low lesions and those where the anal sphincter is intact (as suggested by a well-formed perineal crease and anal dimple) are repaired by a simple pull-through operation (anoplasty). Many will require further treatment to relieve a variable degree of constipation. Lesions above the pelvic muscular sling usually require a defunctioning colostomy and late correction. These, especially if associated with a rectovesical fistula and sacral agenesis, have a guarded prognosis for future bowel continence.

## Biliary atresia

Failure of canalisation or progressive obliteration of the intra- and/or extrahepatic biliary tubules results in biliary atresia in 1 in 10 000 live births. Up to 85% involve the entire extrahepatic ducts, making surgical correction difficult. Biliary atresia is the most important cause of obstructed hyperbilirubinaemia in the newborn, presenting with persistent conjugated hyperbilirubinaemia, pale stools and dark urine, hepatomegaly and failure to thrive. The prognosis improves with earlier diagnosis, and is poor if treatment is commenced after the first 6 weeks of life. The diagnosis is suggested by biochemical evidence of an obstructed jaundice. Biliary atresia must be differentiated from other causes of cholestatic jaundice and neonatal hepatitis. Ultrasonography should exclude a choledochal cyst and other causes of extrahepatic biliary obstruction. Biliary atresia is more likely than neonatal hepatitis if the stools are persistently acholic (pale) and there is no bile on aspiration of duodenal contents. Furthermore, hepatobiliary scintigraphy should demonstrate preserved uptake of isotope tracer by the functioning hepatocytes, but absent excretion into the bowel. With hepatitis, uptake is sluggish but excretion does eventually occur. Ultimately, the diagnosis is confirmed by demonstrating an absence of biliary canaliculi, bile plugs and fibrosis on liver biopsy. In contrast, with neonatal hepatitis there is widespread disruption of the lobular architecture, focal necrosis, and an intense inflammatory response.

Correctable lesions (e.g. a choledochal cyst) should be resected. For biliary duct atresia, a hepatoportoenterostomy (Kasai procedure) is performed, preferably before the eighth week of life, when there is a 90% chance of establishing adequate biliary flow. The operation entails the anastomosis of an isolated loop of small bowel (Roux en-Y) to the porta hepatis, thereby rerouting biliary drainage from residual, small canaliculi into the bowel.

Ascending cholangitis is a serious complication following this procedure, and must be suspected and treated with broad-spectrum antibiotics whenever a fever and increasing jaundice develop. Despite palliation by the Kasai procedure, chronic hepatic inflammation results in cirrhosis and portal hypertension. Ultimately, liver transplantation is the best long-term option for many of these patients.

## Malrotation and volvulus

Infants whose bowel has not developed along the usual embryonic 'anticlockwise' pattern develop bowel malrotation. This predisposes the bowel to twisting on its own axis, constricting the lumen and compromising its

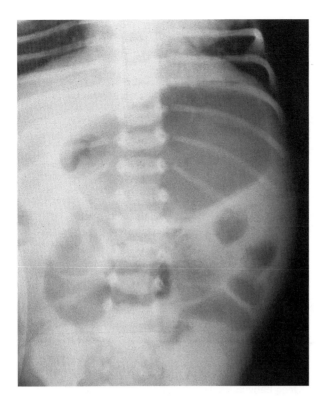

**Fig. 122** X-ray showing dilated bowel loops and fluid levels due to volvulus.

blood supply. In most cases, the caecum lies in a sub-hepatic position and the duodenal–jejunal flexure lies to the right of the midline. The superior mesenteric artery is tethered along a narrow stalk, predisposing to a midgut volvulus. The condition usually manifests acutely in infancy, when signs of bowel obstruction are associated with a rapid deterioration in clinical state (Fig. 122). Surgery to release the volvulus, resect necrotic tissue and place the remaining bowel in its correct alignment (Ladd's procedure) is life saving and should not be delayed. Occasionally, malrotation presents subacutely in preschool children, who fail to thrive and develop intermittent bouts of abdominal pain, distension and vomiting caused by recurrent subacute bowel obstruction. The malrotation can be confirmed by contrast studies of the small bowel, prior to corrective surgery.

## Hirschsprung disease

Hirschsprung disease occurs in 1 in 5000 live births and is more common in boys (4 : 1). It is the most common cause of lower intestinal obstruction in the neonate, and is occasionally associated with other anomalies (e.g. Down syndrome, heart disease). Failure of neuroblast migration from proximal to distal bowel results in an absence of ganglion cells in the submucosa, absent Meissner and Auerbach plexi, and hypertrophied nerve

bundles with increased levels of acetylcholinesterase beyond the submucosa. The aganglionic segment commences at the internal anal sphincter and progresses proximally for a variable distance. It is limited to the rectosigmoid in 75% of patients, but in 10% it affects the entire colon. A gradual increase in neurons is seen in a transition zone that varies in length until normal histological appearances prevail.

Hirschsprung disease should be considered in term babies who fail to pass meconium within 48 hours of birth. Patients usually present in the neonatal period with abdominal distension, which often precedes vomiting. Explosive, foul motions may follow a rectal examination, which may confirm a 'tight' lower rectal segment. If undiagnosed, stasis of bowel contents and mucosal disruption increase the risk of enterocolitis and septicaemia. Occasionally Hirschsprung disease is diagnosed in older children following prolonged, severe constipation and, rarely, is a cause of failure to thrive owing to an associated protein-losing enteropathy.

Confirmation of the diagnosis relies on a lower bowel contrast study showing a microcolon of variable length, rectal manometry (if available) and a punch biopsy of the lower rectum. At operation, several biopsies should be sent for frozen section and the resection margin taken at the site of normal and not transition bowel. Short-segment Hirschsprung disease (i.e. not extending beyond the descending colon) has an excellent prognosis. Those with long-segment disease, particularly those with total colonic Hirschsprung, have a poor prognosis for long-term continence. Rectal pouch refashioning procedures have been designed following total colectomy, but the improvement in loose stool and excessive stool frequency is often short lived.

## Hernias

### Diaphragmatic hernia

Development of the diaphragm is usually completed by the 9th week of gestation. In up to 1 in 4000 births an absence or a defect in the diaphragm allows the herniation of abdominal viscera into the thorax at about 10–12 weeks, when the intestines return to the abdominal cavity from the umbilical cord. In some cases, intrathoracic herniation of viscera may be delayed until the second or third trimester of pregnancy or the early neonatal period. The commonest site of herniation is through the left posterolateral opening (Bochdalek hernia), and very rarely through the oesophageal hiatus (hiatal hernia) or behind the sternum (Morgagni hernia). The latter is always associated with malrotation, often with cardiovascular, neurological, gastrointestinal and major chromosomal abnormalities. The hernial mass prevents adequate lung development on the ipsilateral

a

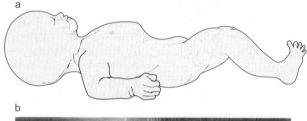

b

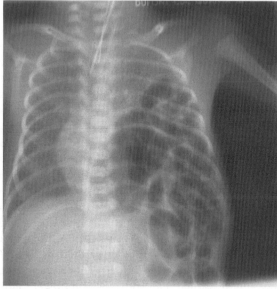

**Fig. 123** Congenital diaphragmatic hernia. (a) Clinical appearance with cyanosis, respiratory distress and scaphoid abdomen. (b) Radiological appearance with bowel loops in thorax, mediastinal shift and a gasless abdomen.

**Box 79** Diaphragmatic hernia

**Signs and symptoms**

| Antenatal (ultrasound) | Polyhydramnios |
|---|---|
| | Demonstration of stomach and intestines (90% of cases) or liver (50%) in the thorax |
| | Mediastinal shift of thoracic contents to the opposite side. |
| Neonatal period | Acute respiratory distress worsened by resuscitation with face mask |
| | Scaphoid (empty) abdomen |
| | Mediastinal shift |
| | Bowel sounds in chest wall |

**Diagnosis (Should almost always be made antenatally)**

| X-ray | Presence of bowel in the thorax |
|---|---|
| | Mediastinal shift |
| | Atelectatic pulmonary tissue |

**Management**

Nasogastric tube to decompress stomach
Intravenous fluids
Intubate and ventilate
Consider prostacyclin or inhaled nitric oxide to reduce pulmonary vascular resistance
Once baby is stable, surgical repair of defect, which may require a prosthetic patch

side, and if there is significant mediastinal shift there can also be significant contralateral pulmonary hypoplasia (Fig. 123; Box 79).

There is significant morbidity and a mortality of about 40% in the early neonatal period. This is related primarily to the severe degree of pulmonary hypoplasia and hypertension. A prolonged period of ventilatory support is often necessary, both pre- and postoperatively. The use of high-frequency oscillation (HFO) ventilation to reduce the risk of barotrauma to the lungs, and nitric oxide (NO) to decrease pulmonary hypertension, may be useful in difficult cases. Currently, research centres on the feasibility of extracorporeal membrane oxygenation (ECMO) and fetal surgery for this condition, although the benefit of this approach is as yet unknown. Long-term survivors have an increased risk of reactive airways disease, developmental delay, gastro-oesophageal reflux, nutritional problems and failure to thrive.

## Inguinal hernia

Inguinal hernias arise following persistence of the processus vaginalis, a primitive protrusion of the peri-toneum through which the testes descend into the inguinal canal. An inguinal hernia is found in almost 2% of children, making this the most common lesion requiring surgery in childhood.

It is commonest in boys (4 : 1) and is almost invariably indirect in type; 10% are bilateral. In boys, it is often associated with undescended testes and presents as an intermittent lump in the groin, scrotum or labia majora, especially during straining or crying. Incarceration develops in 10% of children, but in the majority can be reduced after sedation and gentle palpation. Incarceration should be followed by hernia repair within 48 hours. The risk of strangulation is much greater in the small newborn and in the first year of life, and is suspected if vomiting and abdominal distension develop in the presence of a tender, non-reducible mass. In neonates, surgical repair is best performed prior to discharge from hospital, whereas in the infant age group repair should be effected electively soon after diagnosis. There is less urgency in older children, where the abdominal defect is wide and the hernia is rarely complicated by bowel obstruction. Any associated anomaly, such as undescended testes, should be addressed concurrently. The operative complication rate and recurrence risk for inguinal repair are 1% and 4%, respectively.

## Hydrocoele

Hydrocoeles arise when persistence of the processus vaginalis allows fluid to accumulate in the scrotal sac. The anomaly is usually bilateral and produces painless, cystic swellings that transilluminate brilliantly, sometimes with testicular shadows visible within. Most will resolve spontaneously. Surgery is only indicated when the hydrocoele persists beyond 12 months, and involves ligation of the patent processus vaginalis.

## Gastroschisis

Gastroschisis describes the herniation of loops of bowel not encased within a sac of Wharton's jelly through a defect in the abdominal wall, usually to the right of the umbilicus (Fig. 124a). The diagnosis is usually made on antenatal ultrasound, and naked bowel loops are seen extruding through the abdominal wall at birth. The newborn must be resuscitated and not fed; an NGT is passed and intravenous fluids commenced. The bowel is wrapped in warm plastic film to prevent heat loss and excessive drying prior to surgery. Surgery may necessitate bowel resection if the extruded loops undergo external volvulus and ischaemia. Problems may be encountered on attempting to reinsert the bowel into a relatively small, underdeveloped abdominal cavity, and a staged closure procedure is sometimes required.

## Exomphalos

With exomphalos (omphalocoele) the abdominal contents, including bowel and viscera such as liver and spleen, herniate through the umbilicus in a sac of Wharton's jelly (Fig. 124b). This occurs in approximately 1 in 5000 births. This defect, unlike gastroschisis, may be associated with abnormalities of the karyotype as well as congenital anomalies of the cardiovascular, urogenital and neurological systems. The association of exomphalos with macroglossia, gigantism and neonatal hypoglycaemia constitutes the features of the Beckwith–Wiedemann syndrome.

# Neurological abnormalities

## Neural tube defects and hydrocephalus

These are discussed in Chapter 6.

## Craniosynostosis

The premature fusion of one or more cranial sutures results in an abnormally shaped head and, in some cases, increased intracranial pressure. Craniosynostosis may occur as part of a multiple malformation syndrome, often with autosomal dominant inheritance, e.g. Crouzon syndrome (with proptosis and conductive hearing loss) and Apert syndrome (with syndactyly). The management involves complex, combined maxillofacial and neurosurgical repair.

# Urogenital abnormalities

The primitive kidney develops from the mesonephric duct and migrates upwards along the posterior abdominal wall to lie in the paravertebral gutter beneath the

a

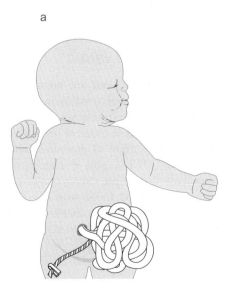

b

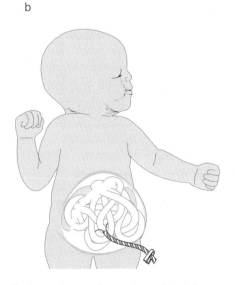

**Fig. 124** (a) Congenital gastroschisis: herniation of naked bowel, sometimes strangulated, in an otherwise normal infant. (b) Exomphalos: bowel and abdominal viscera herniate in a sac of Wharton's jelly; other anomalies may coexist.

overhanging lower ribs. Defects in this embryological process result in congenital anomalies of the renal tracts and are very common, both in isolation and in association with anomalies of other major systems, including the heart, brain, gastrointestinal tract and skeleton. In the *prune-belly syndrome*, renal anomalies are associated with poor renal function, absent abdominal musculature and undescended testes. This condition, like many severe congenital renal anomalies, results in oligohydramnios and secondary pulmonary hypoplasia.

## Hydronephrosis

Obstructions at the pelviureteric junction (PUJ), vesicoureteric junction (VUJ), ureters or urethra can result in retrograde pressure and dilatation of the urinary tract. When the obstruction is complete and occurs early in fetal life, renal hypoplasia and dysplasia ensue. On the other hand, where intermittent obstruction allows for normal renal development, or when it occurs in the second half of pregnancy, hydronephrosis will result and the severity of the renal damage will depend on the degree and duration of the obstruction. Renal pelvic dilatation is therefore often first detected on antenatal ultrasound. Attempts to alleviate the pressure by the insertion of drains antenatally have produced disappointing results, and postnatal procedures are preferable. Postnatal serial ultrasound scans are performed to monitor the progression of the hydronephrosis; micturating cystoureterograms (MCUG) to assess ureteric reflux; and a DTPA (diethylenetriamine penta-acetic acid) or MAG3 isotope excretion scan to assess renal function and the degree of obstruction.

Early surgery is indicated if there is bilateral disease, severe reflux and renal dysfunction. Nephrostomy drainage is beneficial in the short term, pyeloplasty for PUJ obstruction, and ureteric reimplantation for VUJ obstruction. The outcome is related to the degree of obstruction and extent of renal parenchymal dysfunction, especially if both kidneys are involved.

## Duplex system and ureterocoele

A duplex system may be a normal variant and of no consequence. The upper moiety ureter usually drains further down than the upper moiety. If it drains below the urinary bladder sphincter this will result in urinary incontinence (Fig. 125). Cystic dilatation of the lower ureter produces a ureterocoele, commonly associated with duplex systems and which almost invariably results in ureteric obstruction.

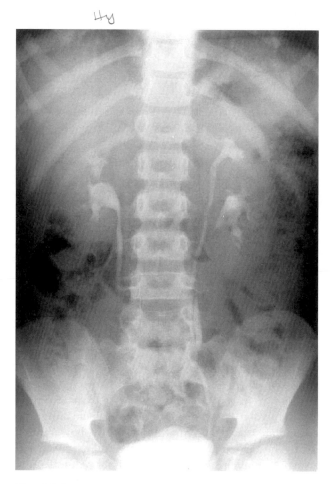

**Fig. 125** Intravenous pyelogram showing hydronephrosis and a duplex left-sided collecting system.

Treatment involves excision and ureteric reimplantation in all but the smallest lesions. If the upper pole of the kidney is dysplastic, a heminephroureterectomy may be performed.

## Posterior urethral valves

Posterior urethral valves are congenital valves that lie within the posterior urethra in boys and result in severe obstruction, with subsequent dilatation of the renal tracts. They are a cause of renal failure in infancy, and early intervention is essential. The diagnosis is confirmed by MCUG and during cystoscopy, when ablation/resection of the valves can be carried out. The prognosis is worse in those with deranged renal function, ureteric reflux and urinary infection. A third of patients go on to develop end-stage renal failure and require renal transplantation.

# Ambiguous genitalia

The surgical treatment of ambiguous genitalia is covered in Chapter 8.

# 12.3 Acquired surgical abnormalities

## Learning objectives

You should:

- know how to examine and manage a baby with pyloric stenosis

- know how to examine and manage a child with appendicitis

- be aware of the clinical manifestations and diagnosis of a child with intussusception

## Obstructive gastrointestinal lesions

### Pyloric stenosis

Pyloric stenosis involves hypertrophic enlargement of the gastric pylorus, resulting in high gastrointestinal obstruction. It typically presents with vomiting and weight loss at around the age of 2–6 weeks (Box 80).

### Hernias

*Umbilical* hernias are usually small (<1 cm) and often resolve spontaneously as the child grows, negating the need for surgical intervention. They are more likely after repair of an exomphalos. Umbilical hernias greater than 1 cm in diameter and which persist beyond the age of 5 years will require surgical closure. *Epigastric* and *supraumbilical* hernias develop above the umbilicus and do not close spontaneously, requiring simple surgical closure. *Inguinal* hernias are discussed above.

### Intussusception

Intussusception is the telescoping or prolapse of one portion of the bowel into an immediately adjacent segment, causing bowel ischaemia and obstruction. It occurs mostly in boys aged between 3 months and 3 years who generally do not have an underlying abnormality in the bowel (Box 81) and the most common site is the terminal ileum (i.e. ileocolic). Once the diagnosis is established, a contrast enema is performed in an attempt to reduce the intussusception. This is contraindicated in those where significant bowel ischaemia or perforation is suspected, when urgent surgery should follow resuscitation. Any gangrenous portions and the leading focus will need to be resected/biopsied, the intussusception undone and the residual bowel reanastomosed.

Despite a small risk of recurrence (10% with hydrostatic and 2% with surgical reduction), the prognosis is excellent provided the diagnosis is suspected and treatment commenced before gangrene is established. If untreated, this condition is usually fatal.

---

**Box 80** Pyloric stenosis

**Signs and symptoms**
Frequent projectile non-bilious vomiting at 2–3 weeks of age
Hungry infant
Constipation
Dehydration
Hypochloraemic alkalosis (from loss of stomach acid)

**Diagnosis**
Palpation of hypertrophied pylorus while baby is being fed
Visible gastric peristalsis
Ultrasound demonstrates an elongated sausage-shaped mass with a pyloric diameter greater than 14 mm, a muscular thickness greater than 4 mm, and a length greater than 16 mm

**Management**
Check electrolytes and haemoglobin
Correct dehydration and hypochloraemia
Correct hypokalaemia if necessary, only after the baby has passed urine
Open or laparoscopic pyloromyotomy
Restart feeding 4 hours post surgery

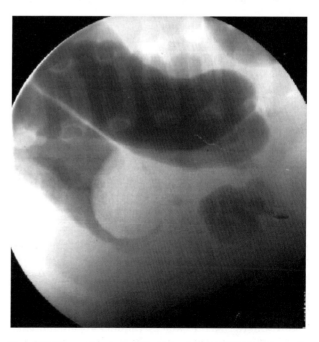

**Fig. 126** X-ray showing dilated bowel loop with clear 'cut-off' suggestive of intussusception.

**Aetiology**
Idiopathic
Enlarged Peyer's patch – recent upper respiratory or diarrhoeal illness
Henoch–Schönlein purpura
Enteric cyst
Cystic fibrosis
Chronic indwelling intestinal tubes
Meckel diverticulum
Intestinal polyps
Blunt abdominal trauma with intestinal or mesenteric haematomas
Haemangioma
Foreign body

**Signs and symptoms**
Sudden onset of acute colicky pain in infant or toddler associated with drawing up of knees and turning pale
Vomiting
Loose or watery stools initially
Later blood or mucous (red currant jelly) stools
Sausage-shaped mass palpable in ascending or transverse colon

**Diagnosis**
Plain abdominal X-ray often shows filling defect and presence of fluid levels in the bowel (indicative of obstruction)
Ultrasound 'target sign' of layers of intussusception

**Management**
Intravenous infusion and rehydration
Nasogastric tube if persistent vomiting
Hydrostatic reduction with air or barium under X-ray screening (also diagnostic)

## Meckel diverticulum

Meckel diverticulum is a small bowel outcrop formed as a remnant of the omphalomesenteric (yolk) sac. It usually measures 3–6 cm and is positioned on the antimesenteric border, 50 cm proximal to the caecum. It is usually an incidental finding at laparotomy. In the majority of symptomatic cases the diverticulum contains ectopic gastric mucosa that secretes acid, resulting in ulceration of the surrounding ileal mucosa and painless rectal bleeding, manifest as brick-red stools. Meckel diverticulum may result in an intussusception and may occasionally become inflamed, presenting in a similar fashion to acute appendicitis. Where the diverticulum is attached to the abdominal wall by a fibrous band, a volvulus and bowel obstruction may ensue. These patients will present with acute or subacute abdominal pain, sometimes localised to the periumbilical region, and vomiting. Acute attacks cannot be differentiated from acute appendicitis, and the diagnosis is often confirmed at surgery. When Meckel diverticulum is sus-

pected in patients with subacute symptoms, the diverticulum can be demonstrated by intravenous injection of a technetium-99m pertechnetate ($^{99m}$Tc)-labelled tracer, which is taken up by the ectopic gastric mucosa, producing a 'hot spot' on imaging. Treatment involves surgical resection of the diverticulum.

## Inflammatory gastrointestinal conditions

### Appendicitis

Appendicitis remains the most common ailment requiring emergency surgery in childhood. It arises through inflammation of the appendix, possibly after blockage of the lumen by a faecolith, occasionally a tumour, foreign body, infection (*Salmonella, Shigella, Ascaris* spp.) or abnormal mucus (e.g. cystic fibrosis). Luminal obstruction and mucus production result in increased intraluminal pressure. Bacteria trapped within the appendiceal lumen begin to multiply, and the appendix becomes distended. Venous congestion and oedema follow next, and by 12 hours after onset the inflammatory process may become transmural. Peritoneal irritation then develops. If the obstruction is left untreated, arterial blood flow to the appendix is compromised, and this leads to tissue ischaemia. Full-thickness necrosis of the appendiceal wall leads to perforation, with the release of faecal and suppurative contents into the peritoneal cavity. Depending on the duration of the disease process, either a localised walled-off abscess occurs or, if the pathologic process has advanced rapidly, the perforation is free in the peritoneal cavity and generalised peritonitis occurs. Because of the difficulty of making the correct diagnosis in childhood, perforation occurs in up to 70% of those aged less than 4 years, compared with 30% in adolescents. Systemic debility, together with generalised abdominal pain, rebound and guarding, is suggestive of peritonitis. Investigations are useful to eliminate other conditions in the differential diagnosis (Table 76), but are unnecessary if the clinical diagnosis is not in doubt.

Acute appendicitis is associated with a mortality of about 0.5%, mainly through missed or delayed diagnosis, resulting in perforation and infection.

### Inflammatory bowel disease

Ideally, surgery is avoided in children with inflammatory bowel disease. It is sometimes necessary to treat localised areas of severe inflammation, bleeding, constriction and chronic fistulation in *Crohn's disease*. However, the risk of recurrence is almost 50% within 5 years of surgery, and surgery may potentiate fistulation,

**Table 76** Differential diagnosis in acute appendicitis

| Diagnosis | Symptoms and signs | Investigation |
|---|---|---|
| **Infection** | | |
| Urinary tract | Urinary symptoms | Urinalysis |
| Gastrointestinal (e.g. *Salmonella*, *Campylobacter*, | Vomiting before pain | Stool, blood culture |
| *Shigella*, *Yersinia*, *Ascaris* spp.) | Diarrhoea dominant | |
| **Inflammatory conditions** | | |
| Mesenteric adenitis | Prodrome, pain not localised | |
| Henoch–Schönlein purpura | Skin, joint problems | Urinalysis, full blood count normal |
| Crohn's, ulcerative colitis | Pain, diarrhoea, weight loss | Contrast meal, biopsy |
| Chemotherapy typhilitis | Drug history, diarrhoea | Neutropenic |
| **Surgical disorders** | | |
| Torsion | Painful testicle | |
| Intussusception | Paroxysmal pain, mass | X-ray, contrast enema and ultrasound |
| Meckel diverticulum | Similar symptoms, signs | $^{99m}$Tc-labelled tracer scan |
| Constipation | Infrequent, firm stool | Plain abdominal X-ray |

**Box 82** Appendicitis

**Signs and symptoms**
Abdominal pain – first periumbilical, then localised to
left iliac fossa (McBurney's point)
Nausea and vomiting
Fever
Coated tongue
Palpate very gently for guarding, rigidity and tenderness
at the McBurney's point
DO NOT ELICIT REBOUND TENDERNESS
Consider digital rectal examination for pelvic appendix if
no other findings

**Diagnosis**
Ultrasound identification of a non-compressible tubular
structure 6 mm or wider in the right lower quadrant.
Often the probe elicits tenderness

**Management**
Intravenous fluids and rehydration
Broad-spectrum antibiotics, including anaerobic cover
Open or laparoscopic appendectomy

stricture, and adhesion formation. Resection should be kept to a minimum to avoid a short-bowel syndrome. Associated abscesses often need surgical drainage in both Crohn's disease and *ulcerative colitis*. In the latter, an acute deterioration in the general condition associated with increased loose bloody stools, abdominal pain, distension and diminished bowel sounds may herald *toxic megacolon* (see Section 5.6). Failure to respond rapidly to conservative management involving intravenous hydration, analgesia, broad-spectrum antibiotics and anti-inflammatory agents is an indication for emergency total colectomy.

## Urological abnormalities

### Obstructive lesions

Acquired hydronephrosis and PUJ and VUJ obstruction require similar treatment to the congenital lesions (see above). Subsequent ureteric stenosis following previous surgery may be alleviated by pyeloplasty techniques employed during cystoscopy. Polyps and tumours – usually botryoid rhabdosarcomas in children – may be found in the bladder and require resection and appropriate chemotherapy and radiotherapy.

### Urinary calculi

Urinary calculi develop in patients with abnormal urine or those with abnormal urinary tracts, especially if this is associated with urinary stasis and recurrent infection. Stones often result in frank or microscopic haematuria, bouts of recurrent renal colic, symptoms of an associated urinary tract infection, and occasionally acute ureteric obstruction. Stones are usually demonstrated on ultrasound imaging and, if calcified, on plain abdominal X-ray film. When found, a full assessment of the urinary tracts is necessary to rule out stasis, obstruction or infection. A screen of the serum and urine will exclude a metabolic disorder predisposing to stone formation (Box 83).

**Management**
Many calculi, both intrarenal and those lying within the collecting system, are small and require medical management aimed at the underlying metabolic disorder and control of infection. Larger calculi (e.g. staghorn calculi) are typically associated with infections, commonly caused by *Proteus* species. Treatment is

---

**Box 83** Causes of urinary calculi

| Abnormal urine and serum | Abnormal urinary tract |
|---|---|
| Excess salts: | Recurrent infection |
| hypercalcaemia, | |
| hypercalciuria, | Pelviureteric or |
| hyperphosphaturia | vesicoureteric junction |
| | obstruction |
| Organic acids: | Duplex systems |
| hyperuricaemia, | |
| hyperoxaluria | Renal tubular acidosis |
| | |
| Amino acids: | |
| xanthinuria, | |
| cystinuria | |

---

directed at ensuring constant diuresis and establishing an appropriate urinary pH to prevent stone precipitation. Occasionally open surgery is required for those stones resulting in severe bleeding, obstruction or recurrent infection. For appropriately sized and positioned stones, lithotripsy can be used.

## Abnormalities of the reproductive organs

### Testes

#### Undescended testes
Undescended testes are found in about 1% of boys during routine examination. Bilateral undescended testes occur in 25% and may be associated with dysmorphic syndromes and chromosomal abnormalities. Undescended testes arise because of incomplete descent along the normal tract, and sometimes can also be found in an ectopic position. Some testes are particularly retractile, and it is important to palpate with warm hands, locating and 'fixing' one side first, before searching for the missing organ throughout the inguinal region down to the scrotum. If located, a gentle attempt should be made to determine the extent to which the testes can be milked into the scrotum. Ultrasound and, if necessary, laparoscopy may locate missing/abdominal testes. Testes lying outside the scrotum will not function normally and, if bilateral, carry a high risk of infertility. In addition, intra-abdominal testes have a 30-fold increased risk of malignant change (usually seminoma) after the third decade of life. Hence, orchidopexy, whereby the testis is untethered and fixed in the scrotum, should be performed between the age of 1 and 2 years. Any associated inguinal hernia and hydrocoele should be treated simultaneously.

#### Testicular torsion
Testicular torsion arises when the testis twists on its vascular pedicle, producing venous congestion and local ischaemia. The condition presents with acute pain and local swelling in preschool and school-aged boys. Examination confirms a tender, swollen scrotal mass associated with bluish discoloration. The testis is often not palpable within the swelling, which does not transilluminate. The differential diagnosis should include torsion of the hydatid of Morgagni, epididymitis and orchitis.

**Management**. Treatment entails analgesia followed by urgent surgical untwisting of the affected organ. In view of the risk of recurrence bilaterally, orchidopexy (fixation) of *both* testes in the scrotum is performed. Surgery within 6 hours of torsion carries a 90% chance of testicular salvage, but a good outcome is unlikely with prolonged delay. Torsion in neonates usually results in infarction and later involution, with loss of the testis. Supportive treatment is appropriate in the first instance, with prosthetic implants later in life and, for those with bilateral infarction, testosterone replacement.

#### Malignant swelling
Malignant testicular swelling is usually caused by leukaemic–lymphomatous infiltration, rarely by primary testicular teratomas. Although biopsy is required in the first instance, total excision is indicated for a primary tumour, followed by chemoradiotherapy as appropriate.

### Penis

Hypospadias, present in 0.2% of newborns, arises when the meatus opens somewhere along the ventral aspect of the penile shaft. Most are glandular and of little consequence; more severe forms result in penile curvature (chordee). Up to 10% are associated with undescended testes and inguinal hernias and, as with those patients with hypospadias resulting in ambiguous genitalia, require karyotype analysis. Treatment entails expert plastic repair to achieve a normal appearance, voiding and sexual function. Circumcision is one of the most commonly performed surgical procedures in boys worldwide, but mostly for cultural and religious reasons. Medical indications include significant meatal obstruction with a poor urinary jet and prepuce ballooning, and recurrent balanitis. Balanitis xerotica obliterans, which never occurs before the age of 5 years, results in scarring of the prepuce and is an absolute indication for circumcision.

## Female reproductive tract

*Imperforate hymen* presents with primary amenorrhoea and requires simple dissection and release of intravaginal contents. All forms of *ovarian cancer* are extremely rare in childhood; they include leukaemic infiltration, teratoma and dysgerminoma. The prognosis is generally poor, except with highly differentiated multicystic teratoma, which is cured by total resection.

## 12.4 Orthopaedic disorders

### Learning objectives

You should:

- know how to examine a baby for a dislocation of the hip
- know the clinical presentation, diagnosis and management of osteomyelitis and septic arthritis
- know the symptoms, signs and management of childhood rheumatoid arthritis

## Congenital abnormalities

### Congenital dislocation of the hip (CDH)

Congenital dislocation of the hip (CDH) has a variable presentation and is probably better termed developmental dysplasia of the hip, to reflect its many facets. The disorder is related to ligament laxity, breech delivery and neuromuscular disease, and has a multifactorial pattern of inheritance. Although unstable (clicky) hips are seen in 1% of all newborns, true dislocation affects 1 in 1000 liveborn infants and is more common in girls (9 : 1). *Subluxatable* hips lie 'loose' and the femoral head slides in the acetabulum. *Subluxated* hips lie away from the floor of the acetabulum. *Dislocatable* hips can be manually displaced from the acetabulum with a palpable clunk. The hip is considered to be dislocated when the femoral head lies outside the acetabulum. The diagnosis of CDH is made by routine physical examination of the newborn, as shown in Figure 127.

Beyond 2–3 months, the characteristic instability of the joints may be lost and there is more likely to be limited abduction of the hip and asymmetrical skin folds. Persistent dislocation and late-onset subluxations are associated with permanent dysplastic changes in the hip, an unstable waddling gait and a positive Trendelenburg test (Fig. 128).

The place of radiology in the diagnosis of CDH is controversial, and currently ultrasound is proving to be more valuable than X-ray as it is able to reveal the cartilaginous areas of the joints and dynamic instability during movement of the hip.

Treatment for dislocated hips should be started at once. The hips are held in at least 90° flexion and 60° abduction using a device (e.g. Malmö splint or Pavlik harness). Dislocations resistant to conservative manage-

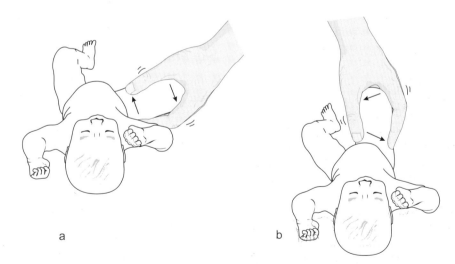

a                b

**Fig. 127** Clinical manoeuvres to detect CDH in the neonatal period. (a) The Ortolani manoeuvre is a reduction manoeuvre to place a hip back into the normal position. The hip is abducted slightly, then, with the index and long fingers over the greater trochanter, the thigh is raised to gently reduce the hip. (b) The Barlow provocative test detects whether the hip is subluxatable or dislocatable. The thumb is placed on the inner aspect of the thigh near the lesser trochanter. The hip is adducted and longitudinal pressure is exerted on the thigh with the thumb pushing it towards the table. In both instances the other hand is used to stabilise the pelvis.

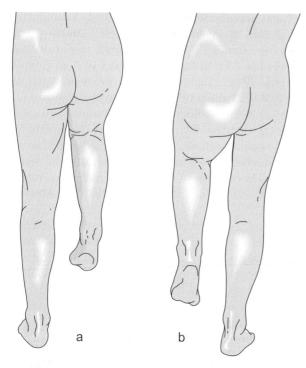

**Fig. 128** Trendelenburg's test. Bearing weight on the normal left leg (a) causes the pelvis to tilt up with elevation of the opposite leg. Standing on the right leg (b) with the unstable hip causes the pelvis to tilt down and the buttock to fall; compensatory scoliosis.

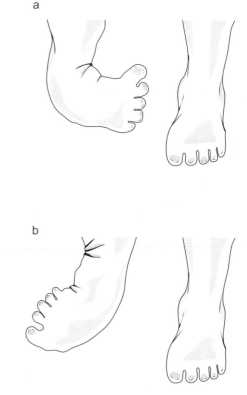

**Fig. 129** (a) Congenital talipes equinovarus and (b) calcaneovalgus.

ment are treated with adductor tenotomies and closed reduction and a hip spica. Abnormalities persisting beyond 18 months of age are difficult to manage and may require open reduction with realigning derotation osteotomies, and possibly acetabular angulation.

## Talipes varus and valgus

Club foot may be caused by neuromuscular imbalance of the lower foot, sometimes by vertical malposition of the talus. It arises in 0.1% of predominantly male births and is bilateral in 50% of patients. Club foot can produce inward, medial deviation of the forefoot (talipes equinovarus, TEV), or abduction at the ankle with external, lateral deviation of the forefoot (talipes calcaneovalgus, TCV; Fig. 129). Although these anomalies may be features of a generalised dysmorphic syndrome, they are usually isolated findings. The severity of the condition is assessed on clinical appearance and the ease by which the foot can be brought into the normal position by simple manipulation. Minor problems resolve with physiotherapy and positioning exercises, which can be taught to the parents. Severe deviation may require serial orthopaedic manipulation, malleable splints, plaster

casts and, if there is no improvement by 3 months, refashioning surgical procedures before normal alignment is achieved.

## Skeletal dysplasias

A multitude of congenital and hereditary conditions result in abnormal bone and skeletal development. Although many of the conditions listed in Table 77 are extremely rare, others are sufficiently common to present in most paediatric and orthopaedic practices.

### Osteogenesis imperfecta

Osteogenesis imperfecta results from abnormal bony moulding and ossification, giving rise to brittle bones. The severe dominant variants are associated with multiple fractures in utero and may be lethal, especially when multiple rib fractures result in a collapsed thorax and significant pulmonary hypoplasia. Recessive forms are more benign, presenting with recurrent fractures after minor trauma, and are associated with blue sclerae. Treatment involves reduction of the fractures and genetic counselling. Bisphosphonates reduce bone turnover and may have a beneficial effect

**Table 77** Skeletal dysplasia and malformations

| Disorders | Inheritance | Description |
|---|---|---|
| **Generalised disorders** | | |
| Osteogenesis imperfecta | AD, AR | Brittle bones, fractures, blue sclerae |
| Multiple exostosis (diaphyseal aclasis) | AD | Disfiguring bony outgrowths |
| Multiple enchondromata (Ollier disease) | SP | Intraosseous expanding chondromas |
| Osteopetrosis (Albers–Schönberg disease) | AR | Dense, brittle, marble bones; loss of bone marrow |
| **Short-limb syndromes** | | |
| Achondroplasia | AD | Short limbs, large head |
| Thanatophoric dwarfism | SP | Short limbs, thoracic hypoplasia |
| Jeune syndrome | AR | Asphyxiating thoracic dystrophy |
| **Isolated patchy disorders** | | |
| Fibrous dysplasia (McCune–Albright syndrome) | SP | Patchy hyperpigmentation, patchy fibrous bony disorganisation |

AD, autosomal dominant; AR, autosomal recessive; SP, sporadic inheritance.

in this condition, although their use so far has been limited.

### Achondroplasia

Achondroplasia is the most common short-limb syndrome, affecting 1 in 2000 live births. It is dominantly inherited, although 80% of new cases are spontaneous mutations. It results in characteristic short limb bones and abnormalities in moulding of the bones at the base of the skull. Subluxation of the cervical atlantoaxial joint makes intubation and manipulation under general anaesthetic potentially hazardous. Other forms of short-limb skeletal dysplasias are rare and often lethal, especially when associated with significant involvement of the thoracic cage.

## Skeletal malformations

### Scoliosis

Scoliosis is usually a primary, idiopathic condition that is slightly more common but often more severe in girls. Occasionally, scoliosis is secondary to a fixed abnormality in the vertebral column (e.g. hemivertebra, skeletal dysplasia), neuromuscular disease, neurocutaneous syndrome and ligamentous laxity (e.g. Marfan syndrome). Functional scoliosis is secondary to disproportionate spasm following a neuromuscular disorder involving the vertebral column and spinal nerves (Box 84).

A full examination is essential to exclude any associated abnormality. The back is examined from behind for symmetry and curvature after correction for any discrepancy in the pelvis, hips and lower limb lengths. Both lateral (scoliosis) and anterior (kyphosis) displacement should be assessed as the patient stands and bends forward. Serial standing X-ray films will confirm and

**Box 84** Causes of scoliosis

**Primary scoliosis**
Idiopathic scoliosis
Congenital scoliosis
  Hemivertebra, unsegmented vertebrae
Spina bifida
As part of syndromes (VATER, neurofibromatosis, Marfan, Klippel–Feil, Sprengel)

**Secondary scoliosis**
Neuromuscular scoliosis
  Cerebral palsy
  Muscular dystrophy
  Spinal muscular atrophy
Compensatory scoliosis
  Muscular strain
  Osteomyelitis in vertebrae
  Spinal, extraspinal tumour
  Lower limb, pelvic discrepancy

monitor the progression of the curve. The risk of progression is greatest in premenarcheal girls with a curve greater than 20°. Often those between 25° and 45° are managed with orthotic devices (e.g. Milwaukee brace), whereas greater curves require surgery, generally entailing posterior spinal fusion with a prosthetic support (e.g. Harrington rod).

### Sprengel shoulder

Sprengel shoulder involves a high-riding and underdeveloped scapula (usually unilaterally) that requires orthopaedic reconstructive surgery.

### Asymmetric limb shortening

Asymmetric limb shortening may be associated with various syndromes (e.g. Russell–Silver), unilateral underdevelopment and limb ischaemia. It may be treated with limb-lengthening procedures.

**Table 78** Infecting organisms in osteomyelitis

| Organism | Patients | Sites | Comments |
|---|---|---|---|
| Staphylococcus aureus | All groups | Any | Commonest organism |
| Haemophilus influenzae type b | <3 years | Any | Becoming rare |
| Group B streptococci | Neonates | Any | |
| Coliforms | Neonates | Any | |
| Neisseria sp. | Neonates | Any | Also sexually active |
| Streptococcal spp. | All groups | Any, foot | |
| Gram-negative bacilli | All groups | Any | |
| Pseudomonas spp. | All groups | Foot | Also immunosuppression |
| Salmonella spp. | Sickle cell disease | Any, vertebrae | |
| Brucella spp. | Older children | Any, vertebrae | |
| Anaerobes | After bites, trauma | Local bones | |
| Mycobacteria (TB) | Older children | Any, spine | Also immunosuppression |
| Fungi | Neonates | Any | Also immunosuppression |

## Acquired inflammatory conditions

### Infective osteomyelitis and arthritis

#### Osteomyelitis

Osteomyelitis is caused almost exclusively by bacterial organisms, except in utero, when osteitis secondary to rubella and cytomegalovirus occurs. Staphylococcal species are the usual infecting organisms, although tuberculous osteomyelitis is still seen, even in developed countries (Table 78). This deep-seated infection is not only a feature of neonates and the immunosuppressed, but is also seen in otherwise normal children who are not at particular risk of infection. Bacteraemia, often without clinical manifestations, results in the 'seeding' of microorganisms in bone, where an indolent abscess develops. A 'spiking' fever with general malaise is usually associated with local erythema, swelling, tenderness over the affected bone, and limitation of movement (pseudoparalysis) because of pain. Neurological signs may arise following spinal compression in those with spinal osteomyelitis and vertebral collapse.

Investigations confirm the site and extent of infection and identify the organism. The white cell count and erythrocyte sedimentation rate (ESR) are usually raised. *Several* blood cultures must be taken, preferably during temperature spikes, when the microbiological yield is likely to be greatest. At times, microbiological confirmation is only successful on culture of a biopsy specimen. X-ray films are usually unremarkable in the early stages of infection, but after 2 weeks show bony irregularities, rarefaction, cystic changes and, eventually, a periosteal reaction with sclerosis and increased ossification. An isotope-labelled scan employing $^{99m}$Tc will show an area of increased uptake ('hot spot') and is essential in children with a high swinging fever and evidence of bacterial sepsis but without an obvious focus.

Treatment entails combination antibiotics given for 6 weeks and administered via the intravenous route for at least 10–14 days. Neonates should be given combination antibiotics to treat *Staphylococcus aureus* and group B streptococci plus Gram-negative coliforms (e.g. methicillin and an aminoglycoside). Children under 5 years are treated for *Staph. aureus* and *Haemophilus influenzae* type b with cefuroxime or ceftriaxone. Older children with proven *Staph. aureus* infection receive flucloxacillin and fusidic acid. Large collections of pus require drainage. Those with sickle cell disease should be given flucloxacillin plus an aminoglycoside, whereas clindamycin is effective against anaerobes. Tuberculous osteomyelitis requires triple therapy with rifampicin, isoniazid and ethambutol.

Subacute infection may become walled off by sclerosis, resulting in a localised abscess (Brodie abscess), typically in the upper tibia. Chronic osteomyelitis that persists for months despite adequate antibiotics results in marked radiological changes, with widespread bone disruption and necrosis, ossification layering beneath the periosteum (involucrum), cystic cavities and sclerotic necrotic bony fragments (sequestrum). Surgical reconstruction with bone graft augmentation may be necessary, especially in those with an adjoining septic arthritis and the development of a Charcot joint. Children with recurrent or multifocal osteomyelitis, especially involving atypical organisms, must be investigated for an underlying immunosuppressions.

#### Septic arthritis

Septic arthritis is often caused by similar organisms to osteomyelitis (Table 78), with *Staph. aureus* being the most common agent in neonates and children over the age of 5 and, until the advent of Hib vaccine, *H. influenzae* in those aged 2 months to 5 years. Up to 30% have an associated osteomyelitis. Patients present with a

**Table 79** Types and clinical features of inflammatory arthritis in childhood

| Arthritis | Characteristics | Outcome |
|---|---|---|
| **Rheumatoid** | | |
| Oligoarthritis | 1–4 large joints; usually RF-negative | Generally excellent |
| Extended oligoarthritis | As above, but progresses to other joints | May be resistant to treatment |
| Polyarthritis | 5+ joints; RF-negative (95%) | 50% remit |
| | 5+ joints; RF+ (5%) | Severe, deforming arthritis |
| Systemic onset arthritis | Fever/PUO, rashes, serositis but no initial joint involvement | 1/3 remit within 3 yrs; 1/3 flare-ups on/off; 1/3 develop polyarticular-type RA |
| **Non-rheumatoid** | | |
| Psoriatic arthritis | With psoriasis; large joints, dactylitis | Lifelong, with varying severity |
| Enteritis-related arthritis | HLA B27 positive, spondyloarthropathies | Lifelong, often back pain |
| Others | Arthritis of unknown cause, aged >6 years | |

fever, swelling, erythema, warmth, pain and limitation of movement in the affected joint, which assumes a position that offers maximal pain relief (antalgic posture). Management is similar to osteomyelitis. Blood cultures are positive in 35% of patients, whereas diagnostic arthrocentesis reveals a positive growth in 75% of infections. The joint must be aspirated and immobilised in its functional position for 72 hours before physiotherapy is started, to prevent permanent contractures and arthrodesis.

## Inflammatory arthritis

Inflammatory arthritides in childhood can be classified as shown in Table 79.

### Transient arthralgia

Transient arthralgia is relatively common in childhood and presents with pain and local limitation of movement following a viral upper respiratory tract infection (URTI). It usually affects the hips and is the most likely cause of an irritable hip. A non-deforming, self-limiting *reactive arthritis* may follow gastrointestinal illnesses, especially those caused by *Salmonella, Shigella, Campylobacter* and *Yersinia*. Joint pain, swelling and restricted movement usually involve the larger joints (e.g. knee, ankle) and may be associated with impressive sterile effusions that require drainage.

Treatment includes analgesia, anti-inflammatory agents e.g. non-steroidal anti-inflammatory drugs (NSAIDs), physiotherapy, and mobilisation as early as possible.

Arthritis and arthralgia are common manifestations of other conditions in childhood, including inflammatory bowel disease, psoriasis, Reiter's disease, systemic lupus erythematosus (SLE) and the vasculitides. The last include a number of rare inflammatory conditions, including Kawasaki disease and polyarteritis nodosa, and more commonly Henoch–Schönlein purpura.

### Rheumatoid conditions

Rheumatoid conditions in childhood are rare, affecting fewer than 1 in 1000 children below 16 years of age, and classified into four main types, as shown in Table 79. Up to 5% of children are rheumatoid factor (RF)-positive, and RF-positive *polyarticular juvenile chronic rheumatoid arthritis* (JCA) is similar to the multiarticular condition seen in adulthood and usually affects girls (80%). The small joints of the hands and feet are predominantly involved; patients present with stiffness and joint pain, particularly in the morning. Chronic, progressive joint deformity develops in 60% of affected patients. RF-negative polyarticular JCA tends to present earlier in childhood, is generally mild, and is rarely associated with complications such as pericardial, pleural and peritoneal involvement and rheumatoid nodules. *Oligoarthritis (pauciarticular arthritis)* is usually RF negative and generally involves fewer than four large joints. *Systemically presenting rheumatoid disease* (Still's disease) is largely associated with extra-articular manifestations. The clinical features are persistent fever (Fig. 130), erythematous rashes, generalised lymphadenopathy, mild hepatosplenomegaly and, occasionally, rheumatoid nodules. Joint involvement is late or initially unimpressive, though up to 25% go on to develop chronic, debilitating arthritis.

Investigations often confirm anaemia with a raised white cell count, sometimes with a striking neutrophilia, raised platelet count, elevated ESR, acute-phase reactants (such as C-reactive protein, CRP) and complement levels (C3, C4). In childhood, RF and antinuclear antigen (ANA) are generally negative (Table 80).

First-line management includes control of the temperature and the use of anti-inflammatory agents such as aspirin and NSAIDs. Disease-modifying drugs such as gold salts, D-penicillamine, hydroxychloroquine and methotrexate are all associated with serious side effects, and their use must be monitored carefully in a specialist centre. Steroids are indicated for severe, unresponsive systemic disease and iridocyclitis. They

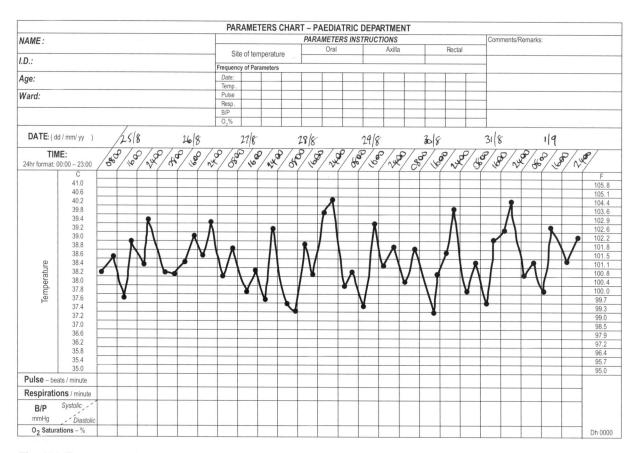

**Fig. 130** Temperature chart showing persistent, spiking temperature in a 4-year-old boy with Still's disease.

**Table 80** Different manifestations of childhood rheumatoid arthritis

| | Polyarticular | | Pauciarticular | | Systemic onset |
|---|---|---|---|---|---|
| | RF– | RF+ | Type I | Type II | |
| JCA (%) | 25 | 10 | 35 | 10 | 20 |
| Female : male ratio | 9 : 1 | 4 : 1 | 4 : 1 | 1 : 9 | 4 : 1 |
| Onset (year) | Any | > 8 | 4–10 | > 8 | Any |
| Joints | Multiple | Multiple | < 4 | < 4 | Variable |
| Sacroiliitis | No | Rare | No | Yes | No |
| Iridocyclitis | Rare | No | 30% | 10% | No |
| Chronicity (%) | 10 | > 50 | 20 | < 10 | 25 |
| RF (%) | – | 100 | – | – | – |
| ANA (%) | 25 | 75 | 90 | 0 | 0 |
| HLA | NS | DR4 | DR5,6,8 | B27 | NS |

RF, rheumatoid factor; ANA, antinuclear antibody; HLA, histocompatibility antigen; NS, non-specific.

can be given as a prolonged course by mouth, when they are likely to be associated with side effects, or intra-articularly for individual problematic joints, or as pulsed intravenous methylprednisolone for acute 'flare-ups'. More recently, tumour necrosis factor (TNF)-blocking drugs such as etanercept and infliximab have shown promising results, and have been included in treatment regimens after a sequential trial of NSAIDs,

steroids and methotrexate. Initial protection of any affected joints should be followed by disciplined physiotherapy, occupational therapy, orthotic advice and early mobilization. The use of special splints can greatly improve function, and orthopaedic procedures are applied to treat severe joint deformities. Ophthalmological input is necessary if uveitis (generally in ANA-positive girls) or iritis (more common in boys) is present.

Extensive disease
Poor initial response to treatment
Prolonged disease activity
RF-positivity
Markedly raised reactive indicators (e.g. CRP, ESR)

Overall, approximately 10% of sufferers will develop severe disability that affects their lifestyle. Features that suggest a poor outcome are listed in Box 85.

## Ischaemia and apophysitis

### Irritable hip

The irritable hip is caused by local painful inflammation in the hip(s) and presents with a limp. It is generally seen in boys aged 3–8 years and may be secondary to a self-limiting, transient synovitis following a viral URTI or local jarring trauma after a fall. Pain and a limp are associated with limitation in abduction and internal rotation. Investigations, including X-rays, should be normal. Treatment is conservative, with analgesia and bed rest, preferably for 7 days.

With similar symptoms in the 5–10 age group, the possibility of *Perthes' disease* must be considered. This is presumably caused by compromise of the delicate blood supply to the growing femoral head, resulting in ischaemic necrosis. Degenerative fragmentation produces distinctive radiological changes, including flattening of the femoral head, sclerosis with cystic changes in both the femoral head and acetabulum, and widening of the femoral metaphysis (Fig. 131). The condition usually affects boys (5 : 1) and is bilateral in 20%. Analgesia should be combined with strict bed rest and abduction stretching exercises until symptoms resolve and regeneration is evident on X-ray film. Although most will recover fully, in others destruction of the femoral head is permanent. This is more likely the greater the degree of initial fragmentation, and in those aged 10 years or more, when prolonged bed rest with hip traction is indicated. Containment of the femoral head is achieved with the use of an abduction cast/orthosis, though the results are better with surgical osteotomy. In severe cases, femoral osteotomy is combined with the insertion of pins to fix the femoral head in the acetabulum, thereby stabilising the joint until regeneration occurs. Osteoarthritis of the affected joint is a late complication.

### Slipped upper femoral epiphysis

Slipped upper femoral epiphysis (SUFE) affects mostly overweight boys over the age of 10. The condition is usually chronic, with symptoms of pain and a limp for

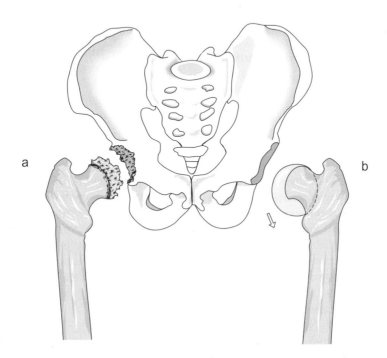

**Fig. 131** (a) Perthes' disease. Destruction of the femoral head with sclerosis, cystic changes and metaphyseal widening. Note similar changes in acetabulum. (b) Slipped upper femoral epiphysis with posterior, downward displacement of the femoral head.

several months. Occasionally slippage is acute, patients presenting with severe pain and inability to bear weight. There is external rotation of the affected limb, with loss of internal rotation, flexion and abduction at the hip. Evidence of posterior displacement of the femoral head is seen on anteroposterior and lateral X-ray films of the hips (Fig. 131b). If analgesia, bed rest and hip traction do not suffice, pinning of the femoral head (epiphysiodesis) in order to prevent further slippage is indicated. The possibility of coexisting hypothyroidism and pituitary disease must be excluded. Severe cases will result in osteoarthritis of the hip joint in early adulthood.

## Trauma

### Fractures

Fractures are extremely common in active children, especially boys. They should be suspected, looked for on X-ray, and reduced with appropriate strapping or plaster. Most fractures in childhood are self-resolving greenstick fractures. However, fractures may be associated with serious complications, especially following major, multiple trauma, as seen with road traffic accidents or a fall from a height. In this instance, the whole child must be examined thoroughly, the general condition stabilised, and organ and soft tissue injuries addressed. The risk of infection with compound fractures is great, and these must be treated aggressively with intravenous antibiotics. Air embolism may complicate open, compound fractures involving the long bones. Non-fusion and pseudoarthrosis may require refracturing and pinning under general anaesthesia.

### Soft tissue injuries

The child with multiple trauma and injury to several major organs presents a major challenge to the paediatric resuscitative team. A thorough detailed assessment must be performed, and repeated as the condition alters. The key to management is identifying all the problems and correcting them in order of urgency. Intravenous access and blood sampling for cross-match are a priority. Major life-threatening problems such as cardiorespiratory failure (e.g. caused by a pneumothorax and tamponade), organ lacerations, transected blood vessels etc. must be corrected urgently. Non-life-threatening injuries (e.g. skin lacerations) and fractures can be addressed once the patient's condition is relatively stable. Support of cardiorespiratory, renal and liver function should accompany attention to normalising haematological and metabolic indices.

## 12.5 Disorders of the ears, nose and throat

### Learning objectives

You should:

- be aware of the causes and problems associated with a cleft lip and palate

- know the clinical presentation and management of child with a foreign body inhalation

## Congenital anomalies

### Cleft lip and palate

Cleft lip and palate are relatively common abnormalities, with an incidence of about 1 in 1000. They may be isolated or form part of a generalised chromosomal abnormality (e.g. trisomy 13) or syndrome (e.g. Stickler syndrome, in association with eye abnormalities). The clefts may be unilateral or bilateral, partial or complete (Fig. 132). They are usually clinically obvious, although small clefts of the uvula may be missed unless a careful examination is made.

Management is best undertaken by an experienced multidisciplinary team. The cleft palate may disrupt feeding, a problem that can be circumvented with the use of special teats. The aesthetically more distressing cleft lip is corrected around the age of 3–6 months. Repair of the palate is delayed to allow for maximal growth, and is carried out once phonation becomes a necessity, usually around 10–15 months. Pharyngoplasty and surgery for midfacial hypoplasia may be required later in childhood.

### Pierre–Robin sequence

The combination of a complete cleft palate with a small lower jaw (micrognathia) results in a major handicap with regard to sucking and feeding. These children are nursed in the prone position on custom-designed frames and require expert nursing care to supervise their feeds. The cleft palate is corrected as soon as possible, care being taken not to disrupt the development of the midface, thereby further compromising the defect.

### Abnormalities above the glottis

Congenital abnormalities above the glottis include a cleft glottis and laryngeal web. They present with stridor from birth and are diagnosed by microlaryngo-

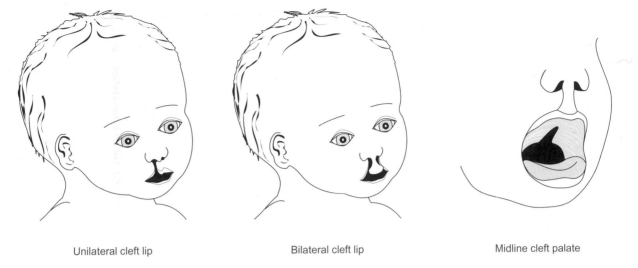

Unilateral cleft lip        Bilateral cleft lip        Midline cleft palate

**Fig. 132** Clinical appearance of cleft lip and cleft palate.

bronchoscopy (MLB). Repair is carried out as early as possible, and follow-up maintained to ensure that stenosis does not develop.

## Abnormalities below the glottis

Larnygotracheomalacia is caused by congenital weakness in the laryngeal and tracheal walls, which partially collapse on inspiration. This is the most common cause of neonatal stridor, and in the vast majority resolves spontaneously as the child grows. Those with severe stridor and airway obstruction requiring repeated intubation may require surgical tracheal reinforcement.

## Acquired infective lesions

Infections of the upper airways are discussed in Chapter 3.

## Problems with foreign bodies

### Foreign body inhalation

The possibility of foreign body inhalation is obvious in those who choke and collapse while eating. In many cases, inhalation of a peanut or similar object follows attempts to swallow these once thrown in the air and then caught 'on the wing'. Temporary airway obstruction results in a minor choking or spluttering episode, which is relieved as the foreign object is displaced distally further down the airway. Later, progressive signs of respiratory distress, breathlessness, cyanosis and fever develop as distal obstruction and incipient pneumonia ensue. An early plain chest X-ray film *taken on expiration* may show early air trapping owing to a

ball-valve effect; later films generally show an area of collapse/consolidation. Most inhaled objects contain organic matter and are not radio-opaque. Severe airway obstruction requires emergency management and is discussed in Section 3.7. Once stabilised, the child should undergo endoscopic examination under anaesthesia and the foreign body should be removed. Antibiotic cover is advisable for almost all cases.

### Foreign body insertion

Children have a predilection for inserting objects such as beads, pencils and rubber erasers into the external auditory meatus or nostrils. If lodged tightly, these require expert removal by the ENT surgeon if further trauma and infection to the area are to be avoided.

## 12.6 Dental problems

### Learning objectives

You should:

• be familiar with the causes and prevention of dental caries

• be familiar with the initial management of avulsed teeth.

## Assessment and clinical examination

At birth, the deciduous teeth are present under the gums, which begin to harden at 3 months of age and become red and swollen around 6 months of age, when

**Table 81** Developmental dental disorders

| Anomaly | Examples |
| --- | --- |
| Timing | Neonatal and natal teeth; delayed eruption and non-eruption |
| Shape | Peg-shaped lateral incisor |
| Size | Megadont central incisor, double teeth |
| Number | Hypodontia or supernumerary teeth |
| **Structure** | |
| Hereditary | Amelogenesis imperfecta |
| | Dentinogenesis imperfecta |
| | Dentine dysplasia |
| Non-hereditary | Fluorosis |
| | Tetracycline staining |
| | Hypoplastic teeth |

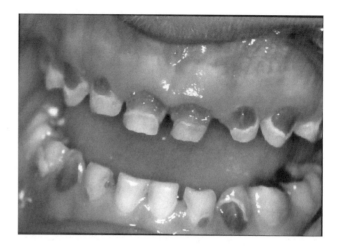

**Fig. 133** Clinical appearance of rampant caries.

the first deciduous teeth (the lower incisors) appear. The preschool child has a set of 20 deciduous teeth, which should have erupted by the age of 2.5 years. Rarely children have a tooth at birth (natal tooth) or soon afterwards (neonatal tooth), and this may hinder breastfeeding and require extraction. At about 6 years the permanent teeth – usually the lower incisors first – will start erupting. The first permanent molars do not replace any deciduous teeth and are sometimes mistaken for deciduous teeth. Delayed or early eruption of either deciduous or permanent teeth is not uncommon and usually needs no treatment. Certain conditions, such as Down syndrome, hereditary ectodermal dysplasia and hypothyroidism, are associated with delayed eruption or hypodontia (missing teeth). Developmental anomalies associated with dentition are listed in Table 81. All children should have their first dental check at around 2 years of age to 'familiarise' them with the dental environment before any treatment becomes necessary. *Orthodontics* is the branch of dentistry that deals with the movement of teeth and the growth of the face and jaws. In children, such treatment is generally carried out between 12 and 14 years, after all the permanent teeth have erupted.

## Dental caries

Dental caries is the most common oral disease in childhood. It results from the demineralisation of dental enamel by acids released by bacteria feeding on sugar substrate present in the microbial plaque on the tooth surface. Dental caries initially appears as a white chalky area on the enamel that later softens and breaks down, forming a carious cavity. If not treated in the early stages, caries progresses towards the pulp, causing pulpitis with resultant toothache and, in some cases, dentoalveolar abscess formation. Management will then require extraction or extensive treatment to save the tooth.

## Rampant caries

Rampant caries (nursing bottle caries; Fig. 133) is decay that spreads quickly, destroying the crowns of many of the erupted deciduous teeth, often with sparing of the lower incisors. Teeth may appear brown or black, and parents are often misled to believe that they have erupted already decayed. Inappropriate nursing habits, such as prolonged or frequent use of a sugary drink in a feeder cup or bottle, are the main cause, typified by children allowed to sleep with a bottle available throughout the night. It is also possible to develop rampant caries from breast milk if feeding is carried out for prolonged periods, and caries has also been associated with late or inappropriate weaning. Milk or water should constitute the majority of drinks given to young children, and sugary drinks should be confined to mealtimes.

### Prevention

Dental caries is a preventable disease, and as dental treatment can be difficult and traumatic for young children, prevention must be a priority.

**Diet control.** The total amount of sugar in the diet, the frequency of sugary drinks, snacks between meals and sugar-containing medicines should all be reduced.

**Plaque control.** Children who brush their teeth at least once a day with a fluoride-containing toothpaste will have less plaque accumulation and less tooth decay. Parents should encourage and help their children to brush their teeth as soon as they erupt, using a 'pea-sized' amount of a low-dose fluoride toothpaste, until they are old enough to brush their own teeth at around 6 years of age.

**Fluoride.** Fluoride, applied topically or taken systemically, most commonly in fluoridated water, is the most effective way to prevent dental caries. The effect of fluoride is to:

- Increase the resistance of the outer enamel to acid attack
- Allow for remineralisation of enamel in the initial carious lesion
- Decrease the growth of bacteria in plaque.

Fluoride tablets, in the appropriate dosage, may be prescribed to children over 3 years of age, if the drinking water is not fluoridated, but should not be given before 6 months of age. Some local authorities have opted for fluoridated milk or salt: these are less effective, but allow for individual choice.

**Fissure sealants.** Fissure sealants are liquid composite resins applied to the occlusal surfaces of susceptible teeth. They fill out fissures and pits in order to eliminate food entrapment and plaque accumulation that can lead to decay. Their use is recommended in cases such as children with a high incidence of caries, or those who are medically compromised.

## Erosion

Erosion is the loss of tooth structure caused by non-bacterial acid attack. There has been a progressive increase in the prevalence of erosion. In 1993 in England and Wales, 50% of 6-year-olds and 23% of 14-year-olds had erosion of their deciduous and permanent dentition, respectively, with dentinal involvement in 2% of cases. When the enamel is eroded the dentine underneath is exposed, which in turn may lead to pain, sensitivity, and eventually pulpitis and tooth loss. *Intrinsic erosion* is related to acid reflux in those with gastro-oesophageal reflux, bulimia and anorexia nervosa. *Extrinsic erosion* is related to the consumption of acidic or carbonated drinks and fruit juices.

## Trauma: anterior teeth

The incidence of trauma to primary teeth varies from 11% to 30%, and usually involves children aged 1.5–2.5 years. Eight percent of 5-year-olds will suffer trauma to their deciduous teeth, and by the age of 15 years 26% of children would have sustained trauma to their permanent teeth. The most common injury to the primary dentition is avulsion, intrusion or subluxation, and the most commonly reported injuries to the permanent dentition include enamel or enamel–dentine fractures and subluxation.

In young children, avulsion of the deciduous incisors is the most common type of injury and these are not replaced, although if intruded there is a possibility of re-eruption. With avulsed permanent teeth the prognosis depends on how long the tooth is out of the mouth and the medium in which it is transported. Ideally replacement is immediate, whereby the tooth is rinsed, not scrubbed, and reimplanted with applied pressure into the empty socket. If the tooth is transported for delayed implantation, the ideal transport medium is milk or saline. Tetanus prophylaxis is essential. Overall, the most common dental injury is a fractured tooth, with the maxillary anterior teeth having the highest incidence of fracture. Both short- and the long-term success of treatment depend on early – preferably immediate – referral to the dentist, as expert intervention may salvage many fractured but otherwise healthy teeth (Fig. 134). Regular review to monitor the vitality of the traumatized teeth is essential. Prevention is the best option and, for example, the use of mouthguards should be advised for contact sports.

a        b

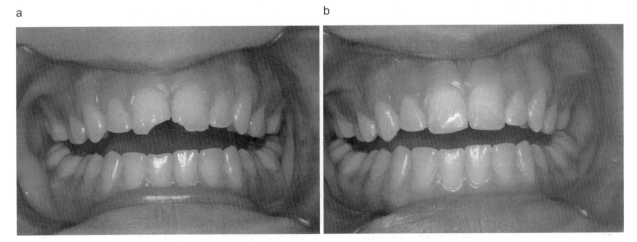

**Fig. 134** Satisfactory treatment of fractured incisor.

# Self-assessment: questions

## Multiple choice questions

1. The following statements describe bowel obstruction:
   a. Vomiting is a feature of upper but not lower gastrointestinal obstruction
   b. Abdominal distension is the most reliable indicator of bowel obstruction
   c. Oesophageal atresia is rarely associated with a tracheo-oesophageal fistula
   d. Duodenal atresia is often seen in children with Down syndrome
   e. High anal atresia has a poor prognosis for future bowel continence.

2. The following statements are true:
   a. Gastroschisis is usually an isolated defect
   b. Exomphalos is a feature of Beckwith syndrome
   c. Diaphragmatic hernias are generally left sided
   d. Diaphragmatic hernia is usually associated with pulmonary hypoplasia
   e. Diaphragmatic hernia is usually an isolated defect.

3. With regard to neural tube defects:
   a. The incidence of spina bifida is reduced by folic acid in the last trimester
   b. A rise in maternal α-fetoprotein may suggest the presence of a neural tube defect
   c. Open lesions should be closed surgically without delay to avoid infection
   d. Hydrocephalus is a good prognostic feature in association with spina bifida
   e. Neonatal hydrocephalus usually follows a congenital not an acquired defect.

4. Hirschsprung disease is characterised by the following:
   a. Bowel obstruction, sometimes from birth
   b. Male preponderance
   c. Normal distribution of neural ganglia in severely affected bowel
   d. A rat-tail appearance on barium enema
   e. Short-segment disease involving the ascending colon.

5. The following statements are correct:
   a. Dandy–Walker cysts result in hydrocephalus due to abnormalities in the third ventricle

   b. Hydrocephalus may follow decreased absorption of CSF
   c. Hydronephrosis may be detected antenatally
   d. Posterior urethral valves are associated with ureteric reflux in most patients
   e. Surgery for ambiguous genitalia is determined by the patient's karyotype.

6. The following statements are correct:
   a. Malrotation arises because of a clockwise twist of the bowel
   b. The inferior mesenteric artery is usually constricted during midgut volvulus
   c. Diaphragmatic hernia is invariably associated with malrotation
   d. Incarceration of inguinal hernias is more common in infants and neonates
   e. Inguinal hernias are usually direct in type.

7. Surgical management of urinary tract obstruction entails:
   a. Resection of posterior urethral valves not before the age of 1 year
   b. Routine antenatal insertion of nephrostomy drains for those with hydronephrosis
   c. Preoperative micturating cystoureterogram for those with megaureters
   d. DTPA scans in children below 1 year with urinary obstruction
   e. Resection and ureteric reimplantation with ureterocoeles.

8. The following statements are correct:
   a. Congenital dislocation of the hip is more common in girls
   b. Most 'clicky hips' resolve by 6 weeks
   c. Talipes equinovarus is generally associated with karyotypic abnormalities
   d. Achondroplasia is inherited in a recessive fashion
   e. Slipped upper femoral epiphyses may be associated with abnormalities in growth hormone.

9. The following are associated with an increased risk of scoliosis:
   a. Hemivertebrae
   b. Paraspinal tuberculous abscess
   c. Spinal dysraphism
   d. Congenital dystrophy
   e. Tuberous sclerosis.

10. The following statements are correct:
   a. A cleft lip is of greater functional consequence than a cleft palate
   b. Testicular torsion in the neonate has a good prognosis
   c. Orchidopexy should be performed bilaterally
   d. Meckel diverticulum is found on the mesenteric border
   e. Meckel diverticulum is easily differentiated from acute appendicitis.

11. The following describe dental caries:
   a. The commonest site is in the occlusal surfaces of the incisor teeth
   b. Bottle feeds can cause caries of the neck of the teeth
   c. Patients with xerostomia are at a higher risk
   d. Reducing the frequency rather than the amount of carbohydrate ingested is more important in prevention
   e. It may be prevented by drinking tea.

## Short notes

Write short notes on the following:

1. The management of a 6-week-old infant with 10% dehydration caused by a pyloric stenosis that has been confirmed on test feed and ultrasound.
2. The investigative approach for a 4-year-old boy who presents with acute pain in the hip.
3. The investigation of a 10-year-old child who develops frank haematuria and passes a stone per urethra.

## Viva voce question

A 10-month-old infant had bacterial meningitis as a neonate and now has a ventriculoperitoneal shunt for postmeningitis hydrocephalus. He presents to A&E with a 24-hour history of increasing lethargy and vomiting. In view of the possible causes for these symptoms, what questions would you ask of his mother, and outline your management.

## OSCE questions

### OSCE 1
i. What is shown on this erect abdominal film (Fig. 135)?
ii. What is this investigation, using contrast medium (Fig. 136)?
iii. What does it show?
iv. How would you manage this child?

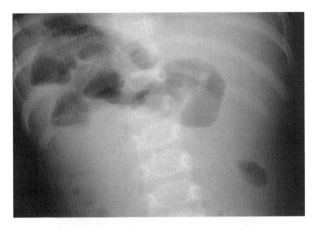

**Fig. 135**

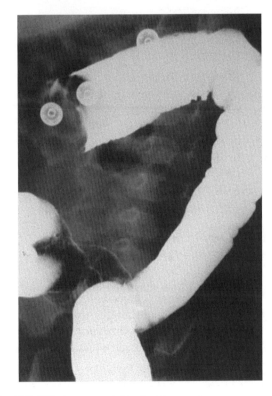

**Fig. 136** (NB: Ignore metal buttons)

**OSCE 2**

Report the abnormalities shown on the intravenous pyelogram (IVP) (Fig. 137).

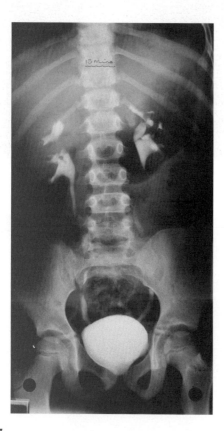

**Fig. 137**

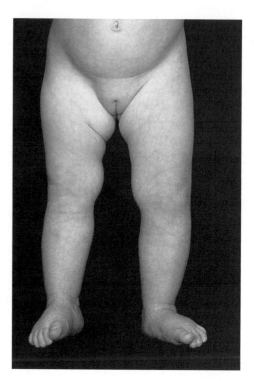

**Fig. 138**

**OSCE 3**

i.   What abnormalities are shown on this photograph (Fig. 138) of the patient standing upright?
ii.  What is the underlying pathological process?
iii. Report the radiological abnormalities on this X-ray (Fig. 139).
iv.  What is the diagnosis?

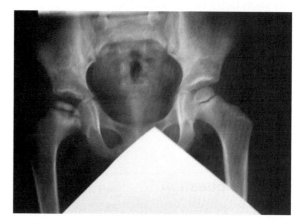

**Fig. 139**

## OSCE 4

i.   What abnormality is shown on Figure 140?
ii.  What immediate steps in management are
     indicated?
iii. Report on this X-ray (Fig 141).
iv.  Name TWO causes for this appearance.

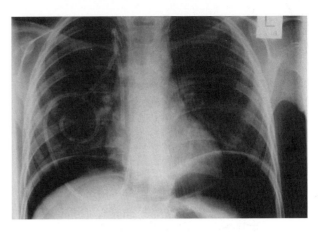

Fig. 141

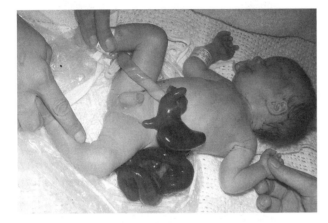

Fig. 140

# Self-assessment: answers

## Multiple choice answers

1. a. **False.** It is a feature of both, although vomiting occurs earlier in upper rather than lower gastrointestinal obstruction.
   b. **False.** Bile-stained vomiting is the most important sign.
   c. **False.** A fistula is present in the huge majority of patients.
   d. **True.** This is the most common congenital abnormality of the bowel in Down syndrome, although it also occurs in newborns without trisomy 21.
   e. **True.** Especially if the atresia extends well above the pelvic levator sling and is associated with sacral abnormalities and fistulae.

2. a. **True.**
   b. **True.** Other features are macroglossia, gigantism (EMG syndrome), organomegaly and neonatal hypoglycaemia.
   c. **True.** Mostly occurs through the left foramen of Bochdalek.
   d. **True.** This arises through pulmonary compression by the bowel in utero and is a major determinant of outcome.
   e. **True.** However, it is sometimes associated with anomalies of the heart and bowel, including tracheo-oesophageal atresia and fistula.

3. a. **False.** Folic acid is given before conception and during early pregnancy.
   b. **True.** Especially with open lesions such as myelomeningocoeles, encephalocoeles and anencephaly.
   c. **True.** The risk of ascending infection leading to encephalitis is very high with open neural tube defects leaking CSF.
   d. **False.** The opposite is true.
   e. **False.** It usually follows intraventricular haemorrhage or infection.

4. a. **True.** Although a physical barrier is not present, the inability of the bowel to undergo normal peristalsis results in a functional obstruction compounded by severe constipation.
   b. **True.** Although *total colonic* disease is more common in females.
   c. **False.** There is a total absence of neural ganglia.
   d. **True.** This describes the radiological appearance

of the transition zone, tapering from dilated upper bowel to small-bore aganglionic bowel below.
   e. **False.** Short-segment disease does not extend beyond the descending colon.

5. a. **False.** Abnormalities are in the fourth ventricle.
   b. **True.** Obstruction of the arachnoid granulations after intraventricular haemorrhage prevents CSF absorption.
   c. **True.** By antenatal ultrasound scanning.
   d. **True.** It occurs in two-thirds of patients.
   e. **False.** The male phenotype may be impossible to achieve despite a 46XY karyotype.

6. a. **False.** The twist is anticlockwise.
   b. **False.** The superior mesenteric artery is constricted.
   c. **True.** With a diaphragmatic hernia, the bowel would not have had the opportunity to rotate anticlockwise and assume its normal position.
   d. **True.** Hence, inguinal hernias must be repaired *before* discharge from neonatal units.
   e. **False.** They are usually indirect.

7. a. **False.** Resection should take place as soon as possible after birth.
   b. **False.** This approach is not effective.
   c. **True.** MCUG will assess the degree of reflux.
   d. **False.** This will assess renal function, but after 1 year of age.
   e. **True.** Ureterocoeles are associated with ureteric reflux and obstruction that will not resolve without surgery.

8. a. **True.** There is a 4 : 1 preponderance.
   b. **True.** Most hip 'clicks' without overt dislocation are simply the result of ligamentous stretching.
   c. **False.** It is usually an isolated defect.
   d. **False.** It is a dominant condition.
   e. **True.** Other features are obesity and hypothyroidism.

9. a. **True.** This occurs in primary, structural scoliosis.
   b. **True.** This is secondary scoliosis.
   c. **True.** Spina bifida.

d. **True.** Myopathies and dystrophies are commonly complicated by progressive scoliosis, which should be looked for on routine examination and spinal X-ray films.

e. **True.** Although tuberous sclerosis is a neurocutaneous condition, scoliosis is more common in neurofibromatosis.

10. a. **False.** A cleft palate results in feeding problems.
    b. **False.** Most will infarct.
    c. **True.** This is because of the risk of contralateral torsion.
    d. **False.** It is found on the antimesenteric border.
    e. **False.** Presentation is usually identical.

11. a. **False.** It usually occurs on the occlusal surfaces of the molar teeth.
    b. **True.** It is also called nursing bottle caries.
    c. **True.** Saliva helps keep the teeth clean!
    d. **True.** Starts at 3–4 months and stops by 2 years.
    e. **True.** Tea contains 100 ppm fluoride, an anticaries agent.

## Short notes answers

1. The infant should be rehydrated, stabilised by correction of the alkalosis, hypochloraemia and hypokalaemia, and prepared for surgery:

   a. Establish intravenous access.
   b. Obtain samples for acid–base status, bicarbonate, chloride and potassium ion levels and cross-match.
   c. Record pulse, blood pressure, urine output.
   d. Commence rehydration using 0.45–0.9% saline with 5–10% dextrose.
   e. Add potassium at 3–4 mmol/kg/day (NB: maintenance 2 mmol/kg/day).
   f. Arrange preoperative anaesthetic review.
   g. Organise surgical pyloromyotomy.
   h. Monitor with apnoea alarm postoperatively because of the increased risk of apnoeas.

2. The most likely cause would be minor ligamentous strain caused by trauma or transient inflammatory arthralgia. An ischaemic insult (e.g. Perthes' disease) is common in this age group, whereas slipped upper femoral epiphysis is unusual. Pauciarticular juvenile arthritis rarely involves a single hip joint, and serious infection (e.g. osteomyelitis), tumour and a haematoma are rare. Hence, a clear history of any preceding events, including trauma, symptoms of infection (especially upper respiratory and gastrointestinal), a family history of arthritis and bleeding diathesis, and drug history must be sought. Examination should focus on evidence of infection, fever, trauma, generalised lymphadenopathy and signs of arthropathy elsewhere. A full assessment of the affected joint should confirm tenderness and limitation in movement. Investigations include a full blood count with differential, erythrocyte sedimentation rate and anteroposterior and lateral X-ray of the hip in the first instance. Several blood cultures must be taken if there is a high temperature. A clotting screen is essential if a diathesis is suspected, rheumatoid factor and antinuclear antibody for rheumatoid disease, and CT scan with biopsy if a tumour is a possibility following the X-rays.

3. Investigation is directed at excluding an abnormal urinary tract and abnormal urine, which could result in an increased propensity for stone formation. Hence comprehensive imaging of the renal tracts is required. A plain abdominal X-ray will detect nephrocalcinosis and radiolucent stones, i.e. those containing calcium and cystine. Ultrasound demonstrates dilatation and congenital/developmental abnormalities of the renal systems, whereas an intravenous urogram may be useful to show stasis, obstruction and filling defects caused by calculi. A micturating cystourethrogram excludes any associated reflux, and functional isotope scanning demonstrates differential renal function (DMSA) and obstruction (DTPA or MAG3).

The urine should be tested for infection and cultures organised. Serum abnormalities such as hypercalcaemia, hyperphosphataemia and hyperuricaemia can result in urinary stones and should be excluded. Serum and urine pH and acid–base balance must be evaluated if renal tubular acidosis is suspected. In addition the 24-hour urine calcium excretion and calcium:creatinine ratio are required in cases of hypercalciuria. Urinary oxalate, xanthine, cystine and uric acid levels can be measured, and many of these amino acids form crystals in the urine that can be visualised on polarising microscopy.

## Viva voce answer

The differential diagnosis includes shunt infection and malfunction owing to blockage or mechanical breakage. Malfunction would result in raised intracranial pressure. The following questions are therefore important:

- Does the child have a temperature, sweats, red painful swelling over the shunt? – indicative of infection.

- Does he seem particularly irritable? Do the vomiting and lethargy show a diurnal variation (e.g. worse in the morning)? – symptoms of raised intracranial pressure.

A full examination is required to exclude any other cause for these symptoms (e.g. acute tonsillitis). The shunt system must be examined for signs of sepsis along the tract (i.e. swelling, erythema, tenderness, discharge), as well as for signs of blockage or shunt breakage (i.e. tense, unyielding reservoir, palpable kinks or gaps along the shunt tubing). Investigation should include an assessment of the white cell count, acute inflammatory indices (e.g. ESR and CRP) and blood cultures. An X-ray of the shunt system and review by the neurosurgical team are required before a sample of CSF is taken for microscopy and culture. Fractured or displaced shunts require surgical replacement. Infected shunts must be removed and prolonged intravenous antibiotics given until the CSF is sterile and a new shunt inserted. In the interim, raised intracranial pressure must be controlled by the insertion of a temporary, exteriorised shunt system.

## OSCE answers

### OSCE 1
i.   Dilated transverse loop of bowel
     No air proximal to dilated loop
     Fluid levels
ii.  Barium/Gastrografin/contrast enema

iii. Hold-up at hepatic flexure or intussusception
iv.  Resuscitate/stabilise
     Rehydrate/fluids
     Analgesia
     Antibiotics
     Surgical/radiological reduction

### OSCE 2
Bilateral hydronephrosis (left > right)
Hydroureters

### OSCE 3
i.   Right short limb, externally rotated, additional crease on right
ii.  Congenital dislocation of hip
iii. Cystic changes, collapse and increased opacification of femoral head
     Flattening of acetabulum
iv.  Perthes' disease

### OSCE 4
i.   Gastroschisis or herniation of bowel through abdominal wall
     Exomphalos
ii.  Resuscitate; fluid replacement; cover bowel loops to keep warm and prevent fluid loss; analgesia; antibiotics; surgical opinion
iii. X-ray showing free air under the diaphragm.
iv.  Perforated viscus
     Abdominal trauma
     Post laparotomy

# 13 Behavioural disorders, social paediatrics, injuries and ethics

| | | |
|---|---|---|
| **13.1** | Introduction | 291 |
| **13.2** | Behavioural disorders | 291 |
| **13.3** | Psychiatric disorders | 294 |
| **13.4** | Social paediatrics | 295 |
| **13.5** | Accidental injury | 296 |
| **13.6** | Non-accidental injury | 298 |
| **13.7** | Medical ethics and paediatrics | 301 |
| | Self-assessment: questions | 303 |
| | Self-assessment: answers | 306 |

## Overview

This chapter covers the main issues relating to behavioural problems in childhood and the impact of social factors on child wellbeing. Accidental injury, often in the home and during recreational activities, is common and often avoidable with simple precautions. The primary management of these children, as well as the basic management of accidental poisoning, is reviewed. Similarly, the warning signs indicating the possibility of non-accidental injury must be recognised. These, together with the steps required in the initial, emergency management of these children, are outlined. Finally, given the increasing complexity of social paediatrics and paediatric care, a basic understanding of the guiding principles of appropriate ethical practice is extremely important.

## 13.1 Introduction

An ever-increasing workload in paediatric health services is devoted to disease and problems stemming from social deprivation. In underdeveloped nations 'social paediatrics' is largely related to widespread poverty, starvation, overcrowding, infectious diseases and child labour. In developed countries, social deprivation is primarily concentrated in inner cities, where poverty, poor family structure and criminal activities, often related to illicit drug abuse and associated crime, abound. It is a sad indictment of 'modern society' that child abuse in various forms is an all too common problem, presenting with depressing regularity. Furthermore, this problem is likely to continue to increase as the family unit continues to disintegrate, leaving young, unsupported single parents to cope with the rigours of everyday life as well as young children. The situation is compounded by the intermittent presence of non-biological parents – often the abusers – and a lifestyle complicated by financial deficiencies, unemployment, drugs, parental ill-health and depression. All too often social services are poorly funded or inadequate to meet the increasing demands of deprived children. Indeed, in many countries worldwide, social services are at best rudimentary, if not totally non-existent.

## 13.2 Behavioural disorders

### Learning objectives

You should:

- be able to differentiate between normal and abnormal behavioural patterns
- be able to appreciate the different types of eating disorders
- know the management of a child with enuresis

### Normal behavioural patterns

#### Habits

*Thumb sucking* is seen in almost all children and may persist for several years, eventually petering out during the early school period. Only 10% still suck their thumbs at 5 years of age. This habit commonly recurs in those children who regress for whatever reason, especially during a serious prolonged illness. *Repetitive mannerisms* such as finger clicking and guttural noises are voluntary movements usually seen in boys and exacerbated during times of stress. They are used to irritate parents and usually disappear when the child is gainfully distracted. Another example of repetitive behaviour is *head banging*, *head-rolling* or *body rocking*. This is seen in 20% of normal toddlers as well as those with developmental problems. In normal children, this behaviour is harmless and usually disappears over a period of months and is rarely seen after 3 years of age.

## Breath-holding

The voluntary cessation of breathing in a child, who becomes deeply cyanosed, can be a frightening experience for the uninitiated. This behavioural tactic is generally the culmination of a bout of crying or a tantrum, following an attempt to discipline a stubborn child aged 6 months to 2.5 years. Forced expiration and apnoea follow a cry. Breath-holding usually stops once cyanosis is established, and is followed by further howling or sobbing. Some children hold their breath to the point of syncope, sometimes with brief tonic–clonic jerks, after which breathing resumes, cyanosis disappears and recovery ensues. Management is aimed at ensuring the diagnosis by taking a graphic history of the 'episodes', confirming normality on examination, and reassuring the parents. Tacit ignoring of the episodes is the best ploy, but in practice is easier said than done!

## Tantrums

Children learn acceptable behaviour by testing the limits of adult tolerance. If thwarted, they may opt for an extreme form of attention seeking whereby they fly into an uncontrolled, sustained rage. Such temper tantrums are more likely during periods of fear, pain and illness. They generally arise in children aged 1–4 years. Recurrent tantrums persisting beyond 5 years, especially those exceeding 15 minutes more than three times a day, may imply an underlying neurodevelopmental disorder. Parents should handle these episodes with a firm disciplinary approach, care being taken to avoid conflicting, inconsistent and reinforcing messages. Corporal punishment is rarely better than non-corporal punitive measures.

## Abnormal behaviour

### Enuresis

Daytime bladder control commences by 18 months onwards, and nappies are no longer required during the day by approximately 2–3 years and at night by 3–5 years. Indeed, only 7% of boys (and less for girls) bed-wet at 5 years of age. Up to 75% of affected children have never been dry (primary enuresis), whereas 25% regress after at least a year of dryness (secondary enuresis). Often a family history of primary enuresis can be elicited. The majority result from minor inadequacies in

toilet training, with over- or under-emphasis on rigid bladder control imposed on the child. These problems resolve spontaneously and require little investigation other than to rule out urinary tract infection. Others, especially secondary enuretics, experience underlying psychological stress, and the possibility of family discord, bereavement, socioeconomic disadvantage and problems at school should be explored. The prognosis is good, once the stressful trigger is eliminated. Organic causes are rare, but continuous day and night-time dribbling is suggestive of an ectopic ureter. The enuretic child should be made to feel involved in treatment, which is directed at achieving an empty bladder at bedtime. This involves avoiding drinks 2–3 hours before bedtime, voiding before going to bed, and again when woken when the parents retire. These practices, when coupled with star charts and a reward for dry nights providing positive reinforcement, are generally successful in 80% of children.

The definitive treatment for enuresis is through the use of conditioning alarms (bell or buzzer). These wake the child as soon as dribbling commences; the child can then empty their bladder. Drug therapy, such as imipramine and desmopressin (DDAVP), is useful for more resistant cases but generally only offers temporary relief. In those under 7 years of age only the behavioural approach is effective, and drugs are not recommended.

### Encopresis

Encopresis is the lack of bowel control, during either the day or the night, beyond the age of 3 years. It generally affects 1% of boys and, like enuresis, may be primary or secondary. Many of these boys are emotionally disturbed and suffer with associated constipation and overflow. The latter must be controlled and a programme of toilet training commenced within the framework of child and family psychotherapy.

### Sleep disorders

*Minor sleep disturbances* are commonplace and usually a result of anxiety in the child regarding such things as fear of school or parental conflict. *Nightmares* are terrifying dreams that result in waking and are remembered; they usually occur in anxious schoolgirls. *Night terrors* are more common in boys, may be associated with sleepwalking, and result in an anxiety state that wakes the child who, nevertheless, cannot recall the dream. Establishing a period of calm before bedtime (e.g. quiet reading of favourite book) or providing a nightlight may be effective therapy. Calm reassurance is usually all that is required following the event. Occasionally light night-time sedation is required, but addictive agents such as tricyclics and benzodiazepines should be avoided.

## Eating problems

### Feeding problems in infancy

*Possetting* – the regurgitation of small amounts of milk – is normal in infants below the age of 6 months, when gastro-oesophageal reflux is common. When severe, repeated 'winding', placing the infant on the right side after a feed, milk thickeners and, occasionally, a prokinetic agent (e.g. domperidone) can be tried. *Underfeeding* results in irritability and poor weight gain, whereas *overfeeding* is characterised by recurrent vomiting and excessive weight gain. Both are usually secondary to inadequate maternal skills and are easily corrected with sympathetic counselling.

Stool frequency is variable and true *constipation* is characterised by firm stool that is difficult to pass. Constipation is becoming increasingly common in 2–4-year-olds. Anal fissures and strictures should be excluded on examination. Infants receiving formula milk often have constipation, and a careful review of the correct reconstitution and volume content of the milk is indicated. Increasing the amount of fluid in the milk is often sufficient in the first few months, followed by increasing fibre later on. Suppositories and mild enemas are sometimes necessary for short periods.

*Colic* arises in infants before the age of 3 months. It results in paroxysms of abdominal pain manifest as inconsolable crying for several hours, often with striking regularity each evening. It follows intestinal distension owing to swallowed air, but rarely is secondary to overfeeding, intestinal fermentation of excess carbohydrate and maternal stress. A careful examination is mandatory to rule out serious pathology. Simple advice regarding over-/underfeeding, regular 'winding' and reassurance is usually all that is required. Paracetamol and various anti-colic medications can be tried: most have little impact on the course of events. In severe cases where family anxiety is intolerable, a mild sedative can be given to settle the child.

### Pica

The ingestion of non-nutrient substances, including dirt and faeces, is common in young children. Although iron deficiency is a common cause of this symptom, persistence of this behaviour beyond the age of 2 years is suggestive of mental retardation, psychological maladjustment and severe family discord and requires investigation. Children who regularly indulge in pica are at an increased risk of parasitic infection and lead poisoning.

### Anorexia nervosa

Anorexia nervosa affects 1 in 300 teenage girls; such girls have an abnormal body image, an intense fear of obesity, and strive to lose weight by any means. Affected girls are very intense, preoccupied with eating, and become emaciated. Hypotension, bradycardia, poor temperature control and amenorrhoea are common clinical findings, and evidence of hypothalamopituitary–ovarian axis and bone marrow failure is seen on investigation. Death from electrolyte disturbance, arrhythmias and heart failure occurs in 10%. Stepwise nutritional rehabilitation and correction of electrolyte disturbances are combined with psychotherapy and, if indicated, treatment of depression.

### Bulimia

Girls with bulimia also have an abnormal body image and fear of obesity. They strive to lose weight by bingeing, followed by self-induced emetic purges, intermittent restricted diets and excessive use of laxatives. The treatment for this disorder is similar to that of anorexia nervosa.

## Learning and cognitive behavioural disorders

### Attention deficit disorders

Attention deficit/hyperactivity disorder (ADHD) is seen in about 4% of school-aged children and is the most common cause of academic underachievement. ADD is characterised by overactivity, short attention span and poor impulse control. These children are generally fidgety, impatient, noisy and sometimes aggressive. As a result, they have difficulty learning and making friends. Treatment involves a multidisciplinary approach involving medical, psychological and educational services. Disciplining such children can be extremely frustrating and exhausting, and parents should be encouraged to reinforce acceptable behaviour while patiently ignoring misbehaviour. The help of a specialised child psychologist and self-help groups is often invaluable. Tricyclic antidepressants and psychostimulants (e.g. methylphenidate, dextroamphetamines) can be used with careful supervision, especially in those with severe hyperactivity. Dietary manipulation and vitamin supplements are ineffective.

### Autism

Autism is characterised by poor verbal and non-verbal skills and a low concentration span, together with repetitive ritualistic behaviour which, if interrupted, often precipitates a tantrum. Patients lack empathy, fail to make friends, adhere to stereotyped, solitary play, and indulge in verbal repetition (echolalia). Autistic features may follow neurological injury, though the aetiology is usually unknown. Asperger syndrome is a mild form of the social impairment of autism. Although these children have near-normal speech development, they have severe impairments in reciprocal social interaction, all-absorbing narrow interests, imposition of routines on self and others, and non-verbal communication problems. Management entails speech therapy and behaviour modification using psychological conditioning programmes. Neuroleptics play a useful role in those with aggressive tendencies and dangerous behaviour. The prognosis is better for those with less destructive behaviour, reasonable intelligence and language development.

## 13.3 Psychiatric disorders

### Learning objective

You should:

- know the common presentations of psychiatric illnesses in children

### Neuroses

#### Anxiety states

Anxiety following a worrying life event is relatively common in childhood and generally resolves with sympathetic counselling. Anxieties related to specific situations (phobias) are less common and require behavioural therapy. School phobia may be a manifestation of underlying depression or problems at school.

#### Depression

Depression manifests as apathy, inactivity, anorexia and failure to thrive in preschool children, and tearfulness, withdrawal, eating, clinging and behavioural disorders in school children. Depression is most common in adolescent girls, who may report fatigue, feelings of sadness, worthlessness and suicidal intentions. The last merits emergency admission to a paediatric psychiatric unit where expert counselling, together with appropriate antidepressants (e.g. tricyclics, serotonin-reuptake inhibitors), can be provided. The prognosis is worse with no clear precipitating insult (which can be eliminated), associated psychotic features, psychomotor retardation and a positive family history. The risk of relapse during childhood is high,

and many of these children continue to suffer with depression in adulthood.

### Psychoses

#### Manic–depressive psychoses

Depressive symptoms together with hallucinations and delusions (often paranoid) are indicative of a psychotic bipolar disorder. Bouts of depression alternate with periods of excessive, unfocused activity, sometimes with inappropriate euphoria (mania). This condition is rare and best treated with lithium carbonate.

#### Schizophrenia

Schizophrenia is rarely seen in childhood. It manifests with thought disorders, chaotic thought processes, flattened affect, paranoid delusions, hallucinations, poor integration in society and disastrous interpersonal relationships. Many go on to suffer with schizophrenia in adulthood. Neuroleptics must be combined with multidisciplinary behavioural therapy if these children are to integrate successfully in a normal childhood environment.

### Suicide and parasuicide

#### Parasuicide

Parasuicide is the unsuccessful attempt to kill oneself. It occurs in 1% of adolescents, is more common in girls, and is often announced beforehand as a *cri du coeur*. The ingestion of tablets is the preferred method. All attempts at suicide, however innocuous, must be considered seriously and require admission to hospital. A trained psychiatrist must review all patients prior to discharge. The seriousness of intent can be gauged by the probability of rescue when seen from the child's point of view. All patients should be given follow-up counselling, and all precipitating factors in their psychosocial background explored. Any conflict, anger and resentment in the family must be addressed.

#### Suicide

In some developed countries suicide is the second most common cause of death in adolescents. It is more common in white males, especially in those who carefully plan the attempt (e.g. with suicide notes etc.), rather than those who have a sudden impulse to inflict self-harm. The increasing incidence of suicide is related to increasing substance abuse, increasing marital breakdown, depression, social isolation, and the availability of weapons. Violent methods are more common in boys, whereas drug overdose is the preferred method in girls. A reduction in the alarming increase in suicides will only follow radical changes in modern lifestyle. Nevertheless, up to 40% of successful suicides follow a previous attempt, so that the importance of heeding any *cri du coeur* cannot be stressed enough.

## 13.4 Social paediatrics

### Learning objective

You should:

- be aware of the different types of substance misuse in children and adolescents

## The social impact of a modern society

The *family unit* consisting of two parents and close relatives living within the same household or nearby is fast disappearing. As a result, many children are brought up by a single, unsupported parent who may herself/himself be very young. This, in itself, may not result in any problems and is preferable to living with squabbling parents whose relationship is beyond salvage. The situation may be compounded by distant, inaccessible friends and relatives, unstable relationships with intermittent partners who are not the biological parent, unemployment, and financial hardship. Little familiarity with indifferent neighbours increases social isolation. The strain within such a disjointed framework can be considerable and increases the risk of failure to cope, substance abuse, depression and child abuse. Furthermore, modern mobile society incurs multiple house moves through job changes, divorce and remarriage. These impose involuntary readjustments in the children with regard to the family, friendships, schooling and the community. These problems are particularly severe for migrants moving from one society to another with a completely different culture and language.

## Social services for children

In many countries social services are rudimentary at best, at worst non-existent. Developed countries have social workers especially devoted to the needs of children. Their work includes advising on financial support, allowances, the provision of adequate housing, fostering services, and the investigation and management of child abuse. They are aided by several child-support agencies and adoption services, and work in close collaboration with drug abuse agencies and the Police Child Protection Unit.

## Illicit substance abuse

The widespread availability of illicit substances, combined with peer pressure, adolescent 'escapism and exploratory urges', results in the worrying statistics listed in Table 82. There is growing evidence of illicit substance abuse by a significant number of pre-adolescent children in the UK – up to 5% of pre-teens currently report the use of illicit substances, and an appreciable number also admit to the use of hard drugs such as heroin.

Up to 70% of teenagers drink alcohol regularly, 5% on a daily basis. Thirty per cent smoke tobacco daily, and although the trend is declining in males, the opposite is true for females. Marijuana was extremely popular until recently, and although its use is declining, that of crack cocaine and Ecstasy is increasing. Intravenous heroin addicts still number approximately 1% of adolescents (4% for inhaled heroin), whereas 4% of adolescents admit to taking anabolic steroids, 15% non-prescription stimulants, and 30% of females have a lifetime prevalence of taking diet pills.

Drug addicts are often unemployable or uninterested, and turn to crime or prostitution to finance their habit. Consequently, drug-related crime is one of the greatest problems in large cities. 'Kicking the habit' once established is considerably more difficult than avoiding it in the first place. Prevention is best achieved through widespread education on the risks involved, together with limiting drug availability. The acute management involves detoxification specific to each individual substance, followed by long-term psychosocial support.

**Table 82** Use of illicit substances in adolescents in developed countries

| Illicit substance | Trend | Male : female ratio |
| --- | --- | --- |
| Alcohol | Increasing/steady | Approaching 1 : 1 |
| Smoking | Increasing in girls | Approaching 1 : 1 |
| Illicit drugs: | | |
| Marijuana | Decreasing | Both |
| Cocaine | Increasing | Male > female |
| Crack cocaine | Increasing | Male > female |
| Ecstasy | Increasing | Both |
| Heroin | Increasing/steady | Male > female |
| Stimulants/ steroids | Steady/declining | Male > female |
| Diet pills | Steady | Female > male |
| Solvents | Decreasing | Male > female |

## 13.5 Accidental injury

### Learning objectives

You should:

- be aware of the differences between accidental and non-accidental injury

- know the assessment and management of child with burns

- know the management of children with paracetamol or salicylate poisoning

### Burns

**Scalds** are typically seen in children below the age of 4 years and are the cause in 85% of admissions following burn injury (Fig. 142). *Flame, chemical* and *electrical burns* make up the remaining 15%. Prevention is extremely important. Adherence to strict laws pertaining to non-flammable clothing, upholstery, toys and water heating settings is responsible for the reduction in fatalities. Indeed, most burn patients survive the ordeal; death usually follows severe smoke inhalation and cerebral anoxia. The site and depth of the burn(s) should be documented (Table 83) and the extent of the affected areas calculated as a percentage of the body surface area (SA) from designated paediatric 'burn charts' (Fig. 143). Burn patients should be examined for other injuries, evidence of respiratory embarrassment and signs of shock – especially likely with more than 15% burns. Resuscitation should include the safeguard of the airway with intubation and artificial ventilation if necessary, and the establishment of good venous access.

Rehydration is commenced at 4 mL/kg body weight for every per cent SA burnt, with half this requirement being replaced in the first 8 hours. Electrolyte imbalance, hypoalbuminaemia and anaemia must all be corrected while adequate analgesia with opiates is provided. Burnt areas must be covered with sterile dressings and kept clean with a topical bacteriostatic agent. Dead tissue is debrided and large denuded areas grafted by a team specialised in this work. Nutritional support, if necessary with total parenteral nutrition, is essential to minimise the catabolic effects of a major burn and encourage healing. Antibiotics are not started unless there is clear evidence of infection, or with subsequent fever and positive cultures. Psychological support may be necessary for those with disfiguring injuries, especially to the face.

**Smoke inhalation** results in pulmonary epithelial sloughing, alveolar destruction, oedema, degradation of surfactant and atelectasis. Mortality is as high as 50% in severe incidents, and survival depends on intensive-care support of the airway and lungs with artificial

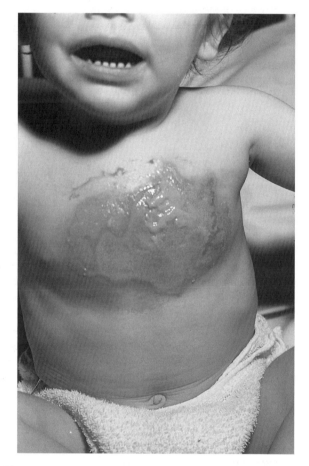

**Fig. 142** Characteristic scald from spilling hot tea.

**Table 83** Classification of burns

| Type of burn | Symptoms, signs | Outcome |
|---|---|---|
| First degree: epidermis only | Pain, erythema | Healing without scars |
| Second degree: epidermis and dermis | Very painful, blisters | May heal with scars, moderate fluid loss |
| Third degree: full thickness | Painless, little bleeding | Contractures, scars, severe fluid imbalance, require grafting |

Ignore simple erythema

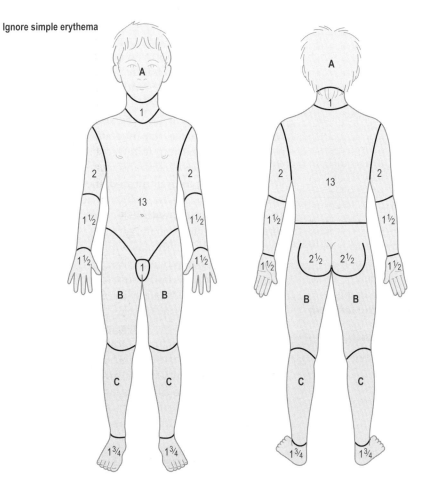

| | Partial thickness loss (PTL) |
| --- | --- |
| | Full thickness loss (FTL) |

| | % | |
| --- | --- | --- |
| Region | PTL | FTL |
| Head | | |
| Neck | | |
| Ant. trunk | | |
| Post. trunk | | |
| Right arm | | |
| Left arm | | |
| Buttocks | | |
| Genitalia | | |
| Right leg | | |
| Left leg | | |
| Sub-total | | |
| **Total** | | |

**Relative percentage of body surface area affected by growth**

| | Age (years) | | | | | |
| --- | --- | --- | --- | --- | --- | --- |
| Area | 0 | 1 | 5 | 10 | 15 | Adult |
| **A** = $\frac{1}{2}$ of head | $9\frac{1}{2}$ | $8\frac{1}{2}$ | $6\frac{1}{2}$ | $5\frac{1}{2}$ | $4\frac{1}{2}$ | $3\frac{1}{2}$ |
| **B** = $\frac{1}{2}$ of one thigh | $2\frac{3}{4}$ | $3\frac{1}{4}$ | 4 | $4\frac{1}{2}$ | $4\frac{1}{2}$ | $4\frac{3}{4}$ |
| **C** = $\frac{1}{2}$ of one leg | $2\frac{1}{2}$ | $2\frac{1}{2}$ | $2\frac{3}{4}$ | 3 | $3\frac{1}{4}$ | $3\frac{1}{2}$ |

**Fig. 143** Typical burns assessment chart.

ventilation and, with upper airway burn involvement, a tracheostomy.

## Accidental ingestion

Accidental ingestion of medication or toxic agents is usually seen in children under 6 years of age; older children, especially teenagers, often overdose intentionally. The precise agent(s), amount(s) ingested and time lapse since ingestion must be ascertained. Unless you are very familiar with the substance involved, immediate telephone contact with the nearest *poison centre* will establish the potential toxicity and urgency of the situation.

If there is any doubt, all children must be admitted for 24 hours for observation. Those in a critical state require resuscitation and transfer to a life-support unit. A few agents have an *antidote* (Table 84); otherwise, general supportive measures are instigated. These include intravenous access, maintenance of blood pressure with fluid and, if necessary, inotropic support.

**Induced emesis** with ipecac has a poor recovery rate of ingested material, is useless at 4 or more hours after ingestion, and is contraindicated in those under 6 months of age or if comatose. Prior to emesis, the airway should always be protected by placing the child in the left lateral position.

**Table 84** Specific treatment/antidote for ingested substances

| Ingested agent | Antidote/treatment |
|---|---|
| Carbon monoxide | Oxygen |
| Cyanide | Sodium nitrite + thiosulphate, or hydroxycobalamin + thiosulphate |
| Iron | Desferrioxamine |
| Nitrobenzene | Methylene blue |
| Opiates | Naloxone |
| Organophosphates | Atropine |
| Paracetamol | N-Acetylcysteine |

**Gastric lavage** is rarely used in children and is only effective if attempted within an hour of ingestion.

**Activated charcoal** placed into the stomach or swallowed prevents further absorption of many agents.

**Forced diuresis** is only indicated in specific forms of poisoning.

**Haemodialysis** is ineffective in many instances because of the volume of distribution and poor clearance rates of most drugs.

## Specific poisoning

**Paracetamol overdose** results in nausea and vomiting, followed by abdominal pain and liver dysfunction by 48 hours. The liver dysfunction peaks at around 80 hours before resolving slowly. Serum paracetamol levels should be measured at 4 hours post ingestion and compared with standard nomograms, administering N-acetylcysteine if the level is elevated above the 'treatment' line. Liver function, including prothrombin time, must be assessed daily.

**Salicylates** in overdose cause hyperventilation, vomiting, tinnitus and lethargy. Respiratory alkalosis is replaced, after an initial 12-hour phase, by hypokalaemia, lactic acidosis and progressive dehydration. The peak plasma level is best ascertained in a sample taken 6 hours after ingestion and compared with a nomogram. Dehydration and acid–base and electrolyte imbalance should be corrected by administering appropriate fluid, bicarbonate and potassium. Forced diuresis may compound pulmonary oedema and, like haemodialysis, is reserved for severe toxicity not responsive to alkalinisation and rehydration.

Excess **iron** ingestion results in gastrointestinal irritation with pain, vomiting and diarrhoea (sometimes with blood), followed by apparent recovery after about 6 hours, only to be replaced by hypoglycaemia, acidosis, and potentially fatal liver failure between 2 and 4 days later. Pyloric stenosis may follow local mucosal damage and is manifest 3 weeks after the event. Total serum iron levels are elevated and exceed the total iron-binding capacity. Forced emesis, lavage and charcoal are seldom effective. Treatment is largely supportive, together with intravenous desferrioxamine and haemodialysis if renal failure complicates the overdose.

**Antidepressants** are widely prescribed for adult patients and, unfortunately, are frequently found and ingested by children. Tricyclic antidepressant ingestion results in tachycardia, dry mucous membranes, drowsiness and hypertension, followed later by hypotension. Arrhythmias, convulsions and coma may lead to death. Forced emesis is contraindicated, though activated charcoal may be useful in reducing absorption. Patients should be admitted, with ECG monitoring. Acidosis is corrected with bicarbonate, seizures with diazepam and phenytoin, and arrhythmias with lignocaine (lidocaine). Renal dialysis is rarely effective.

**Acids** and **alkalis** both cause local damage to the gastrointestinal tract. Alkaline agents cause oesophageal necrosis and strictures, whereas acids irritate the oesophagus and gastric pylorus, causing necrosis, perforation and late strictures. Oral irritation is associated with drooling and dysphagia. If tolerated, water and milk should be drunk in the first instance. Endoscopy should be attempted 24 hours later. Clear, neutral fluids are continued until all symptoms abate. There is no place for ingested acid or alkaline antidotes.

## 13.6 Non-accidental injury

### Learning objective

You should:

- know when to suspect non-accidental injury and what to do next

### Suspicion of non-accidental injury

In the majority of cases accidents are bona fide, resulting from the everyday rough and tumble of childhood. The onus is on the examining doctor to first suspect, then investigate, an injury as *non-accidental* (NAI). A sensible approach is required to avoid over-diagnosis and unnecessary emotional trauma to the family, while ensuring no case is missed. *The benefit of doubt must always be given to the child.* Inconsistencies in the history, implausible explanations, outright untruths and delay in presentation raise the possibility of NAI. A forever-changing history is a hallmark of NAI, the perpetrators embarking on a 'fishing expedition' whereby several explanations are offered in the hope that one will be accepted. A non-committal approach should be adopted, allowing the history to be delivered at will with few leading questions. Suspicious findings on examination include multiple injuries, often of differing ages, injuries incompatible with the history obtained, and injuries that could only result from excessive force being applied to the child (e.g. whip marks). The injury must be assessed in the context of the history and age of the child: hence, a fracture of the humerus may be explicable in a boisterous 6-year-old falling off a fence but is highly suspicious in a 4-month-old infant.

Whenever suspected, the child should be fully examined and any suspicious areas investigated (e.g. X-ray examination of swollen limbs). The child should be admitted, any injuries attended to, and investigated as appropriate. It is well to remember that many of these cases will end up in a court of law. Hence, it is of paramount importance that detailed notes are made, including drawings of any injuries, with measurements, discoloration and estimated age clearly documented. Investigations should be kept to a minimum whenever possible, in order to avoid further trauma to the child. A platelet count and clotting profile are necessary in those with bruises/haematomas (if only for legal reasons), and a skeletal survey in children presenting with fractures. Skull X-ray and a CT scan of the brain are indicated following non-accidental head injury.

Overt cases of child abuse are, in some ways, easier to manage. All hospitals will have local guidelines as to the correct procedures and the people who need to be contacted. There is no doubt that the child must be kept in a place of safety, in most cases an acute hospital ward. Social services must be informed as soon as possible, and in cases of grievous harm or death the police are also contacted. If the child's carers refuse admission, an emergency magistrate's order (or its equivalent, according to country) can be obtained to appoint the child a ward of court. The magistrate will then instruct where the child, as well as any other sibling at risk, is to be nursed (e.g. ward, temporary foster home). It is not the remit of the medical professionals to be judgmental. They should concentrate on treating and safeguarding the child while referring the case to the relevant authorities whose job it is to direct allegations, accusations and arrests.

Many cases of suspected abuse are less clear-cut. Although there may be an inconsistent history and unusual injuries, these may not be tantamount to flagrant abuse. Reference to the local children's *At Risk Register* and discussion with social services may heighten one's suspicions if previous concerns have already been noted. If in doubt, it is best to admit the child and observe and/or investigate over the subsequent few days. A *case conference* attended by all relevant personnel (e.g. medical, nursing, social services, police, school and legal representatives) should review all cases of NAI/suspected abuse. During the conference, deci-

sions regarding the placement of the child (e.g. own home, foster home), the addition of his or her name to the *At Risk Register* and prosecution must be taken. Most children are returned to their biological parents, for whom social service support is organised. Varying degrees of supervision can be imposed by law, depending on the severity of each case. All local authorities have an Area Child Protection Committee (ACPC). This is the key inter-agency forum for child protection, comprising representatives from all the relevant statutory organisations and representing the voluntary sector.

## Specific forms of child abuse

Child abuse can take many forms and produce a range of clinical manifestations of non-accidental injury (Fig. 144).

### Burns

Accidental burns are common in children. However, scalds affecting the buttocks, lower back, the posterior aspects of the lower limbs and feet suggest an *immersion* injury (Fig. 144d). Likewise, multiple small ring- or target-like burns suggest *cigarette burn* injuries (Fig. 144c) and, like clearly demarcated burns from a hot iron, are highly suspicious.

### Bruises

Bruises of varying sizes and ages on the shins of active schoolboys are of no consequence. However, similar bruises distributed over other parts of the body, including the trunk and head, especially if associated with other injuries, should alert one to the possibility of repeated battering (Fig. 144a). It is important to age the bruises (preferably photograph the lesions) and attempt to account for each one from the history. Small mirror-image bruises arranged in a semicircular pattern suggest *bite marks* (Fig. 144b), whereas multiple linear, criss-cross bruising and lacerations indicate a *whipping* injury (Fig. 144h). *Haematomas* often accompany bruises: they should be aged and measured, and, if large and associated with significant pain and limitation of movement, may herald an underlying fracture.

### Fractures

Except in those with osteogenesis imperfecta or with a history of major trauma (e.g. a road traffic accident), *multiple fractures* are always suspicious. This is especially so if the fractures are old, of different ages and in characteristic sites, e.g. rib, skull and spiral fractures of long bones (Fig. 144f, i, j).

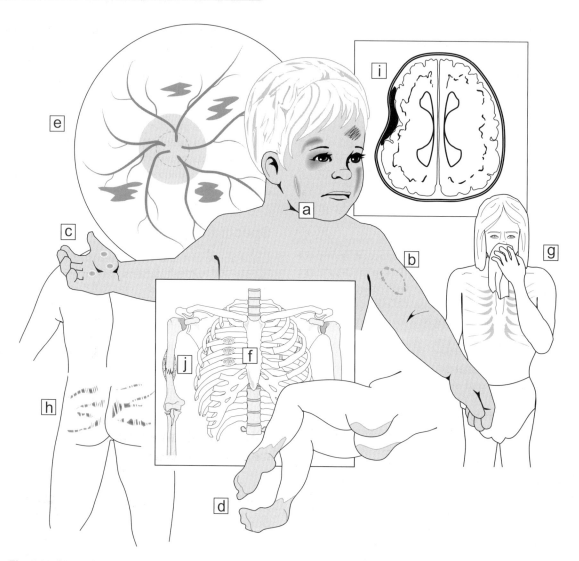

**Fig. 144** Clinical manifestations of non-accidental injury. (a) Multiple bruises, lacerations of different ages; (b) bite mark; (c) cigarette burns; (d) immersion burn injury; (e) retinal haemorrhages; (f) old rib fractures with callus formation; (g) severe emaciation following neglect; (h) whip marks; (i) depressed skull fracture with haematoma; (j) spiral long bone fracture.

## Head injuries

The most common and potentially lethal NAI of the head in small babies without adequate head control involves intracerebral haemorrhage and oedema following a *shaking* injury. *Depressed skull fractures* (Fig. 144i) are seen in older children and present with inconsolable crying, swelling, bruising over the site of trauma, and coma in those with significant underlying brain damage.

## Munchausen syndrome by proxy

Munchausen syndrome by proxy is a much publicised but rare form of child abuse that occurs when a psychi-

atrically unwell guardian – almost always the mother – falsifies illness in her child. This may involve the fabrication of symptoms and signs, the actual causation of illness by exposure of the child to toxins, and alteration of laboratory results. These individuals obtain gratification through the attention focused on themselves as a result of their child's illness. Many such parents have had some medical or nursing background, and can be extremely clever at disguising the fictitious nature of their child's illness. The abused children are invariably too young to implicate their mother as the true offender. They may present with quite bizarre features that, as with smothering and intentional poisoning, may persist in hospital. However, an improvement in symptoms and signs may follow a period of planned, close observation without the mother present, and may clinch what can be a very difficult diagnosis to prove. The parent should be seen by a sympathetic physician and the child social and legal services alerted.

## Emotional deprivation and neglect

Child abuse emanating from chronic physical and emotional neglect may present with non-organic failure to thrive (Fig. 144g) and short stature. These children are often unkempt. Their chronic exposure to an inappropriate mother–child relationship and inattention results in behavioural abnormalities such as apathy, frozen watchfulness, food obsession and autoerotic activity, as well as delayed developmental milestones. However, the last improves on admission to hospital, where the child's initial aloof and reserved nature gives way to a ravenous appetite, clinging behaviour and a need for comfort. A history of rejection, neglect and NAI in the mother is common.

## Sexual abuse

Sexual abuse constitutes any activity with a child below the age of consent that is carried out for the gratification of the adult. In the majority of cases the offender is usually a male family member or friend known to the child. Sexual abuse constitutes approximately 15% of child abuse and is reported in 1–2 of every 1000 children. The increased incidence since the 1970s is partly the result of increased reporting. However, given that 20% of adult females and 5% of males admit to being abused as children, this incidence is still an underestimate of the true size of the problem.

Sexual abuse is an extremely delicate paediatric problem and can only be dealt with by experienced, sympathetic professionals. Occasionally a distressed child presents in a dishevelled state, partially clothed, with evidence of a recent assault amounting to rape or sodomy (usually by a stranger). More often (especially with family perpetrators) there is no associated violence and the possibility of sexual abuse is raised by a chance comment or abnormal or inappropriate sexualised or seductive behaviour. Abused victims may develop non-specific manifestations such as enuresis, poor school performance, truancy, depression, tantrums and sleep and eating disorders. Perineal discomfort, erythema and discharge may be absent or non-specific.

Experienced interviewers should obtain the history, with representatives of the medical, social, legal and police services present unobtrusively. A video recording can help to limit the number of traumatic interviews. Any suspected or alleged case of a penetrating assault should be examined with a view to excluding other physical injuries. In a girl, unless there are signs of severe bleeding or peritonitis, examination of the genitalia must be left to the gynaecology–paediatric–forensic team and, if necessary, carried out under general anaesthesia. Lacerations, scratch marks, bruises, tears of the hymen must be documented and, whenever possible, photographed. Samples for culture, semen analysis and blood typing should be obtained. Injuries should be dealt with and any bleeding stanched. The involvement of an experienced child counsellor and careful follow-up is required to address any psychoemotional sequelae.

## Child exploitation

Child labour was commonplace in Victorian times but, sadly, together with slavery, prostitution and involvement in pornographic practices, it remains a way in which adults exploit children even today. These problems are more prevalent but certainly not exclusive to developing countries. Their long-term eradication will only become a reality with improved respect for human rights worldwide, international cooperation between police forces, and stricter penalties for offenders.

## 13.7 Medical ethics and paediatrics

### Learning objective

You should:

- know the procedures for obtaining consent and breaking bad news

Ethical problems are common in child care, rarely present with a simple solution, and have a significant impact on the individual, their family and, at times, society. An ethical code of practice is essential and should respect confidentiality and the autonomy, physical and mental competence of every child, regardless of age. This code should incorporate honesty and beneficence (doing 'good'), aiming for realistic goals while avoiding conflict and a paternalistic approach.

### Medical decisions

Medical decisions may be difficult enough, but invariably those spanning ethical issues are particularly difficult. Certain criteria listed in Box 86 can help to ensure that the best ethically acceptable decisions are taken which, ultimately, are in the interest of the child. Nevertheless, decision taking is rarely straightforward and,

**Box 86** Requirements for ethically acceptable decision making

| | |
|---|---|
| Omniscience | *all the facts* |
| Omnipercipience | *all points of view* |
| Disinterest | *no bias* |
| Dispassion | *no emotions* |
| Consistency | *reproducibility* |

for example, it is almost impossible to remain totally dispassionate (lacking in emotions) when confronting decisions relating to the discontinuation of life-sustaining therapy in a patient whom you have looked after for several years.

## Bioethics and the non-competent patient

Young children and those with a significant mental disability may not be able to take a meaningful role in the decision-making process, and in this regard are 'non-competent'. Ideally, all patients should be considered to be equal, with an equal right to healthcare, regardless of age and disability. In practice, however, healthcare has limitations, including financial constraints, resulting in 'rationing'. This, in turn, may advantage the 'more deserving' patient while introducing bias against the less competent. All those involved in child care should safeguard against this potential bias.

## Informed consent

Achieving 'truly' free and informed consent that is not based on coercion, bias or vested interest in the 'non-competent' child may be particularly difficult. Invariably, third parties are involved, and although the vast majority do have the child's true interest at heart, this may not always be the case. Lengthy, sometimes exhaustive, discussions are necessary with parents or guardians to ensure that they fully appreciate the problem at hand, with all the potential options and outcomes, and are able to take a meaningful decision which is in their child's interests. Any medical bias, prejudice or vested interest such as research involvement must be excluded from the discussion process. In the United Kingdom, for children under 16 years of age, the parent is required to give consent for treatment or procedures.

However, if the treating physician deems that the child is of sufficient maturity and understanding, or 'Gillick competent', then consent or its refusal may be obtained from the child and the physician will need to respect confidentiality.

## Quality of life

Ultimately, the quality of life (QOL) is paramount, but this is a highly subjective concept that may vary enormously from one individual to another, let alone between social, racial and religious groups. For the individual child, both under- and over-treatment are wrong. Hence, the aim would be to treat appropriately where there is an appreciable chance of success and the likelihood of a meaningful QOL, while avoiding extraordinary or futile therapy in those where there is virtually no hope for a reasonable outcome.

## Children and research

Ongoing research generally benefits future patients not study subjects, a concept that may be impossible for most children to grasp. Moreover, children as study subjects pose problems with informed consent, and great care is required in counselling parents and guardians. Individual vested interests, commitments to fund holders, support groups and benefactors should never influence the enrolment of children into research trials. In practice, all paediatric research should be assessed and first approved by a designated *Ethics Committee*. The latter generally comprise many experts and laypersons representing various walks of life (e.g. the medical field, law, ethnic, religious groups etc.).

## Death and the dying process

Even when death is inevitable and extraordinary measures are not instigated, much can still be done to alleviate suffering and abolish pain, thereby preserving quality (rather than quantity) of life. The decision to discontinue or not to embark on further 'active' therapy for the terminally ill child does not mean that treatment stops, but rather it represents a shift to palliative care. Indeed, many units dealing with children where death is relatively common employ a team of palliative carers. Wherever possible, all health carers should respect the child's and the family's wishes and, ultimately, strive to ensure dignity in death.

# Self-assessment: questions

## Multiple choice questions

1. The following statements describe behavioural disorders:
   a. Thumb sucking at 3 years is indicative of a psychosocial disorder
   b. Breath-holding does not result in seizure activity
   c. Severe tantrums are best managed by intense psychotherapy
   d. Overfeeding suggests a problem with mothering rather than the child
   e. Pica is pathognomonic of iron-deficiency anaemia.

2. With regard to anorexia and bulimia nervosa:
   a. Anorexia is more common in girls, bulimia in boys
   b. Patients are usually happy-go-lucky extroverts who forget to eat
   c. Amenorrhoea is a common complication
   d. Death occurs in 1% of patients
   e. Misuse of laxatives is a common association.

3. The following constitute appropriate therapy:
   a. Dietary manipulation for attention deficit disorders
   b. Psychological conditioning for autism
   c. Behavioural therapy for school phobia
   d. Major psychotropics for anxiety-related depression
   e. Lithium for manic psychosis.

4. With regard to illicit substance abuse:
   a. Abuse generally starts in late school-aged children
   b. The use of crack cocaine is on the increase
   c. Smoking is decreasing in both sexes
   d. Drug abuse is the major cause of crime in teenagers and young adults
   e. Drug taking is the commonest cause of HIV infection in children.

5. The following statements describe accidental ingestion:
   a. It usually occurs in school-aged children
   b. It is rarely fatal
   c. Most cases should be managed at home
   d. Forced emesis is indicated except in comatose patients

e. Haemodialysis is a useful last resort in severe cases.

6. The following increase the risk of child abuse:
   a. The presence of a live-in, non-biological father
   b. Social deprivation
   c. Parents who were abused as children
   d. Specific cultural or racial origins
   e. Prematurity.

## Case histories

### Case history 1

A 4-month-old boy is brought to A&E by his 18-year-old mother, who noted a swelling of his right elbow over the preceding 24 hours. Examination confirms marked swelling of the elbow, overlying green-brown discoloration and painful limitation of movement. The boyfriend felt that the child had caught his arm between the cot sides.

How would you manage this case?

### Case history 2

A baby is born at 37 weeks of gestation to a young woman who was on a registered drug-abuse programme with the local social services and taking a regular supply of methadone. She had suffered repeated beatings from her violent boyfriend, who had disappeared early during the pregnancy. She had attended all antenatal clinics, had stopped smoking tobacco, but was still on methadone at the time of birth. At 12 hours of age the infant was noted to be jittery, with a shrill cry.

1. What is the most likely cause for this baby's symptoms?
2. What other clinical manifestations may develop over the next few hours?
3. What treatment is indicated?

The child remains very jittery over the next 36 hours and has at least two brief, generalised convulsions. Following a thorough examination you are confident that the general clinical condition has not deteriorated, but order some investigations.

4. What investigations would be appropriate at this point?

The child is eventually discharged (without any medication) and followed-up regularly in the outpatient department.

5. What steps would you take prior to discharge?

After a 3-month period of excellent progress, the mother and child start to default from clinic appointments. After several attempts, the social services are finally able to visit and note that the mother looked dishevelled and has several bruises on her arms, as well as a black eye. She claims to have tripped and fallen downstairs. She is coaxed to attend the next paediatric clinic. During the visit it is obvious that the child had not been bathed for several days, has a severe nappy rash and has lost weight.

6. What may have accounted for the apparent change in mothering skills?
7. What action would you take following the last clinic visit?

## Case history 3

A 5-year-old boy is brought to A&E by his mother because he has been crying inconsolably for several hours. On examination you notice several green and brown bruises over the left forehead, right chest wall and back, a circle of five red-brown bruises over the left thigh, and diffuse, tender swelling of the right arm.

1. What other important questions would you ask of his mother at this stage?

In answer to your questioning, his mother reported that he had fallen down a flight of stairs 4 hours before being brought to A&E.

2. In the light of this statement, what is your clinical diagnosis and why?
3. What is the likely cause for the bruising on the left thigh?

The mother then suddenly remembers that her own brother tended to bruise easily, and she believed that he suffered with some rare form of bleeding disorder. She appeared worried that her son may have the same problem. You had already suggested that he required an X-ray of the right arm, but agree that he needs further investigation and arrange for some tests to be carried out in A&E.

4. What additional investigations would you request (apart from the X-ray of the right arm)?

The X-ray revealed a partly displaced spiral fracture of the right humerus with early osteoid formation.

5. What comment would you make in the light of this finding on X-ray?

At this point the mother's boyfriend barges into A&E, smelling of alcohol and holding the 3-year-old sister in his arms. Amid a barrage of foul language, he claims that the boy was 'fine' but just 'too stupid to walk downstairs without falling over'. He insists on taking everyone home and offers to give the boy regular paracetamol.

6. What course of action would you adopt at this point?

## Short notes

Write short notes on truancy.

## OSCE questions

### OSCE 1
Figure 145 was taken from a 2-month-old infant admitted as an emergency in coma.

i.  What is the diagnosis on fundoscopy?
ii. Name TWO causes of this problem.

### OSCE 2
A boisterous 11-year-old lost his footing and was injured following a fall of 1 m from railings (Fig. 146).

i.  Report this X-ray.
ii. Name TWO complications that may develop following this injury.

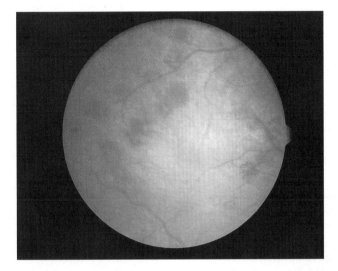

**Fig. 145**

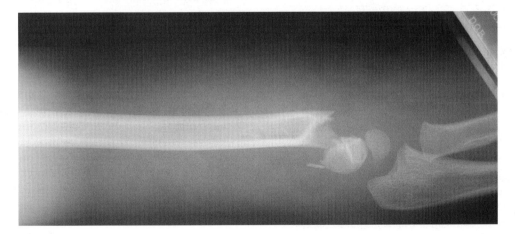

**Fig. 146**

# Self-assessment: answers

## Multiple choice answers

1. a. **False**. It is a normal behavioural pattern at this age.
   b. **False**. It may result in hypoxia-related seizures.
   c. **False**. The best ploy is to ignore the episodes.
   d. **True**. It is usually simple over-anxiety.
   e. **False**. Though it may be associated with iron deficiency.

2. a. **False**. Both are far more common in girls.
   b. **False**. Patients are usually introverted, shy, anxious types.
   c. **True**. Both primary and secondary amenorrhoea occur.
   d. **False**. Death occurs in 10%.
   e. **True**. Laxatives are used in an attempt to purge the body of 'excess calories' from the lower end.

3. a. **False**. This is an ineffective approach.
   b. **True**. This forms the basis of autistic rehabilitation programmes.
   c. **True**. Therapy is used to help relearn appropriate behaviour and suppress the phobia.
   d. **False**. These are rarely required; counselling, reassurance and simple anxiolytics generally suffice.
   e. **True**. As for therapy in adults.

4. a. **False**. Teenagers are the usual starting group.
   b. **True**. Cocaine is becoming more popular and widely available.
   c. **False**. Smoking is increasing in girls.
   d. **True**. Most crime in adolescents centres on illegal activities in order to fund an illicit drug habit.
   e. **False**. Perinatal transmission accounts for most cases of AIDS in childhood; an ever-decreasing number acquired the disease from contaminated blood products received during the period 1970–1986. Household contacts of HIV-positive parents have very little or no risk of contamination. Sexual and drug-related transmission is becoming more common, but presents in late adolescence and early adult life.

5. a. **False**. It is more usual in preschool children.
   b. **True**. Most are innocuous and simply require observation.
   c. **False**. Almost all should be admitted for overnight observation.
   d. **False**. Emesis is often unsafe and rarely effective.
   e. **False**. Few ingested agents are effectively removed by dialysis.

6. a. **True**. He is usually (although not invariably) the abuser.
   b. **True**. This compounds a poor social framework and is a scenario that encourages child abuse.
   c. **True**. It is a sad fact that abused parents are more likely to abuse their own children.
   d. **False**. Abuse knows no cultural barriers.
   e. **True**. This is a well-documented statistic.

## Case history answers

### Case history 1

The findings suggest a significant injury to the elbow with the development of a haematoma and the possibility of an underlying fracture. The first stage in management is to confirm the extent of the injury, reduce any fractures, relieve a haemarthrosis and provide adequate analgesia. An X-ray of the elbow joint and orthopaedic opinion are indicated in the first instance. There are a number of discrepancies in the story: a 4-month-old cannot sustain such an injury simply by getting caught in cot sides, and the age of the bruising is inconsistent with the history. Indeed, as seen in Table 85, green-brown discoloration arises after 7–10 days. Therefore, this case is suspicious and must be assumed to be one of child abuse. The infant must be admitted to the ward (place of safety), all injuries carefully documented (and photographed), and a skeletal survey plus clotting screen performed. The social services must be contacted, the *Child Abuse Register* consulted, the Police Child Protection Unit informed and a case conference organised. Clear

**Table 85** Guide for 'dating' bruises

| Day | Colour |
|-----|--------|
| 1 | Red |
| 3 | Blue |
| 5 | Purple |
| 7 | Green |
| 9 | Yellow |
| 11 | Brown |
| 13–21 | Resolves |

**Box 87** Clinical features of the neonatal withdrawal syndrome

- Tremor, jitteriness, irritability, convulsions
- Hypertonicity, hyperreflexia
- Persistent and high-pitched cry
- Excessive sleepiness or wakefulness
- Hyperventilation, irregular respirations, apnoeas
- Nasal stuffiness, repeated sneezing
- Excessive yawning, hiccups, mouthing movements, fist sucking
- Diarrhoea, repeated vomiting, poor feeding.

decisions regarding placement of the child, supervision of the family and further investigation into the case must be taken before discharge can be contemplated.

## Case history 2

1. The most likely diagnosis is neonatal withdrawal syndrome following methadone use by the mother. Withdrawal occurs in around 50% of babies whose mothers take methadone during pregnancy, especially if taken within 24 hours of parturition.
2. Clinical manifestations of neonatal withdrawal are similar regardless of the drug abused, and are listed in Box 87.
3. Treatment involves the administration of methadone to the infant. This is titrated according to a standardised scoring system based on the presence or absence of the above symptoms and signs. High scores on consecutive recordings result in an increase in the dosage (in a controlled fashion) until a plateau is reached. Once stable, the methadone is gradually reduced over a period of several weeks or months (necessitating prolonged hospital stay). If the logistics of giving a controlled drug to such infants is problematic, the infant can be treated with chlorpromazine, again in increasing dosage until the symptoms of withdrawal abate.
4. Although these complications are almost certainly related to methadone withdrawal, sepsis, including neonatal meningitis and metabolic derangements, in particular hypoglycaemia and hypocalcaemia, must be considered. Serum glucose, calcium and electrolytes are mandatory, and a septic screen performed if there is sufficient clinical suspicion.
5. Close collaboration with social services is required before discharge. You must ensure that the housing and social environment is adequate, and all support

services that may be required are in place. Close liaison with the illicit drug rehabilitation unit is also necessary. Clear follow-up and supervision arrangements must be defined beforehand.

6. Given the sudden change in 'attitude' and the recurrence of bruises on the mother, it is likely that the boyfriend has reappeared. The mother is probably being subjected to physical abuse. The implications of this situation on her own drug problem and the repercussions on the welfare of the child are now brought into serious doubt.
7. The mother needs to be confronted with your fears and social services alerted immediately. If necessary, it may be appropriate to involve the police at this stage. At any rate, the child is no longer in a place of safety and alternative accommodation must be found as a matter of urgency. In view of the child's weight loss and general state, admission to hospital for a short period is required. Following this, the child may be transferred, preferably together with the mother, to a safe place of refuge while the case is investigated (and any charges brought) by the social services and police. Regular medical follow-up must continue to monitor the child's growth and neurodevelopmental progress.

## Case history 3

1. How had he sustained the various bruises?
   When did these injuries occur?
   Ask whether he has been able to use the right arm? How long for?
   Has he had previous injuries/bruises?
   Ask about the family members/history/set-up/ dynamics.
   Ask about the social history, housing, employment.
2. Non-accidental injury.
   History is not compatible with clinical findings in terms of causality and timing.
3. A forceful grip/clutching injury OR bite mark.
4. Other X-rays/skeletal survey.
   Clotting profile/screen.
   Platelet count
5. Fracture cannot be just a few hours old: early osteoid formation suggests at least 10–14 days.
6. Attempt gentle persuasion for accepting admission to hospital.
   Contact social workers urgently.
   Inform senior colleague.
   Prevent removal of both children from hospital (police intervention if required).
   Arrange admission to place of safety (hospital for boy; suitable placement for sibling).
   Consult orthopaedic team/reduce fracture.

## Short notes answer

Truancy is absenteeism or running away from school without a valid reason (e.g. ill health). It is not an extension of normal developmental behaviour and generally signifies an underlying problem. The child may be running away from a distressing situation at school, or be attempting to draw attention to a similarly distressing situation at home. Hence, truancy follows problems in certain areas of the child's life.

### Problems at school

- Anxiety about fear of teacher, fear of peers, teasing and bullying
- Failure to cope with humiliation, learning difficulties, inability to match peers.

### Problems at home

- Anxiety about separation from parents or siblings, parental discord, family strife, disagreement with parents
- Social problems resulting from family disorganisation, unstable family environment, criminal, illicit activities at home
- Child abuse including physical, sexual, emotional abuse or neglect.

### Problems with the child

- Personality problems
- Inadequacy
- Psycho-emotional problems.

The management involves an in-depth investigation into the above possibilities during a series of sympathetic interviews with the child, teachers and family. The underlying cause should be addressed and eliminated. Child psychologists and social services should be involved where appropriate, and supportive behavioural therapy instigated, depending on the cause.

## OSCE answers

### OSCE 1
i.  Retinal haemorrhages
ii. Non-accidental injury/shaking injury
    Bleeding diathesis

### OSCE 2
i.  Displaced, comminuted/supracondylar fracture of lower humerus
ii. Vascular injury, ischaemic necrosis, non-alignment, nerve injury

# Index

Question and Answer Sections are indicated in the form 16Q/18A
References to tables and boxes are in italics

**A**

Abdominal distension, 26
Abdominal epilepsy, *107*
Abdominal migraine, *107*
Abdominal pain, 106–*107*
Abdominal palpation, 52
Accidental injury
  burns, 296–7
  ingestion of medication/toxic agents, 297–8, 303Q/306A
Achondroplasia, 166
Acid peptic disease, *107*
Acidaemias, organic, 195
Acidosis, 154
  metabolic, 201Q/203A
  renal failure, 154
Acids, accidental ingestion, 298
Acute lymphoblastic leukaemia (ALL), 245–6
Acute myeloid leukaemia (AML), 245–6
Addison disease, 173, 182Q/186A
Adenosine deaminase (ADA) deficiency, *198*
Adrenal gland, disorders, 173–5
Adrenal tumours, 175
Agammaglobulinaemia, X-linked, *198*
Airways, upper, 52
Albers-Schönberg disease, *275*
Albinism, *166*
Alkalis, accidental ingestion, 298
Alpha1-antitrypsin deficiency, 196
Alpha-fetoprotein, maternal serum, 201Q/203A
Alport syndrome, 152
Amino acid metabolism, disorders of, *195–7*
Amniocentesis, *25*, 200
Anaemia(s)
  233–40, 252Q/256A
  aplastic, 237
  autoimmune haemolytic, 252Q/256A
  congenital, 236
  congenital hypoplastic, 235–6
  hypochromic microcytic, 251Q/255A
  iron-deficiency, 235–6
  malarial, 221
  megaloblastic, 236
  physiological, of infancy, 234
  in renal failure, 146, 154
Anal atresia, 263, 264
Angelman syndrome, 192
Anorexia nervosa, 170, 293

Antenatal diagnosis, invasive procedures for, *25*
Antenatal screening, 24
Anterior horn cell disease, viruses causing, 224Q/228A
Antibiotic prophylaxis
  endocarditis, *91*
  indications, *149*
Antibiotic therapy, immunocompromised child, 211
Anticonvulsants, *132*
Antidepressants, accidental ingestion, 298
Antidiuretic hormone (ADH) secretion, 179–81
Antiepileptic drugs
  blood tests while on, *132*
  interactions, *133*
  side effects, 137Q/141A
Antireflux (AR) feeds, 9
Antiretroviral therapy, highly active, (HAART), 221
Antiretroviral therapy (ART), 220–1
Anxiety, 294
Aortic incompetence, 83
Aortic stenosis, 83
Apert syndrome, 267
Apgar score, 29, *30*
Apnoea, newborn, 29, 31
Appendicitis, 270
  differential diagnosis, *272*
Arrhythmias, 75, 88–9
Arthralgia, transient, 277
Arthritis
  inflammatory, 277–9
  juvenile chronic, 277–9
  reactive, 277
  septic, 216, 276–7
  types and clinical features, *277*
Asperger syndrome, 294
Asphyxia, birth, 29–30
Aspiration syndromes, 62–4, 66Q/69A
Asthma
  57–60, 65Q/68A
  treatment, 58, *59*–60
Ataxia-telangiectasia, *198*
Atrial septal defect, 78–9
Atrioventricular septal defect, 81–2
Attention deficit disorders, 293
Auscultation, 52
Autism, 293–4

**B**

Bacterial endocarditis, 90–1
Bacteriuria, 156Q/159A
Barlow provocative test, 273
Barrel chest, 51
Becker muscular dystrophy, 136

Beckwith-Wiedemann syndrome, 249, 267
Behavioural disorders, 291–4, 303Q/306A
Berger nephropathy, 152
Beri-beri, 16
Biliary atresia, 264
Bilirubin conjugation, defects, 196
Bioethics, and non-competent patient, 302
Bipolar disorder, 294
Birth asphyxia, 29–30, 40Q/43A
Birthweight, low, 37–9
Bite marks, 299
Bitot spots, 16
Bladder
  distended, 146
  polyps and tumours, 271
Blalock-Taussig shunt, 85, 86
Bleeding disorders
  240–4, 251Q/255A
  diagnosis, *243*
Blood loss, 233–4
Blood pressure
  change with age, *75*
  measurement, 75
  in renal disease, 146
Bochdalek hernia, 265
Bone
  age, 166
  tumours, 249–50
Bone marrow
  failure, 235–7, 242
  transplantation, 250
Bowel
  inflammatory disorders, 111–14, 270–1
  malrotation/volvulus, 264–5
  obstruction, 261–3, 284Q/288A
Bradyarrhythmias, 88
Bradycardias, 88
Brain
  abscess, 130
  damage, imaging assessment in newborn, 30
  tumours, 249
Breastfeeding, 8, *9*
Breath holding, 292
Breathing *see* Respiration
Breathlessness, 95Q/99A
Brodie abscess, 276
Bronchiectasis, 51, 56
Bronchiolitis, 54, 65Q/68A
Bronchopneumonia, 222
Bronchopulmonary dysplasia *see* Chronic lung disease
Brudzinki's sign, 129
Bruises
  'dating' guide, 306
  non-accidental, 299
Bruton's disease, *198*

Buccal mucosa, ulceration, 117Q/120A
Bulimia, 293
Burkitt's lymphoma, 246
Burns, 296
    classification, *296*
    non-accidental, 299

**C**
Calcitonin, 175
Calcium
    deficiency, 176
    homeostasis, 175–7
Calculi
    renal, *107*
    urinary tract, 271–2
Candidal infection, 222
    newborn, 33
Cardiac abnormalities, examination, 75
Cardiomyopathy, 202Q/204A
Cardiorespiratory arrest, 91–4
Cardiovascular disease, 73–5
Cardiovascular system, 73–94
    examination summary, *77*
Catheters, indwelling, 211
Central nervous system (CNS)
    tuberculosis, 218
    tumours, 247–9
    viral infections, 224Q/228A
Cerebral palsy
    127, 137Q/141A
    types, *127*
Charcoal, activated, 298
Chemoprophylactic drugs, 225Q/229A
Chest infections, recurrent, 117Q/120A
Chest wall, 51, 52
Chest X-rays, 50
    aspiration syndromes, 63
    cardiac silhouette, 95Q/99A
    coarctation of the aorta, 83
    congestive heart failure, 89
    cyanotic CHD, *87*
    cystic fibrosis, 61–2
    pneumonia, 56
    tuberculosis, 57
Chiari defect, 125
Chickenpox, 219–20
Child abuse, 299–301, 303Q/306A
Child exploitation, 301
Chlamydia infection, 222
Cholecystitis, *107*
Cholelithiasis, *107*
Chorionic villus sampling, *25*, 200
Christmas disease, 243
Chromosome, 22 microdeletion, cardiac
        malformation, 78
Chromosome
    analysis, 199
    anomalies, 201Q/203A
    breakage, 201Q/203A
    disorders, 192–4
Chronic granulomatous disease, *198*
Chronic lung disease, newborn, 32
Chronic myeloid leukaemia (CML), 246
Cirrhosis, 115–16
Cleft glottis, 280
Cleft of lip and/or palate, 192, 280,

284Q/289A
Club foot, 274
Clubbing, digital, 51, 66Q/69A
Coagulation factors, *242*
Coarctation of the aorta, 83–4
Coeliac disease, 112
Cognitive behavioural disorders, 293–4,
        303Q/306A
Colic, 293
Complement deficiencies, *198*
Congenital abnormalities
    27–9, Q40/A43
    ear, nose and throat, 280–1
    hip dislocation (CDH), 27
    nervous system, 124–7
    orthopaedic, 273–5
    surgical, 261–7
    urinary tract, 146
Congenital adrenal hyperplasia (CAH),
        164–5, 168, 175
Congenital heart defects, frequency, 77–8
Congenital heart disease
    77, *78*–87, 95Q/99A, 192
    cyanotic, 84–7, 96Q/99–100A
Congenital hypoplastic anaemia, 235–6
Congenital infections, 26, 33–4
Congestive cardiac failure *see* Heart
        failure, congestive
Conjunctivitis, newborn, 32–3
Constipation, *107*, 108, 293
Continuous ambulatory peritoneal
        dialysis, 154
Convulsions
    *see also* Seizures
    febrile, 133, 137Q/141A
    neonatal, 37
        types and aetiologies, *37*
Corneal reflex test, 124
Cough, 50–1
Cranial nerves
    abnormalities, 137Q/141A
    assessment in infants, *124*
    examination, 123–4
Craniosynostosis, 126, 267
Crigler-Najjar syndrome, 196
Crohn's disease, 14, 113, 117Q/120A, 271
Croup (laryngotracheobronchitis), 51, 54,
        65Q/68A
Crouzon syndrome, 267
Cushing syndrome, 174–5, 182Q/186–7A
Cyanosis, 51, 74–5
    confirmation, 77
    in congenital heart disease, *78*
    newborn, 31
Cystic fibrosis
    51, 60–2, 65Q/68–9A, 66Q/69A
    complications, *61*
    genetics, 65Q/69A
Cytomegalovirus infection, 33–4
Cytotoxic agents, side-effects,
        251Q/255–6A

**D**
Data interpretation, 3
Dawn phenomenon, 179
Death and dying, 302

Defects, single primary, 27
Deformation, 27
Dehydration, 110
    assessment, *111*
Dental caries, 282–3, 284Q/289A
Dental problems, 281–3
Denys-Drash syndrome, 249
Depression, 294
Development
    abnormal, 13
    milestones, 13, *14–15*, 18Q/21A
    normal, 13, 18Q/21A
Diabetes insipidus, 180
    cranial, 183Q/187A
    nephrogenic, 183Q/187A
    renal, 155
Diabetes mellitus, insulin dependent,
        177–9
Diabetic mothers, infants of, 26
Diamond-Blackfan syndrome, 235–6
Diarrhoea, 108–111
    acute, 109
    bloody, 117Q/120A
    chronic, 111
    infective causes, *109*
    osmotic, 109–10
    persistent, 117Q/120A
    postinfectious, 111
    secretory, 110, 117Q/119A
DiGeorge syndrome, 176, 198
Digestion, 117Q/120–1A
Digestive system, 105–22
Diuresis, forced, 298
Diuretics, cardiac failure, 89–90
DNA, 189
    rearrangement, 201Q/203A
    restriction analysis, 199–200
Dobutamine, 90
Dopamine, 90
Down syndrome, 192–4
    cardiac malformation, 78
    clinical features, *193*
    risk and maternal age, *193*
Dravet syndrome, 131
Drug abuse, *295*
Drug therapy, and opportunistic
        infections, 211
Dubin-Johnson syndrome, 196
Duchenne muscular dystrophy, 135
Duodenal atresia, 262
Duplex system, 268
Dysmorphic syndromes, 146
Dysmorphology, 190
Dystrophy, myotonic, 136, 192

**E**
Ear, nose and throat disorders, 280–1
Eating problems, 293, 303Q/306A
Ebstein's anomaly, 88
Echocardiogram, 89
Echolalia, 294
Edwards syndrome, cardiac
        malformation, 78
Eisenmenger syndrome, 80
Electrocardiogram (ECG), 88, 93–4
    abnormalities, *88*

Emesis, induced, 297
Emotional deprivation, 301
Empyema, 51
Encephalitis, 129–30
Encephalopathy, hypoxic-ischaemic, 30, 37
Encopresis, 108, 292
Endocarditis
    antibiotic prophylaxis, 92
    bacterial, 90–1
Endocrine system, 163–81
Endotracheal intubation, 93
Energy requirements, 8
Enteral feeding, 8
    contraindications, 9
Enteritis, regional see Crohn's disease
Enterotoxins, 214
Enuresis, 292
Epiglottis, 54
Epiglottitis, 51, 216
Epilepsy
    abdominal, 107
    myoclonic, 107
Epileptic seizures, 130–2
    types, 131
Erythroblastopenia of childhood, transient, 237
Erythrocytes see Red blood cells
Ethics, 301–2
Ewing's tumour, 249–50
Examinations, 1–4
    technique, 4–5
Exomphalos, 26, 267
Extracorporeal membrane oxygenation, 266

F
Facioscapulohumeral dystrophy, 136
Failure to thrive, causes, 10
Fanconi anaemia, 236
Feeding/Feeds, 7–10
    elemental, 9
    enteral/parenteral, 8
    formula, 8
    intravenous, 9–10
    nutritional requirements, 7–10
    problems in infancy, 293
    soy-based, 9
    specialised, 9
Femoral epiphysis, upper, slipped, 279–80
Fetal alcohol syndrome, 26
Fetus, 24–6
    blood sampling, 25
    tissue sampling, 25
Fever, 207–9
Fibrosing alveolitis, 51, 64
Fibrous dysplasia, 275
Fluid balance, renal failure, 153
Fluid restriction, renal failure, 154
Folic acid deficiency
    251Q/255A
    treatment, 236
Foreign body
    inhalation, 281
    insertion, 281

Formula milks, 8
Fractures, 280
    non-accidental, 299
Fragile X syndrome, 192, 199
Friedreich's ataxia, 192
Fructose
    excessive ingestion, 107
    hereditary intolerance, 196

G
Gait assessment, 124
Galactosaemia, 195
Gangliosidosis, 196
Gastric lavage, 298
Gastro-oesophageal reflux, 107–8
Gastrointestinal tract
    atresia, 261–2
    congenital abnormalities, 261–4
    examination, 105
    genetic/inflammatory disorders, 111–14
    normal features, 105
Gastroschisis, 267
Gaucher's disease, 196
Genes, 190
    therapy, 200
    trinucleotide repeats, 192
Genetic counselling, 200
Genetic disorders
    diagnosis, 199–200
    molecular basis, 189
Genetic variations, 189–90
Genetics, cystic fibrosis, 60
Genitalia
    ambiguous, 163–4, 182Q/186A
    neonatal assessment, 26
Gilbert syndrome, 107, 196
Glandular fever, 220
Glomerulonephritis, 151–2, 215
    SLE related, 152
Glucose, 6-phosphate dehydrogenase, 237
Glucose, 6-phosphate dehydrogenase deficiency, 251Q/255A
Glucose homeostasis, disorders of, 177–9
Gluten-sensitive enteropathy, 112
Glycogen storage disorders, 196
Goodpasture disease, 152
Gram-negative organisms, drugs for, 224Q/228A
Growth
    see also Stature
    assessment, 165–6
    constitutional delay, 168
    definitions, 23–4
    fetal, 165
    linear, 11, 165
    normal, 10–12, 18Q/21A
Growth hormone
    deficiency, 167–8
    excess, 168
Guillain-Barré syndrome, 135, 137Q/141A

H
Haematological values, 234
Haematomas, 299
Haematopoiesis, development, 233

Haematuria
    151–3, 156Q/159A
    idiopathic, 152
    non-renal causes, 153
    tubular causes, 152–3
Haemodialysis, 298
Haemoglobins, 234
    abnormal, 237–8
Haemolytic uraemic syndrome, 152
Haemophilia, 243–4
Haemophilus influenzae infections, 216
Haemorrhagic disease of newborn (HDN), 17
Handicap, 127–8
Hashimoto disease, 172
Head injuries, non-accidental, 300
Headaches, tension, 133–4
Hearing impairment, 128
Heart, anatomy, 73
Heart block, 88
Heart disease, clinical assessment, 73–5
Heart failure, 73–4
    congestive, 89–90, 96Q/100A
    symptoms and signs, 89
Heart murmurs and diagnoses, 77
Heart sounds, 75–6
Height, assessment, 165–6
Heimlich manoeuvre, 63
Henoch-Schönlein purpura, 107, 241
Hepatic failure, 201Q/203–4A
Hepatic viruses, 114
Hepatitis
    chronic, 115
    infectious, 114–5
Hepatitis B infection, newborn, 35
Hepatolenticular degeneration see Wilson's disease
Hepatomegaly, 52, 76
Hepatosplenomegaly, 201Q/203A
Hernias
    107, 284Q/290A
    diaphragmatic, 265–7, 284Q/290A
    epigastric, 269
    inguinal, 266
    supraumbilical, 269
    umbilical, 269
Herpes simplex infections, 220
    newborn, 35
Herpes zoster, 220
Herpesvirus, 6 infections, 225Q/229A
Hiatal hernia, 265–6
Hip
    congenital dislocation (CDH), 27, Q40/A43, 192, 273–4, 284Q/288A
    dislocatable, 273
    irritable, 279
    subluxatable, 273
Hirschsprung disease, 192, 263, 265, 284Q/288A
HIV infection
    220, 224Q/228–9A
    lymphoid interstitial pneumonitis, 64
    paediatric categories, 221
    perinatal, 34, 41Q/44A
    Pneumocystis carinii, 57

Hodgkin's disease, 246
  clinical staging, *248*
Homocystinuria, *166*, 169
Hunter syndrome, 191
Huntington's disease, 192
Hurler syndrome, 197
Hyaline membrane disease *see* Surfactant
  deficiency
Hybridisation, 199
Hydrocephalus, 38, 125–6, 284Q/290A
Hydrocoele, 267
Hydronephrosis, 268, 271
Hymen, imperforate, 272
Hyperbilirubinaemia
  conjugated, 36
  unconjugated, 36
Hypercalcaemia
  176–7, 183Q/187A
  infantile, 182Q/187A
Hypercholesterolaemia
  familial, 197
    combined, 197
Hyperkalaemia, 154
Hyperlipidaemia, 197
  secondary, 201Q/204A
Hyperphosphataemia, 154
Hypertension, renal, 154
Hyperthyroidism, 173
Hypocalcaemia, 176
  renal failure, 154
Hypoglycaemia, 179, 201Q/204A
Hypoglycaemia test, 168
Hypogonadotrophic hypogonadism, 170
Hyponatraemia, 154
Hypoparathyroidism, 176
Hypoplastic left heart syndrome, 86
Hypospadias, 272
Hypothyroidism, 171–2
  congenital, 182Q/186A
Hypoxic-ischaemic encephalopathy, 30,
  37

**I**
Idiopathic thrombocytopenia purpura,
  241
IgA deficiency, selective, *198*
IgA nephropathy, 152
IgM, hyper IgM syndrome, *198*
Ileostomy, 263
Immunisation, 212–14
  special risk groups, 212–13
Immunity, 212
Immunodeficiency
  chest disorders, 56
  investigations, *205*
  and lung, 64
Immunodeficiency disorders, *198*
  opportunistic infections and, 209, *211*
Immunoglobulins, immunisation, 212
Impetigo, bullous, 214
Imprinting, 192
Infancy, physiological anaemia, 234
Infantile spasms, 131
Infections, 207–27
  bacterial, 214–18
  chemotherapy, 225Q/229A

congenital, 26, 33–4
  features suggestive of, *34*
  fungal, 225Q/229A
  in newborn, 32–5, 41Q/44A
  parasitic, *107*
  respiratory tract, 53–7
  urinary tract, 146–9
Infectious mononucleosis, 220
Inflammatory bowel disease, 270–1
Informed consent, 302
Infradiaphragmatic drainage, 85
Ingested substances, treatment, *298*
Inhalation devices for asthma, 59–60,
  65Q/68A
Inheritance
  autosomal dominant, 190
  autosomal recessive, 191
  autosomal recessive diseases,
    201Q/203A
  co-dominance, 191
  cytoplasmic, 192
  Mendelian diseases, 201Q/203A
  Mendelian patterns, 190–2
  mitochondrial/cytoplasmic, 192
  multifactorial, 192
  sex-linked, 191
  X-linked dominant disorders, 192
Injuries
  accidental, 296–8
  non-accidental, 298–301
  soft tissue, 280
Insulin
  changes in requirements, 179
  diabetes management, 178
Intelligence quotient (IQ), 137Q/141A
Intestinal polyps, 117Q/120A
Intracranial pressure, raised, 134,
  137Q/141A
Intrauterine growth retardation (IUGR),
  25, 37–8, 39
Intussusception, 269–70
Iritis, 287
Iron
  deficiency, 15–16
    anaemia, 235
  deficiency/supplementation,
    251Q/255A
  excess ingestion, 298
Isolation, infectious diseases, 224Q/228A

**J**
Jaundice
  newborn
    35–6, 41Q/44A
    symptoms and signs, *36*
Jeune syndrome, *275*
Joint position, testing sense of, 124
Jugular venous pressure, 75
Juvenile chronic arthritis, 277–9

**K**
Kartagener syndrome, 64, 66Q/69A
Kasai procedure, 264
Kawasaki disease, 222–3
Kernig's sign, 129
Ketoacidosis, diabetic, *107*, 177, 178

Kidneys
  *see also* Renal
  congenital abnormalities, 146
  ectopic, 146
  horseshoe, 146
Klinefelter syndrome, 169, 194
Kwashiorkor, 15
Kyphosis, 275

**L**
Lactose intolerance, *107*, 111
Ladd's band, 262
Ladd's procedure, 265
Laryngeal web, 280
Laryngomalacia, 51
Laryngotracheobronchitis (croup), 51, 54
Laryngotracheomalacia, 281
Lead poisoning, *107*
Learning disorders, 293–4
Leber optic neuropathy, 192
Lennox-Gastaut syndrome, 131
Leukaemia
  acute, 245–6
  acute lymphoblastic, 245–6
  acute myeloid, 245–6
  chronic myeloid, 246
Life support
  advanced, 93–4
  basic, 91–2
Limb girdle dystrophy, 136
Limbs, short, 275
Lipid absorption, 117Q/121A
Lipid metabolism, 197
Lipid storage disorders, 196
Liver disorders, 114–16
Liver enzyme deficiencies, 195–6
Low birth weight, 166
Lungs
  auscultation, 52
  consolidation and collapse
    radiographic features, *55*
    signs, *55*
  immune defects and, 64
  lobar consolidation, 65Q/68A
  palpation and percussion, 52
Lymphogranuloma venereum (LGV), 222
Lymphoid interstitial pneumonitis, 64
Lymphomas, 246

**M**
McCune-Albright syndrome, 171, *275*
Malaria, 221–2
Malformation syndromes, 190
Malformations, 27
  multiple, 190
Manic-depressive psychoses, 294
Maple syrup urine disease, 195
Marasmus, 15
Marfan syndrome, 169
Maternal abnormalities, disorders
  associated with, 25–6
Maternal factors and fetus, 24, *25*
Maturity assessment, 27
Measles, 218–19
Meckel diverticulum, 270
Meconium aspiration, 31, 41Q/44A

Meconium ileus, 263–4
Medical decisions, 301–2
Medication assessment, 53
Medulloblastoma, 249
Meningitis
    128–9, 137Q/141A, 215
    viral, 129
Meningococcal infections, 216
Mental retardation, 202Q/204A
Metabolism, inborn errors, 194–7
Methylmalonic acidaemia, 195
Microcephaly, 126
Migraine, 134
Milk, intake with weight and age, 8
Milk feeds, 8–9, 18Q/21A
Mobility assessment, 124
Morgagni hernia, 265
Moro reflex, 13, 27
Mortality rates
    24, 40Q/43A
    neonatal, 24
    perinatal, 24
Mosaicism, 193–4
Mosquito-borne illnesses, 224Q/229A
Mucocutaneous lymph node syndrome,
    222–3
Mucopolysaccharidoses
    clinical features, 197
    types, 197
Mucositis, 211
Mucous membranes, neonatal
    assessment, 27
Mumps, 219
Munchausen syndrome by proxy, 300–1
Muscle power, grading, 124
Muscle tone, assessment, 124
Muscular dystrophies, 135–6
Mutations, 189–90
Myasthenia gravis, 136
Mycoplasma infection, 222
Myelomeningocoele, 27
Myocarditis, 90, 96Q/100A
Myoclonic epilepsy, 131
Myopathies, 136
Myotonic dystrophy, 136, 192

N
Nebulisers, 59–60
Necrotising enterocolitis (NEC), 38–9,
    41Q/44A
Neglect, 301
Neonates see Newborn
Neoplastic disorders, 244–50,
    251–2Q/255–6A
Nephroblastoma, 248–9
Nephrotic syndrome, 150–1, 156Q/159A,
    249
Nervous system
    congenital abnormalities, 124–7
    examination, 123–4
    infections, 128–30
    peripheral neuropathy, 137Q/141A
Neural tube defects, 125, 192, 284Q/288A
Neuroblastoma, 248
Neurocutaneous syndromes, 126–7,
    137Q/141A

Neurodegenerative conditions, 127–8
Neurofibromatosis, 126
Neurological assessment, newborn, 27
Neuromuscular disease, 123–36
Neuromuscular maturity, assessment, 28
Neutropenia, 211
Neutrophils, 252Q/256A
Newborn
    assessment, 26–7, 40Q/43A
    causes of death, 24
    fever, 207
    infections, 32–5
    infectious causes of morbidity, 33
    jaundice, 35–6
    normal findings, 29
    resuscitation, 30
Nezelof syndrome, 198
Niacin deficiency, 17
Niemann-Pick disease, 196
Nightmares/Night terrors, 292
Nitrogen washout test, 77
Non-accidental injury, 298–301
Non-disjunction, 193
Non-Hodgkin's lymphoma, 246
    clinical staging, 248
Non-steroidal anti-inflammatories
    (NSAIDs), 108, 207
Noonan syndrome, 82, 194
Nuchal translucency, 25, 193
Nutrition
    disorders, 15–17
    requirements
        7–10, 18Q/21A
        normal, 7–8

O
Obesity, 10
Objective Structured Clinical Examination
    (OSCE), 4
Oesophageal atresia, 261–2
Oligoarthritis, 277
Ollier disease, 275
Orthopaedic disorders
    congenital, 273–5, 284Q/290A
    inflammatory, 276–80
    traumatic, 280
Ortolani manoeuvre, 273
Osteodystrophy, renal, 155
Osteogenesis imperfecta, 274
Osteogenic sarcoma, 249–50
Osteomyelitis, 276
    infecting organisms, 276
Otitis media, 53, 215
Outcome, definitions, 24
Ovarian cancer, 272–3
Oximetry, 52

P
Pain sensation, testing, 124
Pancreatitis, 107, 116
Pancytopenia, 251Q/255A
Paracetamol overdose, 298
Parasite infection, 107
Parasuicide, 294
Parathyroid hormone (PTH), 175
Parvovirus infections, 224Q/-229A

Patau syndrome, cardiac malformation,
    78
Patent ductus arteriosus, 80–2
Peak flow measurements, 52
Penis, abnormalities, 272
Pericardial effusion, 96Q/100A
Pericarditis, 90, 216
Peripheral neuropathy, 137Q/141A
Peritonitis, 116
Periventricular haemorrhage, 38
Periventricular leukomalacia, 38
Perthes' disease, 279
Pertussis, 51, 54–5, 65Q/68A, 216–17
Phenylketonuria, 166, 195
Phototherapy, neonatal jaundice, 36
Physical maturity, assessment, 28
Pica, 293
Picture examination, 3
Pierre-Robin sequence, 27, 29, 190, 280
Platelet/coagulation factor defects, 242–3
Pneumococcal infections, 215–16
Pneumocystis carinii infections, 211, 244–5
Pneumocystis carinii pneumonitis, 57
Pneumonia, 55–6
    newborn, 31, 41Q/44A
Pneumonitis
    lymphoid interstitial, 64
    Pneumocystis carinii, 57
Pneumothorax, newborn, 32
Poisoning, 298
Poliomyelitis, 135, 220
Polyarticular juvenile chronic rheumatoid
    arthritis (JCA), 277
Polycystic kidney disease, 146
Polycystic ovary syndrome, 171
Polycythaemia, 74, 75
Polymerase chain reaction (PCR), 200
Polymorphisms, 189
Porphyria, acute intermittent, 107
Portal hypertension, 116
Possetting, 293
Potter syndrome, 29
Prader-Willi syndrome, 170, 192
Precordium, 75
Prematurity, 37
    complications, 38
Propionic acidaemia, 195
Protein, requirements, 8
Protein-energy malnutrition (PEM), 15
Proteinuria, 149–51
Pseudohermaphroditism, 164
Pseudohypoparathyroidism, 176
Psychosocial emotional deprivation, 167
Pubarche, premature, 171
Puberty
    see also Sexual maturation
    constitutional delay, 168
    delayed, 170, 182Q/186A
    disorders, 169–71
    normal, 169–70, 182Q/186A
    precocious, 168, 170
    staging, 166
Pulmonary atresia, 86
Pulmonary incompetence, 82–3
Pulmonary murmur, 76
Pulmonary sounds, 75–6

Pulmonary stenosis, 81–2
Pulse, 52, 75
  change with age, 75
Pyloric stenosis, 192, 269
Pyrexia of unknown origin (PUO), 208–9

Q
Quality of life, 302

R
Red blood cells
  decreased production, 234–7
  destruction, 237–40
Reflexes
  assessment, 124
  newborn, 13
Rehydration, oral therapy, 111
Renal, see also Kidneys
Renal abscess, 149
Renal agenesis, 146
Renal calculi, 107
Renal dialysis, 154
  indications, 154
Renal dysfunction, 155
Renal dysplasia, 146
Renal failure
  153–5, 156Q/159A
  acute, 153–4
  chronic, 156Q/159A
  end-stage, 154
Renal hypoplasia, 146
Renal transplantation, 154–5, 156Q/159A
Renal tubular acidosis, 155
Renal vein thrombosis, 153
Repetitive mannerisms, 291
Reproductive organs, abnormalities,
    272–3
Research and children, 302
Respiration, work of, 51–2
Respiratory disease, newborn, 31–2
Respiratory distress, pathology, 31
Respiratory distress syndrome see
    Surfactant deficiency
Respiratory rate, 52
  infantile, 26
Respiratory system, 49–64
Respiratory tract, 49–50
  lower, infections, 54–7, 73–4, 75
  upper, infections, 53–4
Restriction analysis, 199
Restriction endonucleases, 199
Restriction fragment length
    polymorphisms, 199
Resuscitation
  cardiorespiratory arrest, 91–4
  neonatal, 30
Retinoblastoma, 250
Reye syndrome, 116
Rhabdomyosarcoma, 250
Rheumatic fever, 215
Rheumatoid arthritis, manifestations, 278
Rheumatoid disease, 277–9
Rickets, 16, 176, 182Q/187A
Rifampicin chemoprophylaxis,
    224Q/228A
Ritter disease, 214

Rotor syndrome, 196
Rubella, 219
  maternal, 219
  newborn, 34
Russell-Silver syndrome, 166, 275

S
Sacrococcygeal teratoma, 27
Salicylates, 298
Sarcoma, osteogenic, 249–50
Scalded skin syndrome, 214
Scalds, 296
Schizophrenia, 294
Scoliosis, 51, 275, 284Q/288–9A
Screening, tuberculosis, 57
Scurvy, 14, 17
Seizure-like disorders, 133
Seizures
  see also Convulsions
  absence, 131
  epileptic, 130–2
  generalised, 131
  multiple, 131
  non-epileptic, 133
  partial, 131
  tonic-clonic, 131
Self-appraisal, 4–5
Sensorimotor neuropathies, 135
Sensory examination, 124
Septicaemia, pneumococcal, 215
Sequence of errors, 27
Severe acute respiratory syndrome
    (SARS), 224Q/228A
Severe combined immunodeficiency
    disorder (SCID), 198, 200
Sexual abuse, 301
Sexual differentiation, disorders of, 163–5,
    182Q/186A
Sexual maturation, 11, 12
  see also Puberty
Shaking injury, 300
Shock, septic, 209
Short bowel syndrome, 118Q/121A
Shunts, cardiovascular, left-to-right,
    77–81, 95Q/99A
Sickle cell syndromes, 237–8
Single nucleotide polymorphism, 200
Skeletal dysplasias and malformations,
    274–275
Skin
  neonatal assessment, 27
  neurocutaneous syndromes, 126–7
  pustules, newborn, 33
  vesicular lesions, 225Q/229A
Skull, depressed fractures, 300
Sleep disorders, 292–3
Slide examination, 3
Small bowel atresia, 263
Smoke inhalation, 296–7
Social paediatrics, 295
Social services, 295
Soft tissue injuries, 280
Somogyi effect, 179
Sorbitol, excessive ingestion, 107
Sotos syndrome, 169
Southern blot, 199

Spastic diplegia, 38
Speech, motor disorders, 124
Spherocytosis, hereditary, 237
Spina bifida, 27, 125
Spinal cord compression, 134
Spinal muscular atrophy, 134–5
Spinocerebellar ataxia, 192
Sprengel shoulder, 275
Staphylococcal infections, 214,
    224Q/228A
Stature
  see also Growth
  disorders of, 165–9
  short
    166–8, 182Q/186A
    endocrine causes, 167
    investigations, 166
    systemic causes, 167
  tall, 168–9
Status epilepticus, 133
Still's disease, 277
Still's murmur, 76
Stomach, ulcers, 108
Stools
  normal, 105
  watery, 108
Streptococcal infections, 214–215
  group B, newborn, 34–5
Stridor, 51
Subacute sclerosing panencephalitis
    (SSPE), 219
Subarachnoid bleed, 134
Substance abuse, 295, 303Q/306A
Suicide, 294
Supradiaphragmatic drainage, 85
Supraventricular tachyarrhythmias,
    88–9
Supraventricular tachycardia, 96Q/100A
Surfactant deficiency, 31, 41Q/44A
Surgery
  acquired abnormalities, 269–73
  congenital abnormalities, 261–8
Syndrome of inappropriate ADH secretin
    (SIADH), 180–1
Syphilis, congenital, 34
Systemic inflammatory response
    syndrome (SIRS), 209
Systemic lupus erythematosus,
    glomerulonephritis related, 152
Systolic murmurs, grading system, 76

T
Tachyarrhythmias, 88–9
Talipes calcaneovalgus, 274
Talipes equinovarus, 274
Tantrums, 292
Tay-Sachs disease, 196
Teeth
  assessment and examination, 281–2
  erosion, 283
  trauma, 283
Temperature, sensation of, testing, 124
Testes
  malignant swelling, 272
  torsion, 272
  undescended, 266, 272

Tetralogy of Fallot, 86–7, 95Q/99A
Thalassaemia syndromes, 239–40
Thelarche, premature, 171
Thermogenesis, non-shivering, 207
Thrombocytopenia, 251Q/255A
Thumb sucking, 291
Thymic hypoplasia, *198*
Thyroid gland, disorders, 171–3
Thyrotoxicosis, 168–9, 182Q/186A
Tonsillopharyngitis, 53–4, 225Q/229A
Total anomalous pulmonary venous
    drainage (TAPVD), 85
Total parenteral nutrition (TPN), 10
Touch, assessment, 124
Toxic megacolon, 271
Toxic neuropathies, 135
Toxic shock syndrome, 214
Toxoplasmosis, newborn, 34
Tracheo-oesophageal fistula, 261
Trachoma, 222
Transfusion, exchange, 36
Transposition of the great arteries, 84–5
Trauma, 280
Trendelenburg's test, 273–4
Tricuspid atresia, 85
Trisomy 13, 194
Trisomy 18, 194
Trisomy 21, 192–4
Tuberculosis, 56–7, 65Q/68A, 217–18,
    224Q/229A
Tuberous sclerosis, 126–7
Tumour lysis syndrome, 247
Turner syndrome
    166–7, 182Q/186A, 194
    cardiac malformation, 78
Tyrosinaemia, *166*

**U**
UK immunisation schedule, *212*
Ulcerative colitis
    113–14, 117Q/120A, 271
    cf Crohn's disease, *114*
Ultrasound, 24–5
    abnormalities detected on, *25*
Urea cycle defects, 195
Ureterocoele, 268
Urethral valves, posterior, 268
Urinalysis, 146
Urinary tract, 145–55
    calculi, 271–2
    congenital abnormalities, 146
    infections, 146–9, 147–9, 156Q/159A
    obstructions, 284Q/288A
    obstructive lesions, 271
    signs of disease, 146
    symptoms of disease, 145–6
Urine, altered colour, 202Q/204A
Uveitis, 278

**V**
Vaccines
    225Q/229A
    adverse effects, 213–14
VACTER anomalies, 262
Vagal nerve stimulation, 132
Varicella, 219–20
VATER association, 190
Venous hum, 76
Ventilation
    high-frequency oscillation, 266
    preterm infants, 32
Ventricular hypertrophy, 75
Ventricular septal defect, 79–80

Ventricular tachycardia, 89
Vesicoureteric reflux, 146
Vibration sense, testing, 124
Vibratory murmur, 76
Viral infections, 218–21
Visual impairment, 128
Vitamin A deficiency, 16
Vitamin B1 deficiency, 16–17
Vitamin B2 deficiency, 17
Vitamin B6 deficiency, 17
Vitamin B12, 251Q/255A
Vitamin B12 deficiency, 17
    treatment, *236*
Vitamin C deficiency, 17
Vitamin D deficiency, 16, 175
Vitamin E deficiency, 17
Vitamin K deficiency, 17
Viva voce, 3
Vomiting, 107–8
    bile-stained, 261
Von Willebrand's disease, 243

**W**
WAGR syndrome, 248–9
Waterhouse-Friderichsen syndrome, 216
Weaning, 8–9
Weight gain, 10
West syndrome, 131
Wheeze, 51, 52
Whipping injury, 299
Whooping cough *see* Pertussis
Wilms' tumour, 248–9
Wilson's disease, 115
Wiskott-Aldrich syndrome, *198*
Wolff-Parkinson-White syndrome, 88–9,
    96Q/100A